Early Breast Cancer

Early Breast Cancer
from screening to multidisciplinary management

Edited by

M.W.E. Morgan, FRCS
St Margaret's Hospital
Epping, UK

R. Warren, FRCP, FRCR*
Addenbrooke's Hospital
Cambridge, UK

and

G. Querci della Rovere, MD, FRCS*
Royal Marsden Hospital
Sutton, UK

*Formerly St Margaret's Hospital, Epping, UK

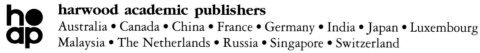
harwood academic publishers
Australia • Canada • China • France • Germany • India • Japan • Luxembourg
Malaysia • The Netherlands • Russia • Singapore • Switzerland

Amsteldijk 166
1st Floor
1079 LH Amsterdam
The Netherlands

British Library Cataloguing in Publication Data
A catalogue record for this book is available from the British Library.

ISBN: 90-5702-469-1

This book is dedicated to the memory of my old and dear friend Mr Ettore Bertazzoni. He was the owner of Bi & Gi Publishers, Verona, Italy who invited and encouraged me to be one of the Editors of this book. Unfortunately his premature and sudden death prevented the completion of the task he had until then so brilliantly accomplished.

G. Querci della Rovere

Contents

9 Foreword
U. VERONESI

11 Preface
G. QUERCI DELLA ROVERE

12 Acknowledgements

13 Contributors

The Background of Breast Cancer Screening

17 The epidemiology of screening for breast cancer
L.J. POINTON, N.E. DAY

29 Genetics and breast screening
D.G. EVANS

34 The biology of breast cancer and its relevance to screening and treatment
J.R. BENSON

42 The organisation of breast cancer screening
E.J. ROEBUCK

49 Clinical aspects of a screening programme
G. QUERCI DELLA ROVERE, D. LOWRY, P. FULTON, J. SPENCER KNOTT, Y. STEEL, R. WARREN

49 a. *The role of the General Practitioner*
D. LOWRY

51 b. *The role of the Radiographer*
P. FULTON

53 c. *The Assessment Clinic*
G. QUERCI DELLA ROVERE, Y. STEEL, R. WARREN

55 d. *The role of the breast specialist nurse in breast screening*
J. SPENCER KNOTT

The Radiology of Breast Cancer

61 Film reading and recall of patients
R. WARREN

64 Radiology of the normal breast and differential diagnosis of benign breast lesions
S. CIATTO, D. AMBROGETTI

75 The radial scar
N. PERRY, I. MORRISON

79 Circumscribed breast masses
A.R.M. WILSON

86 Microcalcifications
R. GIVEN-WILSON

100 Distortion of architecture and asymmetry
C. KISSIN

109 Ultrasound in the diagnosis of small breast carcinomas
E. MOSKOVIC

Tissue Diagnosis

117 Fine needle aspiration cytology
J.G. McKENZIE, J. DALRYMPLE

125 Diagnostic biopsies
M.W.E. MORGAN

129 Pre-operative localization of impalpable breast abnormalities
G. QUERCI DELLA ROVERE, A. PATEL

133 ABBI: Advanced Breast Biopsy Instrumentation
G.A. FARELLO, A. CEROFOLINI

The Pathology of Breast Cancer

139 Normal breast and benign breast lesions
K. AGARWAL

151 Risk factors, prognostic indicators and staging
S.E. PINDER, I.O. ELLIS

161 Premalignant, borderline lesions, ductal and lobular carcinoma *in situ*
C.N. CHINYAMA, C.A. WELLS

176 Invasive carcinoma of breast
     M. LETCHER

189 Cytological and histological correlation
     in breast cytopathology
     P.A. TROTT

196 Radio-pathological correlations
     S. CIATTO, D. AMBROGETTI, S. BIANCHI

Multidisciplinary Management

205 Surgical treatment of minimal breast
     cancer
     R.M. SIMMONS, M.P. OSBORNE

214 The management of the axilla
     M. GRECO, N. CASCINELLI

219 The importance of resection margins in
     conservative surgery
     L. CATALIOTTI, V. DISTANTE, S. BIANCHI

226 Adjuvant therapy of breast cancer
     N. DAVIDSON, A. PATEL

231 Local recurrence after breast
     conservation
     M.W. KISSIN

245 Interval carcinomas
     R. WARREN

Final Remarks

259 Medico-legal aspects
     S. LEVENE

265 The prevention of breast cancer: Recent
     progress and future developments
     T.J. POWLES, J. CHANG

270 Mammographic screening in women
     under age 50: A critical appraisal
     I. JATOI, M. BAUM

277 A critical appraisal of breast cancer
     screening for women aged 50 and over
     J. CHAMBERLAIN

286 Subject Index

Foreword

There has been a great revolution in thought and concepts over the last 20 years regarding breast carcinoma. A few decades ago the idea became widespread that in most cases breast cancer was a disseminated disease from its inception so that the most important efforts should only be directed towards systemic medical treatment and that local management of the disease did not deserve great attention. On the one hand, this conception helped surgeons to explore and experience less mutilating procedures, on the other it went against the principles of early detection as a most important means of controlling the disease.

As a matter of fact, for many years screening programs appeared to be difficult to implement in many countries and were not without opposition. But results of randomised population-based studies in different parts of the world demonstrated the ability of screening programs to significantly reduce breast cancer mortality rates. At the same time, the revolution in imaging through new advances in mammography, ultrasound and magnetic resonance techniques has brought surgeons an increasing number of cases of minimal, often non-palpable, carcinomas with curability rates up to 95 percent showing beyond doubt that breast carcinoma, when detected very early, is a *local* disease. Today, in any European institution where some decades ago early breast cancer (say less than 2 cm) was an uncommon event, the situation has completely changed with such tumours representing 60% of the total, one-third of which are clinically non-palpable. In light of this situation, the strategy to fight the disease must be reconsidered and rewritten.

This objective, in brief, represents the content of this beautiful book which focuses attention on this new condition which will become more and more widespread in the near future. All aspects of early breast cancer are carefully considered in a logical sequence so that the reader is led to draw conclusions through the wide-ranging analysis of the diagnostic, pathological and therapeutic aspects of small mammary carcinomas.

A book of this kind was absolutely necessary. Its educational value will be evident from its reading and its impact on the medical profession dramatic. All those involved in oncology and senology must realise that early detected breast cancer is a disease with an excellent prognosis and that most breast cancer mutilations could be avoided, that many axillary dissections are unnecessary, and that heavy systemic adjuvant chemotherapy regimens are often recommended without reason. Those women aware of breast cancer issues and who participate in early detection programs should be rewarded with gentle and appropriate care and not punished with heavy and often unjustified treatments. This is the message of this book and I firmly hope that it will reach the largest possible audience.

Umberto Veronesi

Preface

In 1987, the National Health Service Breast Screening Programme (NHSBSP) was introduced in the United Kingdom. Initially the experience was obviously limited. After a learning period and with dedication and determination, most Screening Centres have been able to produce excellent results and have improved beyond the forecast of the Forrest Report with regard to recall of patients and benign/malignant biopsy ratio. The success of the NHSBSP should be measured not only on the percentage mortality reduction achieved in breast cancer patients, but also on the greatly increased quality of the management of women with breast problems. Before the advent of breast screening, most breast diseases were relegated to the end of a busy operating list in the hands of a junior doctor.

Breast Screening has promoted and stimulated a multidisciplinary approach in the diagnostic and therapeutic fields, where radiologists, cytopathologists, surgeons and medical oncologists cooperate to provide the best possible management of the patient. Radiographers and Breast Nurse Specialists are essential members of the team; the Screening Programme has produced a group of Breast Specialists.

This book is based on the experience accrued during 10 years of breast screening. The various specialist sections are not intended for the specialist's own discipline; they are written by professional radiologists, pathologists and medical/surgical oncologists and aimed at the other members of the medical and nursing team. The multidisciplinary approach has been the key to the success of the NHSBSP. However by tradition, training is compartmentalised into specialist disciplines, with scant knowledge gained in parallel branches of medicine dealing with the same pathology. It is imperative that each member of the team knows as much as possible of all the specialised fields of diagnosis and treatment of breast diseases. In the future the Breast Specialist will be a doctor trained in radiology, pathology and medical and surgical oncology of the breast. Such a specialist will have a more comprehensive understanding of the problem of breast cancer and will overcome present management decision biases that result from training in different medical specialities rather than a training covering various specialities in one field of pathology.

G. Querci della Rovere

Acknowledgements

We would like to thank Mrs S. Firman, Mrs J. New and Miss C. Price for their secretarial help; Mr Peter Bird, FRACS for his contribution in reviewing the text. Mrs Maria Rosa Udeschini and Bi & Gi Editori, Verona for their excellent work in preparing the book and promptly agreeing to the sale; Harwood Academic Publishers for rescuing the book after Mr Bertazzoni's sudden and tragic death.

Contributors

Agarwal K.
Department of Pathology, St Margaret's Hospital, Epping, Essex, UK

Ambrogetti D.
Centro per lo Studio e la Prevenzione Oncologica, Florence, Italy

Baum M.
Department of Surgery, University College Hospital, London, UK Formerly Academic Unit, Royal Marsden Hospital, London, UK

Benson J.R.
Department of Surgery, Royal Marsden Hospital, Sutton, Surrey, UK

Bianchi S.
Istituto Istologia e Anatomia Patologica, University of Florence, Italy

Cascinelli N.
Istituto Nazionale per la Cura e lo Studio dei Tumori, Division of Surgical Oncology "B", Milan, Italy

Cataliotti L.
Istituto di Clinica Chirurgica e Terapia Chirurgica I, University of Florence, Italy

Cerofolini A.
Department of Surgery, City Hospital, Schio, Vicenza, Italy

Chamberlain J.
Cancer Screening Evaluation Unit, Institute of Cancer Research, Section of Epidemiology, Cotswold Road, Sutton, Surrey, UK

Chang J.
Department of Medical Oncology, National University Hospital, Singapore, Formerly Department of Medicine, Royal Marsden Hospital, London, UK

Chinyama C.N.
Department of Histopathology, St Thomas' Hospital, London, UK

Ciatto S.
Centro per lo Studio e la Prevenzione Oncologica, Florence, Italy

Dalrymple J.
Department of Pathology, St Margaret's Hospital, Epping, UK

Davidson N.
Radiotherapy Department, North Middlesex Hospital, London, UK

Day N.E.
MRC Biostatistic Unit University, Forvie Site, Cambridge, UK

Distante V.
Istituto di Clinica Chirurgica e Terapia Chirurgica I, University of Florence, Italy

Ellis I.O.
Department of Histopathology, City Hospital NHS Trust, Nottingham, UK

Evans G.D.
Christie Hospital, Manchester and St Mary's Hospital, Manchester, UK

Farello G.A.
Department of Surgery, City Hospital, Schio, Vicenza, Italy

Fulton P.
Breast Screening Unit, St Margaret's Hospital, Epping, Essex, UK

Given-Wilson R.
Department of Radiology, St Georges Hospital, London, UK

Greco M.
Istituto Nazionale per la Cura e lo Studio dei Tumori, Division of Surgical Oncology "B", Milan, Italy

Jatoi I.
Brooke Army Medical Center, Fort Sam Houston, Texas and Uniformed Services University of the Health Sciences, Bethesda, Maryland, USA

Kissin C.
Jarvis Breast Screening Centre, Stoughton Road, Guildford, Surrey, UK

Kissin M.W.
Royal Surrey County Hospital and Jarvis Screening Centre, Guildford, Surrey, UK

Letcher M.
Department of Pathology, St Margaret's Hospital, Epping, Essex, UK

Levene S.
199 Strand, London, UK

Lowry D.
General Practice Surgery, The High Street, Epping, Essex, UK

McKenzie J.G.
Department of Pathology, St Margaret's Hospital, Epping, Essex, UK

Morgan M.W.E.
Department of Surgery, St Margaret's Hospital, Epping, Essex, UK

Morrison I.
Department of Radiology, St Bartholomew's Hospital, London UK

Moskovic E.
Department of Radiology, Royal Marsden Hospital, London, UK

Osborne M.P.
Department of Surgery, Strang Cancer Prevention Center, New York Hospital, USA

Patel A.
Department of Pathology, St Margaret's Hospital, Epping, UK

Perry N.
Department of Radiology, St
Bartholomew's Hospital,
London, UK

Pinder S.E.
Department of Histopathology,
City Hospital NHS Trust,
Nottingham, UK

Pointon L.J.
MRC Biostatistic Unit, University
Forvie Site, Cambridge, UK

Powles T.J.
Breast Unit, Royal Marsden Hospital,
Sutton, Surrey, UK

Querci della Rovere G.
Breast Unit, Royal Marsden Hospital,
Sutton, Surrey, UK
Formerly St Margaret's Hospital,
Epping, Essex, UK

Roebuck E.J.
National Breast Screening Training
Unit, Nottingham, UK

Simmons R.M.
Department of Surgery, Cornell Medical
Center, The Strang, Cornell, Breast
Center, New York Hospital, USA

Spencer Knott J.
Breast Screening Unit, St Margaret's
Hospital, Epping, Essex, UK

Steel Y.
Breast Screening Unit, St Margaret's
Hospital, Epping, Essex, UK

Trott P.
Department of Pathology, Royal
Marsden Hospital, London, UK

Warren R.
Breast Screening Unit, Addenbrooke's
Hospital, Cambridge, UK

Wells C.A.
Department of Histopathology, St
Bartholomew's Hospital, London, UK

Wilson A.R.M.
Breast Screening Unit, City Hospital
NHS Trust, Nottingham, UK

The Background of Breast Cancer Screening

The epidemiology of screening for breast cancer

L.J. Pointon, N.E. Day

Introduction

Breast cancer is the leading cause of death from cancer among women in the UK and as such presents a major public health problem. In 1992, there were 13,663 deaths from breast cancer in England and Wales. The aetiology of the disease is not fully understood and although the risk is known to be associated with reproductive and family history,[1] there is as yet no preventative therapy available. Screening for breast cancer has been shown to advance the diagnosis of the disease which can lead to more successful treatment and therefore reduced mortality.

The natural history of breast cancer is fairly well documented.[2] The disease is believed usually to have a pre-invasive stage where the carcinoma cells are confined to the duct system within the breast. This may then become invasive and begin to invade the surrounding tissue, and thereafter possibly spread to the lymph nodes or other secondary sites within the body. Breast tumours may disseminate at different stages in their natural history. In some women, and for some types of tumour, this could take years, whilst in others metastatic spread may take only weeks, depending on the aggressiveness of the cancer. Ideally, screening should detect tumours while they are still small and before any metastases have developed.[3] In order for screening to be effective, the disease must have a recognisable early stage. In the case of breast cancer this is the pre-clinical detectable phase where a tumour can be seen on a mammogram but before it becomes palpable (about 1cm in diameter). Tumours in this phase are more likely to be non-invasive or, if already invasive, less likely to have local regional or distant spread.

For screening to be beneficial, treating breast cancer at this earlier stage must also improve the prognosis compared to more advanced cancers. It is not, however, sufficient to compare the survival of women with screen detected cancers with those who present symptomatically without removing the effect of various biases. Figure 1 illustrates the stages the disease passes through as it progresses. Lead-time bias occurs because survival is measured from time of diagnosis. As screening will advance the date of diagnosis, the survival time will automatically be longer even if there is no effect on the actual date of death. Also, less aggressive, slower growing cancers will spend more time in the pre-clinical detectable phase than will fast growing cancers which are more likely to present symptomatically. Screening will therefore detect proportionally more of the slow growing, or non-invasive cancers which in turn have a better prognosis.

This is known as length bias. There is also the problem of selection bias in which those who attend for screening are more likely to be health-conscious individuals than those who refuse and would probably have a better prognosis anyway. These biases can be removed by comparing mortality in a population which was offered screening with that in a population which was not offered screening, in the context of a randomised controlled trial.

The suitability of any screening test depends on its accuracy. It must be able both to detect the majority of women who have breast cancer (high sensitivity) and therefore give few false negative results, and also to eliminate the majority of women who do not have the disease (high specificity) thereby minimising the number of false positive results. Sensitivity is defined as the proportion of all those with breast cancer present who test positive; specificity is defined as the proportion of all those without the disease who test negative. Ideally, both sensitivity and specificity would be 100% but there is an inevitable compromise as no test is perfect and the two are inversely related to one another. Different screening modalities will be discussed in more detail later.

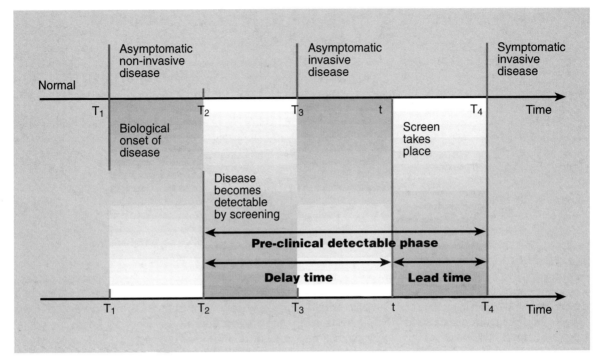

Fig. 1. Model of disease progression.

For public health, the acceptability of a screening test by the general population is of paramount importance. The acceptability will be reflected by the rate of compliance with invitation to screening. A level of 70% compliance has been shown to be effective in reducing breast cancer mortality in the target population.[4] This seems to be an achievable level in the UK[5] and levels of between 80% and 90% have been seen in Sweden.[6]

Another important consideration in a screening test is that it should do no harm, either physical or psychological. The potential physical hazards from screening by mammography are the risk from ionising radiation (X-rays) and unnecessary surgical procedures resulting from overdiagnosis of tumours which may never have become invasive in the lifetime of the patient. The radiation risk from mammography has been very much reduced in recent years. Due to technical advances the maximum dose is now about 0.15 cGy (compared with 2-3 cGy in the past).[7] There is no evidence that this level of radiation induces breast cancer but from the excess breast cancer incidence seen in women exposed to higher doses, it has been inferred that modern mammography may induce one breast cancer in a population of two million women above the age of 50, after a latent period of 10 years. When compared to the expected natural breast cancer incidence of 1,400 cases per million women per year at age 50 and 2,000 cases per million women per year at age 65, the risk is consid-

ered to be insignificant compared to the potential benefits. High quality screening techniques and highly trained technical and radiological staff should minimise the risk of overdiagnosis. Ideally, the recall rate should be as low as possible. It is also important that adequate assessment and treatment facilities exist to ensure that women are seen as quickly as possible. In addition, there is a range of non-invasive investigative techniques which stop short of open biopsy which should be employed to reduce the risk of unnecessary surgery. These include spot views, micro-magnification, fine needle aspiration and possibly needle core biopsy. Using these techniques, it is possible to achieve the situation where less than one in ten biopsies have a benign result.[8]

Screening must be repeated at regular intervals to ensure its effectiveness as the risk of developing breast cancer increases with age and the growth rate of the disease is variable. There has to be a compromise taking into account the cost and practicality of screening too frequently whilst aiming to let as few cancers as possible escape detection by screening. In the UK the interval is currently three years although further research is under way in the UKCCCR Breast Screening Frequency Trial, including both assessment of the consequences of more frequent screening for mortality and a parallel economic evaluation.

Screening for breast cancer was introduced in the UK following the recommendations of the Forrest Report in 1986. The programme offers single mediolateral oblique view mammography to women aged 50 - 64 years with an interval of three years,[7] although most screening centres are now using two-view mammography for at least the prevalence screen. Women aged 65 years or over may be screened on demand but the acceptance rate in this age group has been shown to decline with age[5,9] and the benefits of mass screening are therefore reduced.

Screening modalities

There are three basic potential screening tools: mammography, physical examination by trained staff and breast self-examination. Mammography has been shown to be effective in reducing breast cancer mortality. The Swedish Two-County Trial[6] used single medio-lateral oblique view mammography alone and achieved a mortality reduction of 30% in women aged 40-74. The sensitivity was 86% to 95% for women over 50 years, around 60% for women in the 40-49 age group and 82% overall. This may be due to denser breast tissue in younger women and sensitivity could possibly be improved by using two-view mammography. The main reason for using a single view in this case was the perceived need in the 1970s to minimise radiation dose. As has already been discussed, with modern mammography techniques, this risk is now insignificant. A recent study[26] has shown that by adding a second (cranio-caudal) view, the sensitivity of screening during the prevalence round of a population screening programme was increased from 93.9% to 96.1% and 18 additional cancers were detected out of a total of 267. The recall rate was also reduced by the addition of a second view, from 8.9% to 6.7%. In conclusion, mammography, particularly with two views, is highly effective, acceptable and sensitive as a primary screening method.

The effectiveness of clinical examination alone has not been tested, although some trials have used it in conjunction with mammography. In Edinburgh between 1979 and 1981, 45,130 women were entered into a randomised controlled trial in which approximately half were invited to screening.[10] At the prevalence round, the study group were offered two-view mammography and clinical examination. Subsequent screens involved clinical examination alone in years 2, 4 and 6, and one-view mammography plus clinical examination in years 3, 5 and 7. Although the compliance at the initial screen was poor (61%), and fell at subsequent screens, there did not appear to be any difference in the acceptance of clinical examination and mammography. At the first screen, 85 out of 88 cancers (97%) were detected by mammography and 65 (74%) by clinical examination, although in some cases a palpable lump was found only after referral to assessment following a suspicious mammogram. Only 3 (3%) of cancers were discovered solely by clinical examination. The sensitivity for clinical examination was 69% and this rose to over 90% when mammography was included. The Edinburgh data lack statistical power however, and there is no conclusive evidence to show that clinical examination is effective in reducing mortality.

Breast self-examination (BSE) is very difficult to assess as the only intervention possible is education, and failure to practice seems to be a major disadvantage to the use of BSE as a sole screening method. The sensitivity of BSE is very difficult to measure but it is assumed that frequent BSE will enable a woman to detect a cancer earlier than less frequent visits for a professional clinical examination. There is some evidence that BSE may lead to a reduction in tumour size at diagnosis.[7] There is no evidence that BSE contributes to a reduction in mortality but women should not be discouraged from practising it as it may contribute to an earlier diagnosis.

Evidence for mortality reduction from randomised controlled trials

The Health Insurance Plan Study of Greater New York (HIP) was the first trial of breast cancer screening.[4] The population consisted of approximately 62,000 women aged 40-64 years who were selected from 23 of the 31 HIP medical centres. From each centre, two systematic random samples of women with membership in HIP for at least a year were selected and entered into the programme from December 1963 to June 1966. These two groups then formed the study and control populations. The study group were offered screening by clinical examination and two-view mammography firstly at entry to the trial and then yearly for the next three years. The control group were not invited to screening. The compliance at the first screen was 67%, 80% of these women attended the first annual examination, 75% the second and 69% the third. Overall, 40% attended all four screens. Ten years after the start of the trial, the breast cancer mortality reduction in the study group was 30%. After 18 years, the reduction was still 23%.

The Swedish two-county study took place in Östergötland and Kopparberg counties, Sweden.[6] Women aged 40-74 were entered into the programme from 1977 to 1981. The trial population was randomised by population cluster rather than by individual. Later analyses have shown the loss of power to be minimal. In Östergötland, one cluster in each block of two was randomised to invitation to screening and in Kopparberg it was two clusters in each block of three. This resulted in a study group of 77,080 and a control group of 55,985. Women aged 40-49 were invited to screening by one-view mammography alone every 24 months, and those in the age range 50-74 were invited every 33 months on average. The control group were not invited to screening in the initial study. In 1985, after four rounds of screening in the younger age range, three in the 50 - 69 range and two in the 70-74 range, the control group were invited to screening. All breast cancers in both arms of the trial diagnosed between randomisation and the end of the first screen of the controls were included in the final analysis of the trial results. Compliance was good. In women under 70 years, participation was consistent at approximately 90% at all screens. For women aged between 70 and 74 years, the participation rate was 79% at the first screening round and 67% at the second. Consequently no further invitations were issued to this age group. The first results of the study, before the controls were invited to screening, were published in 1985 and showed a mortality reduction in the study group of 31%. In an update, which followed women up to 31 December 1990, the main result of the trial remained the same: the mortality reduction in the study group was 30%.

The Malmö mammographic screening trial started in October 1976 to determine whether breast cancer mortality in women over 45 could be reduced by mammographic screening.[11] All women born in 1908-1932 were identified from the population registry of Malmö, Sweden. Half the women in each birth year cohort were randomly selected as the study group and invited to mammographic screening at intervals of 18-24 months. The remaining women were allocated to the control group and were not offered screening. In the first two rounds, two-views were taken. In subsequent rounds either both views or just the oblique was taken depending on the density of the breasts. The attendance rate was higher in the first round (74%) than in subsequent rounds (70%) and higher among younger rather than older women. The pre-determined end of the trial was 31 December 1986 and by this stage no significant reduction in mortality was seen in the study group. In fact, during the first seven calendar years of the screening programme, the cumulative number of deaths from breast cancer was higher in the study group than in the controls, although by the end of the trial this situation had been reversed. The Malmö study suffered from loss of power due in part to the attendance rate but also to dilution of the control group. A random sample of 500 of the control group showed that 24% had undergone mammography during the study period.

The randomised controlled trial in Edinburgh, Scotland[8] has been described previously in an earlier section. Like the two-county study, population clusters (general practices) rather than individuals, were randomised. Although the mortality reduction was not significant, there was a greater use of conservation therapy for screen detected cancers which is clearly a reflection of smaller tumour size. This can be viewed as a positive result, although it does not have the weight of a significant mortality reduction. Compliance was low in the Edinburgh trial and non-compliance will affect the mortality reduction as non-attenders tend to have increased mortality compared to the controls.[6] There was evidence that the cluster randomisation did not achieve comparability between the two groups in, for example, cardiovascular mortality.

In Stockholm, Sweden, a randomised controlled trial was begun in March 1981 to compare single view mammography with no intervention in women aged 40 to 64 years.[12] Selection was done individually by birth date and 40,000 women were randomised to the study population and 20,000 to the controls. The study group were invited twice to attend for mammography with a screening interval of about 30 months. The compliance was over 80% in the first and second screening rounds with little difference between the age groups. After the second round was completed in 1985, the control group were invited for one screen by mammography where the compliance was approximately 77%. The relative risk of mortality from cancers detected before screening the controls was 0.7 (95% confidence interval 0.4 to 1.2) which is not statistically significant. This may also be due to screening in the control group as 25% of the invited group had mammography in the three years before screening and the control group would be likely to have similar characteristics due to randomisation.

The Canadian National Breast Screening Study (NBSS) was planned in the late 1970s and started screening women in January 1980. The study was in two parts - women aged 40 to 49 years[13] and women aged 50 to 59 years[14] followed different screening regimes. In the younger age group, 50,430 women with no history of breast cancer and who had not undergone mammography in the previous 12 months, were invited to an initial physical examination. At this initial visit, half were then randomly assigned to the MP (study) group who would be offered annual mammography and physical examination and the other half to the UC (control) group who would be returned to usual community care with annual follow-up by mailed questionnaire. The first 62% of the study women were eligible for a four year programme; the remainder were offered a three year

Table I. Randomised controlled trials of breast cancer screening with mammography.

Study	Year started	Age group	Approx. number of subjects (total)	Percentage mortality reduction	95% confidence interval
HIP, New York[4]	1963	40 to 64	62,000	29	(11, 44)
Two-county, Sweden[6]	1977	40 to 74	133,000	30	(15, 42)
Malmö, Sweden[11]	1976	45 to 69	42,000	4	(-35, 32)
Edinburgh, Scotland[10]	1979	45 to 64	45,000	17	(-18, 42)
Stockholm, Sweden[12]	1981	40 to 64	60,000	29	(-20, 60)
NBSS (1), Canada[13]	1980	40 to 49	50,000	-36	(-121, 16)
NBSS (2), Canada[14]	1980	50 to 59	39,000	3	(-52, 38)
Gothenburg[16]	1982	40 to 59	50,000	14	(-37, 46)

programme. All women were taught breast self-examination (BSE). The mean follow-up time was 8.5 years. Over 90% of the women in each group attended the screening sessions or returned the annual questionnaires or both over years two to five. The ratio of the proportions of death from breast cancer in the MP group compared with the UC group was 1.36 (95% confidence interval 0.84 to 2.21) which was not significant. The study concluded that screening with mammography and physical examination had no impact on the rate of death from breast cancer after seven years.

The entry criteria and randomisation techniques were the same in the older age group.[14] In this part of the study, 39,405 women attended the initial physical examination and were randomly assigned to undergo either annual mammography and physical examination (MP group) or annual physical examination only (PO group). The first 62% of the women who entered the study were offered five annual screens and the remainder were offered four. Again, all women were taught BSE at the initial examination. These women were followed up for an average of 8.3 years. Over 85% of the women in each group attended the screening sessions after the initial screen. The survival rates were similar in the two groups. Women whose cancer had been detected by mammography alone had the highest survival rate. The ratio of the proportions of death from breast cancer in the MP group compared with the PO group was 0.97 (95% confidence interval

0.62 to 1.52) which, again, was not significant. The conclusions were similar to those in the younger age group. Unfortunately, no conclusion can be drawn from either Canadian study because the quality of the mammography, as assessed by independent review, was unacceptably poor.[15]

The results from the screening trial in Gothenburg, Sweden have not yet been published but the results are given briefly in an overview of all four Swedish trials.[16] Recruitment of women aged 40 to 59 years started in December 1982. Approximately 21,000 women were randomly allocated to the study group and 29,000 to the controls. The randomisation was done by individual in the age range 40 to 49 years and by cluster from 50 to 59 years, according to day of birth. The study group were invited to two-view mammography at intervals of 18 months. The control group was not invited to screening. The compliance at the first round was 84% and the mortality reduction was found to be 14% although this result was not significant. The controls were invited to screening from November 1987 onwards. The results of all these randomised controlled trials are summarised in Table I.

Age effects

The most important risk factor for breast cancer is age. In addition to screening those most likely to

Table II. Age specific compliance in the Edinburgh trial.[10]

Age	Screening visit		
	1st	2nd	3rd
45 - 49	63.8%	56.8%	55.9%
50 - 54	63.3%	57.0%	55.5%
55 - 59	60.9%	53.9%	52.0%
60 - 64	56.5%	49.7%	47.6%
All women	61.3%	54.6%	53.1%

Table III. Age specific compliance in the Swedish Two-County trial.[6]

Age	Screening visit			
	1st ASP	2nd ASP	3rd ASP	1st PSP
40 - 49	93.2%	89.2%	88.4%	90.4%
50 - 59	91.8%	87.7%	86.2%	87.3%
60 - 69	87.9%	80.9%	77.8%	79.9%
70 - 74	78.7%	66.8%	–	–
All women	89.3%	83.3%	84.0%	85.8%

develop breast cancer, one should also consider those whose prognosis will be improved by early detection. All trials have shown decreasing compliance in the older age groups, i.e. over the age of 65, and this will reduce the effectiveness of mass screening. Tables II and III show the age specific compliance for the Edinburgh and Swedish two-county trials. Furthermore, the disease seems to be less aggressive in older women and the probability of dying from other diseases is greatly increased.

No trial has yet been published which was specifically designed to look at the issue of screening by age. Studies have shown screening to be effective in reducing breast cancer mortality in women over the age of 50 years,[4,6,9,17] but in the 40 to 49 age group there have been no significant results. The NBSS(1) assessed the effect of mammographic screening and clinical examination in this age range. Although the results showed no benefit from screening, the trial has been criticised regarding the technical screening quality, staff training and statistical power, and further research is needed. A meta-analysis conducted by combining results of randomised controlled trials relevant to the 40 to 49 age group excluding the NBSS(1) study have shown a mortality reduction of 15% (95% CI -8 to 32)[18] among women invited to screening as compared with control groups. When the NBSS (1) data is included, this becomes a mortality reduction of 7% (95% CI -15 to 24).[18] A more recent meta-analysis[19] has found a statistically significant mortality reduction in this age range of 21% (95% CI 2 to 36) when the NBSS(1) results are excluded. Inclusion of the NBSS(1) data yields a non-significant reduction of 14% (95% CI -5 to 29). Table IV shows the mortality reduction by age for all the randomised controlled trials discussed so far. This issue is currently being investigated in the UKCCCR Age Trial.

How does screening work?

As neither the cause of breast cancer nor the means of preventing it are known, the only intervention possible at the moment in healthy women to improve mortality from breast cancer is screening. Trials of chemoprevention agents are, however, underway. Although treatment, notably chemotherapy and hormone therapy, has improved, prognosis still deteriorates rapidly with increasing tumour burden. Screening can advance the diagnosis so that the cancer is treated at an early stage with greater chance of success. This is reflected in the earlier stage of tumours detected in the study group in the Swedish two-county trial.[6] The progression of the disease is shown in Figure 1.[20] The lead time is the interval

Table IV. Age (at entry to trial) specific mortality reduction observed in randomised trials.

Study	Age less than 50 years		Age 50 years or more	
	Percentage mortality reduction	Confidence interval	Percentage mortality reduction	Confidence interval
HIP New York[4,20]	24	(-17, 50)	32	(4, 52)
Two-county Sweden[6,16]	13	(-41, 46)	34	(19, 46)
Malmö Sweden[11,19]	49	(-17, 78)	NP	NP
Edinburgh Scotland[10]	22	(-31, 54)	15	(-15, 38)
Stockholm Sweden[12]	-4	(-105, 47)	43	(-10, 70)
NBSS Canada[11,12*]	-36	(-121, 16)	3	(-52, 38)
Gothenburg[16,19]	27	(-97, 73)	NP	NP

NP = not published
* The mammography in the Canadian trials has been found to be unacceptably poor therefore no conclusions may be drawn from these results.

between the time when a prevalent case is detected by screening and the time when that case would otherwise have become clinically incident. The longer the lead time for a given case, the better one would expect the prognosis to be. If the cancer is not detected until it becomes clinically detectable, the lead time is zero. The lead time for an individual case is unobservable but the distribution of lead times is dependent on the distribution of the time spent in the pre-clinical detectable phase (sojourn time). The sojourn time is also unobservable but may be estimated using the method of Walter and Day.[20] The method will also provide an estimate of the sensitivity of the screen and this may be used to estimate the optimum screening regime and the potential gains in terms of mortality. For example, if the sojourn time is long, the maximum possible lead time is correspondingly long. If the sojourn time is short however, the potential benefit from screening is smaller and screening must take place more frequently to increase the probability that the pre-clinical disease is detected before it becomes clinically apparent.

Detection status

In a screening trial, breast cancers can be detected in seven different ways: symptomatically in the control group; after randomisation but before screening; at the first (prevalence) screen; at later (incidence)

Table V. Breast cancer deaths /cases by age group and detection mode and relative risk by detection mode in the Swedish two-county study.[6]

Detection mode	Breast cancer deaths/cases in age group					Relative risk
	40 - 49	50 - 59	60 - 69	70 - 74	Total	
PSP	32/160	73/315	90/419	40/146	234/1040	1.00
Before screening*	1/6	3/5	3/12	1/4	8/27	NK
First screen	5/39	13/102	20/184	10/101	48/436	0.57
Later screens	9/110	12/156	15/183	6/52	42/501	0.69
Interval 0 - 11 months	7/32	3/19	2/23	0/2	12/76	0.80
Interval 12 - 23 months	10/43	7/35	7/36	2/11	26/125	
Interval 24+ months	6/12	10/32	8/34	2/9	26/87	
Interval (time not known)	0/4	0/4	0/2	0/0	0/10	
Refuser	4/10	15/28	20/49	23/50	62/137	1.46
After screening#	0/0	0/0	0/0	8/30	8/30	NK
Total ASP	42/256	63/381	75/523	52/259	232/1419	0.70

* Between randomisation and commencement of screening;   PSP = passive study population, i.e. not invited to screening;
#In women aged 70 - 74 after routine screening ceased in this group;   NK = not known.
ASP = active study population, i.e. invited to screening;

Table VI. Cancer detection rate in the Swedish two-county study.[6]

Screen	Cancer detection rate per 1,000 women screened	Cancers per open biopsy
Prevalence	6.1	0.50
First incidence	3.4	0.75

screens; in the interval between screening; in women who refused screening; or after screening has finished or the control is broken. In a routine screening programme, not a randomised trial, there are three possible modes of detection: at screening, in the interval between screens, and in refusers. In the Swedish two-county trial, a cancer was classified as being in a refuser if it was diagnosed after the woman did not attend a screen to which she was invited but before the invitation to the next. Interval cancers are those that appear symptomatically between screens, after a negative screen. Table V shows the number of deaths from breast cancer by age and detection mode and also the relative risk of mortality by detection mode in the Swedish two-county trial. The cancer detection rate at the first two screens is shown in Table VI by age.

The detection rates are also expressed as multiples of the incidence rate in the control group. Detection rates increase steadily with age. Although the detection rate at the prevalence screen was higher, Table V shows that the relative risk of mortality is lower than for subsequent screens. This is due to length bias. Many slow growing cancers, which may have been present for years, will be detected at the first screen and these will have a far better prognosis than the more aggressive fast growing tumours. After the prevalence screen, this bias can be eliminated by

defining the so-called "unbiased set". The improvement in the cancer to biopsy ratio is partly due to increasing expertise as the trial progresses and partly because, at the first screen, more benign and non-invasive lesions will be picked up. In younger women there is a predominance of deaths from interval cancers whereas in older women there are more deaths in the refuser category. This is due to the fact that interval cancers are more common in younger women and that older women are more likely to be refusers, rather than age variation in case fatalities. A good means for expressing interval cancer rates is to express them as a proportion of the underlying incidence that would be expected in the absence of screening (in a trial this is given by the control group incidence). The Swedish two-county study proportionate incidence rates for interval cancers are shown in Table VII. For women over age 50, these results have been used as targets in the UK national programme. The rates for younger women (under 50) are notably higher than for women over 50.

Both the lower cancer detection rates and the higher interval cancer rates underline the difficulty of effective screening for women under 50. They provide an explanation of the smaller mortality reduction that is generally seen.

Tumour characteristics

The three prognostic factors of a breast tumour which are most commonly considered are its size, nodal status and an underlying measure of malignant potential such as histological grade. The nodal status is an indication of how far a tumour has spread. If the lymph nodes are negative then the tumour is almost certainly still localized to the breast. If it has spread to the lymph nodes the prognosis will

Table VII. Control incidence of breast cancer by age at randomisation, with screening prevalence and interval incidence as a percentage of control incidence, by age, and by screening round in the Swedish two-county study.[6]

Age group	Control incidence*	Interval incidence# in year			Screening prevalence*
		1	2	3 or more	
		First interval			First round
40 - 49	1.05	46	53	–	2.09
50 - 59	1.87	10	28	52	4.67
60 - 69	2.50	17	27	57	8.80
70 - 74	2.99	8	44	48	12.15
		Second interval			Second round
40 - 49	as above	66	41	–	2.65
50 - 59		19	35	62	3.03
60 - 69		9	31	43	4.89
70 - 74		–	–	–	7.50
		Third interval			Third round
40 - 49	as above	22	109	–	2.16
50 - 59		23	40	85	3.74
60 - 69		24	22	26	5.07
70 - 74		–	–	–	–
		Overall			Overall
40 - 49	as above	45	62	–	2.30
50 - 59		17	34	63	3.84
60 - 69		17	27	46	6.41
70 - 74		8	44	48	10.13

* incidence per thousand woman years; prevalence per thousand women.
# As a percentage of control incidence; for ages 40 - 49 only given years 1 and 2+.

be worse; if distant metastases are present, the prognosis is very poor. The grade is a measure of the aggressiveness of the tumour. Grade 1 tumours have the best prognosis as they tend to be slow growing (well differentiated), whereas grade 3 tumours are notably more aggressive (poorly differentiated). However, grade is assigned by the pathologist and, as judgements vary, can be subjective. In the Swedish two-county study, grade was assessed independently by one pathologist in each county and the grade distributions were different. This is more likely to be a reflection of the differences between the two pathologists rather than differences in the tumour populations. However, the effect of grade on prognosis was much the same, suggesting that the pathologists were measuring the same phenomenon but scoring it differently. The prognostic importance of these three factors, when considered together, is given in Table VIII.[21]

In the same study, detection status was found to be significantly related to each of the tumour attributes size, nodal status and grade. Screen detected cancers are more likely to be small and have favourable nodal status and grade, all of which indicate a good prognosis. The tumours in the refusers are larger, more likely to have positive nodes or distant metastases and have worse grades. There is no ap-

parent reason to expect the cancers in the refusers to have a poorer grade than those detected at screening unless the grade is not static for each tumour but deteriorates as the tumour grows. This could be explained if tumours have a mixture of poorly- and well-differentiated cells; the poorly-differentiated cells would be expected to multiply more quickly. In order to test this, an unbiased set was required so that two groups of tumours could be compared whose only major difference was that one was detected at an earlier stage. In the study and control groups, non-invasive (in-situ) cancers were excluded, and also those occurring in women aged 70 to 74 at entry to the trial as they were invited to only two screening rounds. Cancers that occurred before or at the prevalence round were omitted to avoid length bias in the study group.

The tumour characteristics of the two groups were then compared: these are shown in Table IX. The distributions of grade were indeed different in the two groups indicating that grade does deteriorate as tumours grow. When grade was controlled for size however, there was no significant difference between the two groups. One could thus consider the effect of early detection on size to induce the effect on grade. Overall, it was found that size, grade and nodal status are significantly and inde-

Table VIII. Estimates of relative hazard based on proportional hazards regression, with each factor adjusted for the others, and for age and county, in the Swedish two-county study.[21]

Factors/category	Hazard ratio	(95% CI)
Size (mm)		
1 - 9	1.00	–
10 - 14	1.57	(0.94 - 2.63)
15 - 19	1.84	(1.11 - 3.07)
20 - 29	3.23	(1.99 - 5.23)
30 - 49	5.35	(3.28 - 8.74)
50 +	9.97	(6.04 - 16.4)
Lymph node status		
Negative	1.00	–
Positive or		
distant metastases	3.20	(2.6 - 3.9)
Histologic type		
Others*	1.00	–
Ductal grade 1	0.75	(0.45 - 1.27)
Ductal grade 2	1.24	(0.85 - 1.80)
Ductal grade 3	2.06	(1.44 - 2.93)
Ductal grade unspecified	1.56	(0.83 - 2.92)
Lobular	1.19	(0.76 - 1.86)
Medullary	0.94	(0.50 - 1.78)
Missing size,		
lymph node status or type	3.84	(3.21 - 4.58)

CI: Confidence interval
* Others include ductal carcinoma *in-situ*, mucinous carcinoma, tubular carcinoma, and other carcinomas.

Table IX. Percentage distribution of grade, nodal status and size of invasive tumours diagnosed in women aged 40 - 69 in the ASP and the PSP after the prevalence screen in the Swedish two-county study.[6]

Factors/category	Group ASP	PSP	Overall
Grade			
1	21.3	16.8	19.3
2	38.7	34.7	36.9
3	40.0	48.5	43.8
Number of cases	600	493	1.093
Nodal status			
Negative	68.2	54.5	62.0
Positive	27.6	39.8	33.2
Distant metastases	4.2	5.7	4.8
Number of cases	670	558	1.228
Tumour size (mm)			
01 - 09	18.0	7.1	13.0
10 - 14	22.4	15.4	19.3
15 - 19	20.5	19.7	20.0
20 - 29	23.2	29.0	25.9
30 - 49	10.5	20.0	14.9
50 +	5.4	8.8	7.0
Number of cases	704	590	1.294

ASP = active study population, i.e. invited to screening
PSP = passive study population, i.e. not invited to screening

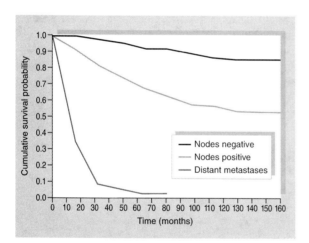

Fig. 2. Cumulative survival probability by nodal status.

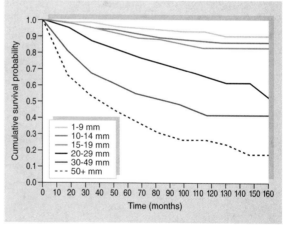

Fig. 3. Cumulative survival probability by size.

pendently related to each other and to detection mode. All three prognostic factors are more favourable in tumours which are detected earlier, but although screen detected tumours tend to have a lower grade, there are still considerable numbers of high grade lesions (grade 3). Figures 2 to 5 show the survival probabilities plotted against time by nodal status, tumour size, grade and detection status.[6] It is clear that all of these factors have a considerable effect on survival.

Targets and monitoring

In the UK, the National Health Service Breast Screening Programme (NHSBSP) is based on the recommendations of the Forrest Report.[7] It is important that it should be closely monitored in order to ensure that it is on course for meeting the Health of the Nation target, which is a 25% reduction in breast cancer mortality, in women of screening age, by the year 2000. The expected reduction in mortality may

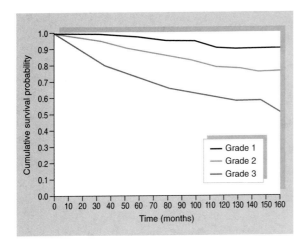

Fig. 4. Cumulative survival probability by grade.

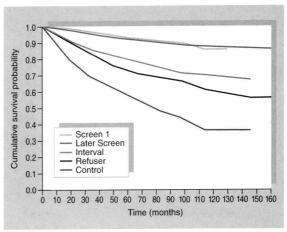

Fig. 5. Cumulative survival probability by detection status.

take ten years to become significant so in the meantime, progress may be measured using short-term surrogate end-points. The most relevant trial results to the UK programme are those of the Swedish two-county study. This is because the screening modality used was mammography alone, and the screening interval in the age range of interest (50-64 years) was 33 months, which is close to the UK interval of three years.

The three main indicators of the success of the programme are the changes in mortality, the changes in the absolute rate of advanced disease and the parameters of the screening process. These parameters incorporate the screening test and any further diagnostic tests that are performed as a result of the screen. They include sensitivity, specificity, the distributions of lead time and sojourn time, and the predictive value for malignancy (i.e. the cancer to biopsy ratio).

The overall effectiveness of the programme will also depend directly on the proportion of the target population who attend for screening. Compliance is therefore another important interim measurement. Every effort must be made to ensure that the population lists used are accurate and that every woman who is invited is both alive and resident in the catchment area.

In a screening programme, there are three possible groups to compare with the target population. The first is to use historical cancer registry data from the same area covering the same age range. There may be secular trends already occurring in the data which should be adjusted for. Secondly, a neighbouring geographical area could be used. This is obviously of limited usefulness in a national programme as it may only be used while the programme is being introduced. Lastly, there is the case-control approach whereby the screened and unscreened women in a population are compared. There will then be the risk of selection bias but the problem of secular trends will be avoided; therefore it may be best to combine this with the historical data approach to strengthen both.[9]

Table X. UK national targets for the NHSBSP.[22]

Measure	Acceptable level
Compliance rate	No less than 70%
Prevalence rate at first screening test	No less than 55 per 10,000 women screened
Rate of interval cancers:	
first year after negative screen	2 to 3 per 10,000 women screened per year
second year after negative screen	4 to 5 per 10,000 women screened per year
third year after negative screen	7 to 8 per 10,000 women screened per year
Stage distribution of screen detected cancers:	
at first test	No more than 40% of stage II or more advanced
at subsequent tests	No more than 30% of stage II or more advanced
Reduction in rate of advanced cancers	No less than 30% in target population, seven years after first invitation sent
Reduction in breast cancer mortality rates	No less than 25% in target population free from breast cancer when first invitation sent, 10 years after programme starts

Table X summarises the target levels for the compliance rate, the prevalence detection rate, the interval rate and the distribution of stage[22] which have been set initially in the UK programme. They are currently under review.

Conclusion

The government objective set out in its "Health of the Nation" strategy in 1993 is to reduce the breast cancer mortality rate by 25% by the year 2000 (from 95.1 per 100,000 population to no more than 71.3 per 100,000 population).[23] Early results for compliance and cancer detection rate at prevalence showed that the national targets were being met.[24] This was a good indication that the NHSBSP was on course to meet the Health of the Nation objective. Interval cancers however, are also an important measure and it is these that have recently become the subject of some debate.

In the North Western region, it has been found that the incidence of interval cancers is higher than the targets set in the NHS Breast Screening Programme guidelines.[22,25] In fact, the incidence approaches that expected in the absence of screening after two years. An unpublished report (in preparation) shows that this is also the case in East Anglia. Preliminary data have also been collected by the National Breast Screening Radiology Quality Assurance Committee suggesting that these results are representative of the country as a whole. In both regions the prevalence round achieved the target rate of over three times the incidence expected in the absence of screening. This may be an indication that the targets, particularly for small cancers, were not stringent enough. It is the small aggressive cancers which, if missed, will grow quickly and present as interval cancers. In East Anglia, there is a deficit of small screen detected cancers which is approximately balanced by the excess of intervals (these figures are not published for the North Western region). There is understandable concern about the sensitivity of the screening test which needs to be improved to increase the detection rate for small aggressive cancers in order to meet the Health of the Nation target.

There are several ways in which sensitivity may be improved. Woodman et al. in the North Western region, concluded that the screening interval should be reduced. This would not however, address the underlying sensitivity problem and would have considerable implications on resources, both financial and staffing. At present, there is a national shortage of suitably trained radiologists. There is currently a national trial being conducted to assess the benefits of more frequent screening. Two-view mammogra-phy and double reading of films have both been shown to improve sensitivity and specificity. Many screening centres are already implementing these measures and a working party of the National Breast Screening Radiology Quality Assurance Committee is currently examining the feasibility of double reading throughout the UK programme. Most centres are now using film with an increased optical density which is more sensitive to small cancers, and a programme to give radiologists additional training is being established.

It is hoped that with these ongoing improvements in the service, the UK NHS Breast Screening Programme will attain the target breast cancer mortality reduction of 25%, in women aged 50 to 64, by the year 2000, based on the evidence from the Swedish two-county trial.

References

1. Petrakis N.L., Ernster V.L., King M.C.: Breast. In: Schottenfeld D., Fraumeni D.F. (Eds). *Cancer Epidemiology and Prevention*. Philadelphia, Saunders, 1982

2. Tubiana M., Koscielny S.: Natural history of human breast cancer: Recent data and clinical implications. *Breast Cancer Res. Treat.*, 1991; 18: 125-140

3. Tabàr L., Fagerberg G., Day N.E., Duffy S.W., Kitchen R.M.: Breast cancer treatment and natural history: new insights from results of screening. Lancet 1992; 339: 412-414

4. Shapiro S., Venet W., Strax P., Venet L., Roeser R.: Selection, follow-up, and analysis in the Health Insurance Plan Study: a randomised trial with breast cancer screening. Natl. Cancer. Inst. Monogr., 1985 May; 67: 65-74

5. UK Trial of Early Detection of Breast Cancer Group. First results on mortality reduction in the UK trial of early detection of breast cancer. Lancet, 1988; 2: 411-416

6. Tabàr L., Fagerberg G., Duffy S.W., Day N.E., Gad A., Gröntoft O.: Update of the Swedish two-county program of mammographic screening for breast cancer. Radiol. Clin. North. Am. 1992 Jan; 30(1): 187-210

7. Forrest A.P.M.: Breast cancer screening. London: HMSO, 1986

8. Warren R.: Team learning and breast cancer screening (letter). Lancet, 1991; 338: 514

9. Collette C., Collette H.J., Fracheboud J., Slotboom B.J., de-Waard F.: Evaluation of a breast cancer screening programme - the DOM project. Eur. J. Cancer., 1992; 28A(12):1985 - 8

10. Alexander F.E., Anderson T.J., Brown H.K., Hepburn W., Kirkpatrick A.E., McDonald C., et al.: The Edinburgh randomised trial of breast cancer screening: results after 10 years of follow-up. Br. J. Cancer, 1994; 70: 542-548

11. Andersson I., Aspergren K., Janzon L., Landberg T., Lindholm K., Linell F., et al.: Mammographic screening and mortality from breast cancer: the Malmö mammographic screening trial. BMJ 1988; 297: 943-948

12. Frisell J., Eklund G., Hellström L., Lidbrink E., Rutqvist L.E., Somell A.: Randomised study of mammography screening - preliminary report on mortality in the Stockholm trial. Breast Cancer. Res. Treat., 1991; 18: 49-56

13. Miller A.B., Baines C.J., To T., Wall C.: Canadian National Breast Screening Study: 1. Breast cancer detection and death rates among women aged 40 to 49 years. Can. Med. Assoc. J. 1992; 147(10): 1459-1476

14. Miller A.B., Baines C.J., To T., Wall C.: Canadian National Breast Screening Study: 2. Breast cancer detection and death

rates among women aged 50 to 59 years. Can. Med. Assoc. J. 1992; 147(10): 1477-1488

15. Baines C.J., Miller A.B., Kopans D.B., *et al.*: Canadian breast screening study: assessment of technical quality by external review. Am. J. Roentgenol., 1990; 155: 743-747

16. Nyström L., Rutqvist L-E, Wall S., Lindgren A., Lindqvist M., Rydén S., *et al.*: Breast cancer screening with mammography: overview of the Swedish randomised trials. Lancet, 1993; 341: 973-978

17. Peeters P.H., Verbeek A.L., Hendriks J.H., van Bon M.J.: Screening for breast cancer in Nijmegen. Report of six screening rounds, 1975-1986. Int. J. Cancer. 1989 Feb. 15; 43(2): 226-230

18. Eckhardt S., Badellino F., Murphy G.P.: UICC meeting on breast cancer screening in pre-menopausal women in developed countries. Int. J. Cancer, 1994; 56: 1-5

19. Smart C.R., Hendrick R.E., Rutledge J.H., Smith R.A.: Benefit of mammography screening in women aged 40-49: current evidence from randomised controlled trials. Cancer, 1995; 75: 1619-1626

20. Day N.E., Miller A.B., (Eds). Screening for breast cancer. Germany: Hans Huber Publishers, 1988

21. Tabàr L., Fagerberg G., Chen H.H., Duffy S.W., Smart C.R., Gad A., *et al.*: Efficacy of breast cancer screening by age. Cancer, 1995 May; 75(10): 2507-2517

22. Patnick J., Gray J.A.M.: Guidelines on the collection and use of breast cancer data. NHSBSP Publication no. 26. Jan 1993

23. Secretary of State for Health. The Health of the Nation. A Strategy for Health in England. London: HMSO, 1992

24. Chamberlain J., Moss S.M., Michell M., Johns L.: National Health Service Breast Screening Programme results for 1991 - 2. B.M.J. 1993; 307: 353-356

25. Woodman C.B.J., Threlfall A.G., Boggis C.R.M., Prior P.: Is the three year breast screening interval too long? Occurrence of interval cancers in NHS Breast Screening Programme's North Western region. B.M.J. 1995; 310: 224-226

26. Warren R.M.L., Duffy S.W., Bashir S.: The value of the second view in Screening mammography. Br. J. Radiol., 1996; 69: 105-108

Genetics and breast screening

D. Gareth Evans

Introduction

Human cancers may follow exposure to particular environmental factors, but it is well established that cancer is, at the cellular level, genetic in origin. Genetic changes associated with initiation and progression are usually acquired "somatic" events. Occasionally one of these genetic changes may be inherited, resulting in a predisposition to cancer. Almost all types of cancer have been reported in familial clusters, but a site commonly involved is the breast.[1]

Inherited cases account for only a small proportion, perhaps 5-10%, of breast cancer. However, those at risk in families may benefit from screening and early diagnosis particularly as they are at risk of developing the disease at a much younger age. Study of families with breast cancer provided the opportunity to localise and clone a breast cancer gene on chromosome 17.[2,3] It is believed that the genetic changes observed in many sporadic cancers and those observed in inherited counterparts are similar.[4] Intense study of the familial forms will therefore be of great general importance, since the more common non-familial forms may result from mutation of the same gene(s), although early signs do not suggest that BRCA1 is involved in sporadic disease. These may nonetheless be of great significance when designing new genetic therapies.

Breast cancer

Complex segregation analysis has been applied to breast cancer to investigate genetic and environmental models of disease transmission in pedigrees and to determine the most likely explanation for familial aggregation considering that breast cancer is probably aetiologically heterogeneous,[5] in that there is more than one gene conferring breast cancer sus-

ceptibility in a population. Newman et al.[6] found that complex segregation analysis of an unselected population-based series of breast cancer patients demonstrated an autosomal dominant model with an incomplete but highly penetrant susceptibility allele as the explanation for transmission of breast cancer within 4% of all breast cancer cases. They reported that lifetime risk may be as high as 40-50% in first degree relatives of those with the gene. Other workers have similarly found a model of a dominant susceptibility gene as the best explanation of the pattern of breast cancer in families.[1] It is often hard to establish that an aggregation of breast cancer in a family is truly hereditary as the disease is so common. However, early age at diagnosis, bilaterality and multiple affected family members would most likely infer a dominant gene.

The breast/ovary gene

Overall it is now certain that breast and ovarian tumours are related genetically, in the light of the well documented breast/ovarian families,[7,8] the now published linkage to chromosome 17q in many families[9] and the more recent cloning of the susceptibility gene, BRCA1.[3]

It appears that the vast majority of families with breast and ovarian cancer are linked to BRCA1 and that mutations will eventually be found in this gene as the cause of the disease in those families. However breast/ovary families are not always caused by BRCA1, as they have been described with BRCA2[10] and p53.[11] Nonetheless if there are two or more cases of epithelial ovarian cancer in a family, that is strong evidence, in itself, that BRCA1 is likely to be involved. There is also now increasing evidence that families with BRCA1 involvement have differing risks of susceptibility to ovarian cancer.[12] Although the overall cumulative lifetime risk across all the linked families is 85% for breast and 60% for ovarian cancer, it is likely that there are at least two subsets of mutation; one causing predominantly an ovarian cancer risk and the other only a relatively low risk of ovarian involvement. It may well be that so-called site specific ovarian cancer families are in fact virtually all caused by BRCA1 mutations. Supportive evidence for this comes from the long term follow up of apparently site specific families,[13] new cancers in families from the UKCCCR familial ovarian cancer study (Ponder personal communication) and linkage analysis in the families.[14]

Other genes predisposing to breast cancer

In addition to BRCA1 there are at least 4 further major susceptibility genes predisposing to breast cancer. The first of these to be implicated was the p53 gene on the short arm of chromosome 17. Mutations were found in the germline of individuals with a rare cancer family syndrome[15] predisposing to sarcoma, glioma and various childhood tumours in addition to extremely early onset breast cancer (20-40 years). The p53 gene which is implicated in programmed cell death (apoptosis) is the most commonly implicated gene in human cancer, but probably accounts for only a small proportion of familial breast cancer (Table I). More recently a gene on chromosome 13 was implicated by linkage studies in families excluded from BRCA1.[10] This may well account for the majority of families with male breast cancer, but it is ovarian cancer that is a part variable of the susceptibility pattern caused by mutations in this gene. Male breast cancer may also be caused by

inherited mutations in the androgen receptor gene (Reifenstein's disease). Family aggregations of breast cancer may also be related to carriage of a mutation in the DNA repair gene causing ataxia telangectasia.[16] However, the risk associated with the heterozygous state is probably insufficient to cause a true dominant pattern of inheritance. In addition to the genes already described there is at least one further locus predisposing to breast cancer as some clear dominant families are not linked to either BRCA1 or BRCA2 (Table I).[10]

How to ascribe risks

Only a small proportion of women seeking advice about their family history will have a definite dominant family history of the disease. Therefore in order to ascribe risks it is necessary to consult large epidemiological studies.[17] Evidence from these studies shows that a woman with an affected mother and sister may be at a 20-fold increased relative risk compared to the general population when the affected cases developed the disease at less than 30 years of age. Clearly, a relative risk of 20 does not mean that a women is at 20 times the general population lifetime risk of one in 12, since the relative risks apply to a particular age. For example the risk of a woman developing breast cancer at age 35 years is 1 in 2,500; 20 times this risk is 20 in 2,500 or 1 in 125; at age 70 the risk for that year is 1 in 400; 20 times this risk is one chance in 20. However, once a woman reaches 60 years her relative risk differs little from the general population. This means that a genetic tendency is likely to have expressed itself by this age, although non-penetrance does occur; the estimated penetrance of the breast cancer genes is

Table I. Hereditary conditions predisposing to breast cancer.

Disease	Other tumour susceptibility	Inheritance	% of familial breast cancer	Location
Familial breast BRCA1	Ovary/prostate	AD	45%	17q
BRCA2	Male breast, ovary	AD	40%	13q
Li-Fraumeni	sarcoma, leukaemia brain, adrenal	AD	1-5%	17p(p53)
Lynch type 2	Bowel (proximal) endometrium, ovary pancreas, stomach	AD	?5%	2p 3p 2q 7p
A-T	HoZ (leukaemia etc) HeZ (?other sites)	AR	?	11q ?others
Cowden's	Skin and other sites	AD	<1%	10q
Reifenstein's	?	?XLR	<1%	X

AD= Autosomal dominant; AR= autosomal recessive; XLR= X-linked recessive; HoZ= homozygous; HeZ= heterozygous.

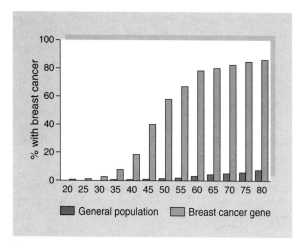

Fig. 1. The breast cancer genes: penetrance of susceptibility.

around 80% from epidemiological studies. A typical penetrance curve for the breast cancer genes is shown in Figure l; it can be seen from this that even those with the gene have little more risk than the general population if they have not already developed breast cancer by the age of 60 years.

It is probably easier for women (and their doctors) to understand cumulative risks. The individual wants to know the risk of developing breast cancer in her lifetime or at least over a fixed period until she is, say, 60 years old. Cumulative risks can be estimated from epidemiological studies where the incidence of breast cancer in families with an affected relative is compared to the incidence in families without an affected relative. The most comprehensive data in this field are derived from the Cancer and Steroid Hormone Study Group (CASH) from the United States.[17] The CASH data is helpful for giving approximate risks to women in clinics.

Dupont and Page[18] have provided useful data concerning the association between proliferative disease of the breast [epithelial hyperplasia, and atypical ductal hyperplasia (ADH)] and family history. They showed that the additional risk of a biopsy finding of ADH in the general population is 5 times and, if a family history is present, 11 times that of someone without a family history with a normal biopsy. If the latter risk was present for a lifetime then the chances of developing breast cancer would be nearly 100% (11 x 1 in 12 lifetime risk). This figure was puzzling until Dupont and Page published a further paper[19] indicating that this risk only held true for about 10 years after the biopsy and then fell substantially. Epithelial hyperplasia and ADH may be a greater risk factor in those with a family history of breast cancer than in those without since it may be a manifestation of a faulty gene in the family.[20] This

supposition was supported by fine needle aspiration cytology of breasts from women with a family history of breast cancer. A segregation analysis confirmed that the proliferative disease was segregating with breast cancer. Other groups have shown positive immuno-staining for the p53 gene product in needle aspirates; the prognostic significance of this requires further study. Use of the high risk clinic and of fine needle aspiration which is a well tolerated procedure are likely to answer questions about early genetic changes in both familial and sporadic disease.

Value of a family history clinic

Referral to a family history clinic allows as precise a definition of risk as possible, discussion concerning the meaning of the risks, the opportunity to institute early detection by mammography and breast examination and the opportunity for women to take part in prevention and other research programmes. Most women when asked, appear to welcome the opportunity to discuss their fears of breast cancer with experts and to feel that they are being incorporated into an ongoing follow-up programme. Women have a conception that they are at increased risk, but it is remarkable how much this varies from woman to woman. We have asked women to estimate their risks by means of a questionnaire given before discussion of their cases with the clinician.[21]

This showed how diverse was the perception of risk amongst a well-motivated, essentially self-referred group of women. Their estimation of population risk varied from "inevitable" to less than 1 in 200; 29% of women underestimated their own risks by more than 50% while 23% exaggerated their risk by more than this.

Those who overestimated risk gained some reassurance that their risks where lower than they thought and were more likely to retain risk figures at follow-up.[22] However, even though a considerable number of women were given higher risk estimates at the clinic than they had originally estimated, this group had a high re-attendance rate, but did not retain information so well and continued to underestimate risk. It is nonetheless reassuring that from early data from psychological evaluation that these women are not made more anxious by coming to the clinic (unpublished results).

Screening

A combination of annual breast examination with mammography from 35 years, or 5 years before the earliest onset cancer, is now standard practise in high risk women. This practise exemplifies the paradox that in many women with a family history their period of greatest risk is below the age of 50 years, ages at which the effectiveness of mammography in the general population is marginal. No data are available on the high risk group, where the detection rates should be much higher. National collaboration between risk clinics co-ordinated through the National Screening Programme is needed to assess the value of screening, but high risk women are unlikely to accept randomisation into non-screened groups. Annual mammography is required because of evidence from the Swedish studies showing that over 60% of breast cancers are detected with annual screening in the under-fifties, but that 70% present with interval cancers if only screened twice-yearly.[23] This approach is, therefore, being used in the UK under-fifties trial. We have found that ultrasound is a useful adjunct to mammography, particularly in the younger age group or when breast cysts are present. There is a national initiative underway in the UK to screen women proven to be gene carriers with MRI annually in addition to mammography to compare the sensitivities of the two techniques in a group of women with a 2% annual risk of the disease. At present there is no genetic or biochemical marker in blood to identify early disease.

Prevention trials

Identification of a group of women at high risk provides the possibility of obtaining sufficient events (development of breast cancer) to make prevention trials worthwhile. Three major groups of trials of prevention are currently in progress, although, apart from an international collaborative trial on tamoxifen, none are in the UK. Tamoxifen has been shown to reduce contralateral breast cancer in treated patients by 30-40% and is also well tolerated.[24] It may also have a beneficial effect on the heart and bones and therefore provides an ideal candidate for prevention trials on what are essentially fit and healthy volunteers. Other studies underway involve reduction in fat intake in Canada, administration of retinoids in Italy and the administration of the anti-oestrogen, tamoxifen, in America, Australasia and mainland Europe.

Preventative mastectomy

Increasingly, women at high risk in the UK are opting for preventative mastectomy. This is likely to increase further when genetic testing is more widely available and women at 80-90% lifetime risk of breast cancer are identified. However, in order to be truly preventative 100% of the breast tissue would have to be removed. Subcutaneous mastectomy may leave up to 10% of the breast epithelium behind and there are significant cancer rates in the retained breast tissue after this procedure.[25, 26]

As BRCA1 carriers have a 60% chance of bilateral disease, leaving 10% of the breast tissue behind may leave a residual lifetime risk of over 20% of developing breast cancer. A more logical approach would, therefore, be a total mastectomy.[27] It is, however, important that women receive adequate counselling before surgery and that they are aware of all the available options.

Genetic testing

Pre-symptomatic testing of unaffected individuals currently requires that the causative mutation has been established in the family or that the family is sufficiently large to allow significant linkage to one of the breast cancer genes. Until all of the genes predisposing to breast cancer have been identified and mutation screening techniques are sufficiently sensitive to detect >90% of the mutations, it will not be possible to reassure an individual that they are not at high risk of developing breast cancer.[28]

Even with the recent isolation of BRCA2,[29] testing of both genes will still not fully reassure a woman at risk.

It is still necessary to undertake family studies and to obtain samples from affected individuals before testing can be performed. It is also important that the individual is aware of the many implications of a high risk result (ethical, insurance), and pre-test counselling is essential.

Conclusions

A small proportion of breast cancer is caused by highly penetrant dominant genes. Family history clinics provide a forum for giving a professional service to women at risk and organising appropriate screening. The cloning of the various hereditary breast cancer genes will allow specific mutation analysis in families and the identification of those who are truly at high risk. Techniques which are likely to be far more accurate, such as MRI with gadolinium enhancement may be a real possibility for this very small group of women at up to 80-90% risk of developing breast cancer. The genetic tests will also allow reassurance of a much larger group of women who have not inherited a faulty gene, with the potential saving of not requiring early screening.

References

1. Claus E.B., Risch N.J., Thompson W.D.: Age at onset as an indicator of familial risk of breast cancer Am. J. Epidemiology, 1990; 131: 961-972

2. Hall J.M., Lee M.K., Newman B., *et al.*: Linkage of early onset familial breast cancer to chromosome 17q21. Science, 1990; 250: 1684-1689

3. Miki Y., Swensen J., Shattuck-Eidens D., *et al.*: A strong candidate for the breast and ovarian cancer gene BRCA1. Science, 1994; 266: 66-71

4. Ponder B.A.J.: Inherited predisposition to cancer. T.I.G., 1990; 6: 213-218

5. Evans H.J.: Genetic predisposition to some common cancer. M.R.C. News, 1990; 49: 46-47

6. Newman B., Austin M.A., Lee M., King M.C.: Inheritance of human breast cancer: Evidence for autosomal dominant transmission in high-risk families. Proc. Natl. Acad. Sci., 1988; 85: 3044-3048

7. Fraumeni J.F., Grundy G.W., Creagan E.T., Everson R.B.: Six families prone to ovarian cancer. Cancer, 1975; 36: 364-369

8. Lynch H.T., Harris R.E., Cuirgis H.A., Maloney K., Carmody L.L., Lynch J.F.: Familial association of breast/ovarian cancer. Cancer, 1978; 41: 1543-1549

9. Narod S.A., Feunteun J., Lynch H.T., *et al.*: Familial breast-ovarian cancer locus on chromosome 17q12-q23. Lancet, 1991; 338: 82-83

10. Wooster R., Neuhausen S.L., Mangion J.: Localization of a breast cancer susceptibility gene, BRCA2, to chromosome 13q12-13. Science 1994; 265: 2088-2090

11. Jolly K.W., Malkin D., Douglas E.C., Brown T.F., Sinclair A.E.: Look A.T.: Splice-site mutation in the p53 gene in a family with hereditary breast-ovarian cancer. Oncogene, 1992; 9: 97-102

12. Easton D.F., Ford D., Bishop D.T.: Breast and ovarian cancer incidence in BRCA1 mutation carriers. Am. J. Hum. Genet., 1994; 56: 265-271

13. Evans D.G.R., Donnai D., Ribeiro G., Warrell D.: Ovarian cancer family and prophylactic choices. J.Med. Genet., 1992; 29: 416-418

14. Steichen-Gersdorf E., Gallion H.H., Ford. D., *et al.*: Familial site-specific ovarian cancer is linked to BRCA1 on 17q12-21. Am. J. Hum. Genet., 1994; 55: 870-875

15. Malkin D., Li F.P., Strong L.C., *et al.*: Germline p53 mutations in cancer families. Science, 1990; 250: 1233-1238

16. Swift M.L., Reitnauer P.J., Morrell D., Chase C.L.: Breast and other cancers in families with ataxia telangectasia. N. Engl. J. Med., 1987; 316: 1289-1294

17. Claus E.B., Risch N., Thompson W.D.: Autosomal dominant inheritance of early-onset breast cancer. Cancer, 1994; 73: 643-651

18. Dupont W.D., Page D.L.: Risk factors for breast cancer in women with proliferative breast disease. N. Engl. J. Med., 1985; 312: 146-151

19. Dupont W.D., Page D.L.: Relative risk of breast cancer varies with time since diagnosis of atypical hyperplasia. Hum. Pathol., 1989; 20: 723-725

20. Scolnick M.H., Cannon-Albright L.A., Goldgar D.E., et al.: Inheritance of proliferative disease in breast cancer kindreds. Science, 1990; 250: 1715-1721

21. Evans D.G.R., Burnell L.D., Hopwood P., Howell A.: Perception of risk in women with a family history of breast cancer. Br. J. Cancer, 1993; 67: 612-614

22. Evans D.G.R., Blair V., Greenhalgh R., Hopwood P., Howell A.: The impact of genetic counselling on risk perception in women with a family history of breast cancer. Br. J. Cancer, 1994; 70: 934-938

23. Tabar L., Faberberg G., Day N.E. *et al.*: What is the optimum interval between mammographic screening examinations? An analysis based on the Swedish two-county breast cancer screening trial. Brit. J. Cancer, 1987; 56: 547-551

24. Powles T.J., Tillyer C.R., Jones A.L., *et al.*: Prevention of breast cancer with tamoxifen on the Royal Marsden Hospital pilot programme. Eur. J. Cancer, 1990: 26: 680-684

25. Price P., Sinnett H.D., Gusterson B., *et al.*: Duct carcinoma *in situ*: predictors of local recurrence and progression in patients treated by surgery alone. Brit. J. Cancer, 1990; 61 :869-872

26. Goodnight J.E., Quagliani J.M., Morton D.L.: Failure of subcutaneous mastectomy to prevent the development of breast cancer. J. Surg. Oncol., 1984; 26: 198-201

27. Evans D.G.R., Fentiman I.S., McPherson K., Asbury D., Ponder B.A.J., Howell A.: Familial Breast Cancer. Brit. Med. J., 1994; 308: 183-187

28. Evans D.G.R.: Genetic testing for cancer predisposition: need and demand. J. Med. Genet., 1995; 32: 161

29. Wooster R., Bignell G., Lancaster J. *et al.*: Identification of the breast cancer susceptibility gene BRCA2. Nature, 1995; 378: 789-792

The biology of breast cancer and its relevance to screening and treatment

J.R. Benson

Introduction

The principles of screening were enunciated by the World Health Organisation (WHO) in 1968[1] and formed the basis for Breast Screening Programmes. Included amongst the pre-conditions for effective population screening was the assumption that the natural history of the disease in question should be "well understood" with a recognisable early stage for which treatment outcome would be enhanced compared to later stages.

Randomised trials of breast screening have now confirmed the efficacy of screening in women over 50 years of age where reductions of breast cancer mortality of between 30-40% are attainable.[2-3] However, despite the apparent success of screening as judged by the end-point of population mortality, it could be argued that the aforementioned screening criteria have not been fully satisfied in relation to breast cancer. For this reason, the underlying mechanism and extent by which advancing the time of diagnosis improves overall survival of a screened population remains unclear. Breast cancer is a heterogeneous disease, both in terms of the cellular composition of different tumours, and of cells within any individual tumour. This biological heterogeneity confers a variable natural history upon breast cancer, and may ultimately undermine and limit the potential impact not only of screening programmes, but also treatment schedules for breast cancer.

Biological models of breast cancer

The essence of breast cancer screening is to detect malignant lesions at an earlier stage in their natural developmental history for which instigation of appropriate therapies will lead to improved outcome. Detection of a lesion at a smaller size *per se* will not necessarily result in reduction of mortality; this could yield an increase in survival by advancing the time of diagnosis – the so-called lead-time bias. In effect, a patient is merely given advance knowledge of her disease. For screening to produce a genuine improvement in survival and reduction of cause specific mortality, there must be an event in the natural history of the disease beyond which prognosis is adversely affected, and for which there is a threshold effect reflected in the size of a detectable lesion. If a lesion progressively increases in size without any such concomitant 'event', then it would be of no consequence whether this was excised at size x or x+1 provided that excision was complete.

There are two events which may occur in the natural history and progression of malignant breast lesions which could account for the efficacy of screening and provide a biological rationale for early detection strategies; a) early dissemination and b) phenotypic progression. Should one or both of these events occur at some stage in neoplastic development which is dependent upon tumour size, then earlier detection and intervention may pre-empt formation of micrometastases and/or a more biologically aggressive primary tumour and so lead to improved prognosis.[4]

Before discussing these issues in more detail, it is perhaps instructive to consider the two dominant paradigms of breast cancer biology which have governed the management of breast cancer over the past century – the Halstedian paradigm and the paradigm of biological predeterminism. Though the latter has become pre-eminent in recent years, both find relevance to the philosophy of breast screening.

a) Halstedian paradigm – Virchow proposed a centrifugal theory for dissemination of breast cancer in which a tumour was considered initially to invade local tissues and subsequently to encroach in a progressive, sequential and predictable manner upon ever more distant structures which lay in anatomical continuity.[5,6] The lymph nodes were thought to act as mechanical filters which formed a circumferential line of defence against such centrifugal dissemination and temporarily impeded the spread of cancer. However, once this filtration capacity was exhausted, cancer cells would then pass into the efferent lymphatics and thence to more distant sites. This model provided the rationale for the Halsted radical mastectomy in which an *en bloc* resection of tumour and loco-regional tissues was performed.[7] As a tumour was believed to spread in a sequential manner with successive involvement of structures in anatomical continuity, such *en bloc* resection was considered to offer the best chance of 'cure'. Though the operation of radical mastectomy provided high rates of local disease control,[8] there was no evidence for improved survival relative to lesser surgical procedures.[9] This implied that some 'event' had occurred prior to mastectomy which pre-determined survival and was unaffected by surgical intervention *per se*. Analysis of survival data for patients undergoing radical mastectomy revealed that fewer than a quarter of these patients shared a similar hazard ratio as an age-matched control population.[10] Therefore radical mastectomy could not be hailed as a general curative procedure for breast cancer, and fostered some doubt in the underlying paradigm.

b) Biological pre-determinism – an alternative paradigm was proposed by Fisher which challenged the concept of progressive centrifugal spread according to anatomical and mechanical criteria. Instead, breast cancer was considered to be largely a systemic disease at the outset as a consequence of cancer cells entering the bloodstream at an early stage in tumour development.[11] In particular, such haematogenous dissemination was not conditional upon lymph node involvement, and regional lymph nodes were not viewed as the instigators of distant metastases. Rather they reflected a tumour – host relationship which favoured dissemination. Experimental models were employed to demonstrate transnodal passage of tumour cells[12] together with destruction of tumour cells by lymph nodes.

These findings repudiated the concept of lymph nodes as passive filters,[13-14] and showed that cancer cells could pass not only directly into efferent lymphatics, but also into the bloodstream via lymphatico-venous communications. Further animal models had shown that dormant tumour cells could develop into overt metastases under appropriate conditions.

These experimental observations formed the basis for an alternative paradigm of biological pre-determinism in which cancer is viewed as a predominantly systemic disease at inception with clinical outcome pre-determined by micrometastases present at the time of diagnosis. Prognosis is ultimately determined by the propensity for these micrometastases to develop into overt metastatic disease. There are important consequences of this hypothesis which have implications both for the potential efficacy of any screening programme and treatment strategies. In terms of therapeutic sequelae, this paradigm of biological pre-determinism would predict that the extent of primary surgery does not influence overall survival, as the latter is dependent upon micro-metastases which are present in all patients irrespective of surgical procedure. Trials of breast conservation surgery have confirmed that lesser surgical resections do not compromise overall survival though they are associated with higher rates of local recurrence.[15-18]

The Guy's trial showed that, for patients with stage I disease, overall survival was similar in patients undergoing radical mastectomy and chest wall irradiation compared to wide local excision with breast irradiation. However, stage II patients had a higher incidence of distant metastases and a corresponding reduced survival.[15] Subsequent trials found no difference in overall survival for either stages I or II disease. Fisher's group compared total mastectomy with lumpectomy either with or without breast irradiation.[16]

Though survival rates were similar in all groups, local relapse was much higher in the non-irradiated breast conservation group.[16] Veronesi compared mastectomy with quadrantectomy, axillary dissection and radiotherapy (QUART) for small tumours ≤ 2.5cm.[17] Once again, this trial and other smaller ones[18] confirmed that overall survival rates were uninfluenced by the extent of primary surgery, and supported the notion of predeterminism based on sub-clinical dissemination of micrometastases.

The second therapeutic sequela of this hypothesis is that initiation of systemic therapies which could destroy these putative micrometastases should improve prognosis. This aspect of treatment would therefore be complementary to loco-regional therapy (surgery±radiotherapy). Clinical trials of adjuvant therapy for breast cancer have provided corroborative evidence for the second prediction of this alternative paradigm.[19] In 1992 the Early Breast Cancer Trialists Collaborative Group (EBCTCG) published the results of a 10-year overview of adjuvant trials of endocrine and chemotherapy involving a total of 75,000 women.[20] Adjuvant polychemotherapy reduced the annual risk of disease recurrence by 28% and mortality by 17% in an unselected group of breast cancer patients. Similarly, adjuvant tamoxifen therapy was most effective in the over 50 age group where risk of local recurrence was reduced by 30% and mortality by 19%.

Application of models to breast screening

The above evidence together with data on the clinical outcome of stages I and II breast cancer indicates that micro-metastases are present in over 50% of cases of 'early' breast cancer at the time of clinical diagnosis. If one adopts the philosophy that all breast cancer is systemic at the outset, then any screening programme is doomed to failure, as earlier detection and treatment of a primary lesion will not reduce mortality if survival has already been pre-determined by micrometastatic disease.

To date there is no conclusive evidence for any subgroup of breast cancer patients who have been 'cured' as defined by either statistical or clinical criteria.[21] Statistical cure[22] can only be claimed if, after prolonged follow-up, a sub-group of patients are found to have an annual death rate from all causes which is identical to an age-matched control population. Several studies, including that of Brinkley and Haybittle (vide supra) have identified sub-groups whose survival approximates to a control group, but in none of these has the ratio of observed to expected deaths been unity.[23-25] Similarly, there is no evidence for a clinically cured group who are deemed to have no increased relative risk of subsequently dying from breast cancer. Most studies reveal that all groups of treated patients remain at relatively increased risk of death from breast cancer and also of developing a contra-lateral cancer.[23,24,26] Though 'cure' cannot hitherto be claimed on strict statistical criteria, there are reports which purport to define sub-groups with a highly favourable prognosis who may be effectively cured. This particularly applies to small tumours and may have some bearing on screening. Thus Hayward has recently analysed long-term follow-up of stages I and II patients treated at Guy's Hospital by mastectomy.[27] Some of these have attained hazard ratios very similar to an age-matched control population. Similarly, patients with a Nottingham Prognostic Index[28] of less than or equal to 3 have been declared to have equivalent survival to a control population. Sigurdson et al. (1990)[29] analysed prognostic factors (% S-phase, progesterone receptor and tumour size) in stage I patients within a screening programme and described a sub-group of approximately 30% who would have a calculated relative survival of 100%. Notwithstanding the pre-eminence of biological pre-determinism, it is implicit from a Breast Screening Programme that a substantial proportion of patients are potentially curable by earlier detection. If it is believed that screening can genuinely reduce mortality, then it probably has to be accepted that all breast cancer is not systemic at the outset. Moreover, it is assumed that dissemination and establishment of viable micrometastases can occur during the pre-clinical phase when a breast cancer is mammographically detectable. The crucial question is what proportion of tumours disseminate between the time of radiological detection and clinical presentation? In other words, what proportion of cancers can be successfully detected mammographically before any development of micrometastases? Is there a threshold of tumour size above which dissemination occurs? As breast cancer is a heterogeneous disease, the answer to this question is unlikely to be consensual, with a range of sizes rather than a single threshold value.

A tumour requires a blood supply to grow beyond the size of a million cells (a few cubic millimetres),[30] but it is quite feasible to propose that a tumour can possess an established vasculature without necessarily showing vascular invasion at these early stages of tumour development. Furthermore, cancer cells could travel to the regional lymph nodes and remain there without entering the circulation via lymphatico-venous communications. In both these scenarios, cure could theoretically be achieved by excision of tumour and regional nodes. Patients who are reported to have microscopic nodal deposits have a similar prognosis to node negative cases.[31,32]

Even if tumour cells gain access to the circulation at a very early stage, these may not necessarily develop into viable micrometastatic foci. The host immune system can destroy rogue cancer cells within the bloodstream and successful establishment of micrometastases will depend upon innate biological properties of the tumour cells, as well as local host factors. From a clinical perspective, it is of greater significance to ascertain the earliest stage in tumour development at which viable metastatic foci can form. Screening programmes would then be aimed at maximising the capacity to detect lesions before this clinical dissemination occurred. The smallest lesion which can be detected mammographically with state-of-the-art technology is approximately 3 mm. By the time a tumour has attained this size, it will probably contain over 1 million cells and therefore have already entered the vascular phase of growth.[31] In experimental models tumours reach a maximum size of only 1-2 mm in the absence of vascularisation, though growth rapidly accelerates upon induction of a vasculature.[30] Despite the tendency for new blood vessels to be 'leaky',[32] it does not follow that infiltration by tumour cells is an obligate phenomenon once neovascularisation has occurred. Therefore detection by screening of smaller tumours which are in the vascular phase of growth could still precede systemic dissemination. Ideally, screening should pick up tumours whilst they are still in the prevascular phase where growth is very slow and there is no opportunity for haematogenous spread.

It was stated in the introductory section that the efficacy of screening could be accounted for by two possible mechanisms. In addition to detection of tumours prior to any systemic dissemination, screening might also pick up tumours with a more favourable grade and biological credentials. There is some evidence that the malignant phenotype evolves and becomes more "aggressive" as a tumour grows,[35] though not all agree with this concept.[36] If cancers can progress to less differentiated forms, then screening might improve prognosis if it permitted detection and removal of lesions prior to such changes.

Relationship between reduction of mortality and changes in size and stage distribution of screen-detected tumours

So to what extent can screening reduce tumour size, and is such a reduction in the size of tumours *per se* related to prognosis? Screening is associated with a reduction in the proportion of larger tumours and metastatic lesions.[37-38] The following section examines how improvements in survival amongst patients with screen-detected cancers can be accounted for by changes in conventional prognostic indices and whether screening can detect lesions prior to any dissemination.

Lymph node status remains the most accurate prognostic indicator for breast cancer,[39, 40] and has yet to be succeeded by newer biological indices such as ploidy, percentage S-phase and abnormal gene expression. Survival is closely correlated with the number of lymph nodes infiltrated by tumour. If there is no axillary nodal involvement, then 5 year survival rates are of the order of 80-90%, falling to approximately 65% if fewer than 4 nodes are positive and 30% if 4 or more nodes are affected. Prognosis is particularly poor if more than 10 nodes are positive.[40] By implication, lymph node status is an indirect indicator of the likelihood of micrometastastic foci pre-existing at the time of primary surgery. Tumour size is related both to lymph node status and the risk of distant metastases[41,42,43,] and there is provisional evidence that a similar relationship appertains to screen-detected lesions.[44]

In the Swedish WE study[45] there was a significant reduction in both size and nodal status of screen-detected invasive cancers. More than half of the tumours were less than 15 mm in diameter and 83% were node negative. Comparison of tumour size with the control group revealed a 26% reduction in tumours more than 20 mm in size and a 40% reduction in those over 30 mm. The observed incidence of node negativity represented a 24% reduction in proportion of patients with positive nodes. This reduction in

tumour size and node positivity was paralleled by an improved survival, presumably reflecting a lower incidence of micrometastases in these screened breast cancer patients.

Hatschek *et al.*[46] reported a very favourable reduction of node positivity for invasive tumours detected in incidence screens from 40% (controls) to 18%, and an increase in small tumours ($\leq$20mm) from 59% to 85%. Of interest, in the Edinburgh trial (EBSB) the node positivity rate remained high for the incidence rounds (28%) and only half of invasive tumours detected were $\leq$ 20mm. As might be expected, this study found more favourable effects on tumour size, lymph node status and histology in the prevalence round, but this was not sustained for the incidence round.[47] Prevalence screens are innately biased towards tumours with better prognostic indices[48] and some have criticised studies based exclusively on prevalence data.[49,50] Crisp *et al.*[50] reported a higher proportion of smaller tumours with less lymph node involvement in a population of 131 screen-detected compared with clinical tumours (7.4 tumours per 1000 women screened). Furthermore, these authors translated these data into predictions of survival using the NPI and concluded that screening conferred a survival advantage of 26.5% at 5 years consistent with a 30% reduction in mortality. These data suggest that screening can lead to a change in stage distribution of invasive breast cancers. This so-called 'stage drift' may represent detection of cancers at an earlier biological stage. However, the relationship between reduction in tumour size and lymph node positivity may be more complex apropos screen-detected lesions; an increased proportion of smaller tumours may not necessarily be accompanied by predicted changes in nodal status based on data from clinical tumours. Abernathy *et al.*[51] reported that following introduction of a mass screening programme in Colorado involving over 15,000 patients, there was an increase of approximately 20% in the fraction of tumours less than 2 cm.[51] However, an interesting finding of this study was an increase in the proportion of tumours between 2-5 cm with positive lymph nodes. At first, this anomalous result might appear to indicate a reversed stage drift! The authors have suggested that screening detects lesions at a smaller size, and facilitates their removal before they can develop into node negative tumours within this size range. This implies that increasing tumour size does not invariably lead to a stage shift involving a progression to node positivity. Screening will tend to be biased towards these node negative tumours because they are likely to be slower growing – length time bias *(vide infra)*. Therefore the effects of screening on nodal status and hence precise stage distribution may be inherently more complex than previously thought. Even if there is a genuine stage shift,[52] screening methods must ultimately be capable of detecting lesions prior to any haematogenous dissemination; node negativity does not equate with absence of micrometastases, but rather reflects a relationship between tumour and host in which the chances of dissemination are minimised.[11] The goal of screening practice is therefore not to achieve stage I status *per se*, but to detect tumours at a size which precedes the threshold for haematogenous dissemination. The fundamental problem is that this threshold size will vary between tumours, and the precise proportion of lesions which are detected at this pre-dissemination stage will be dictated not only by the natural history of individual tumours, but also technical nuances of mammographic screening. There are no specific mammographic features which correlate with the biological behaviour of an invasive tumour and its propensity to metastasise, though some correlation between mammographic densities and increased risk of non-invasive proliferative lesions has been reported.[53]

Screening provides information on size and local extent of a tumour only. Techniques are currently being developed to extract maximal prognostic information from cytological samples, and these may help predict which screen detected lesions are likely to have already metastasised.

The above studies on screen-detected lesions have revealed changes in distribution not only of tumour size and nodal status, but also histological type and grade. Some studies claiming that breast screening detects less aggressive cancers have been confined to prevalence screens only,[49] and should perhaps be interpreted with caution. Nonetheless, others have found a persistent change in the histological grade and 'malignant potential' of incidence screen detected tumours.[45-47,50-54,55]

Indeed, in the Swedish two-counties trial referred to above, improved survival could not entirely be accounted for by reduction in tumour size and proportion of node positive tumours. Screen detected tumours were also of more favourable histological grade, and when taken together with these other 2 factors, differences in survival between screened and control groups could be fully accounted for.[56]

Most studies have revealed a significantly higher proportion of special tumour types amongst screen detected lesions compared to symptomatic cancers.[47,50,55,57] Approximately 8% of the latter are of special histological type, whilst these have constituted between 12.5%[50]-25%[55] of screen-detected invasive lesions.

The value of 12.5% reported by Crisp et al.[50] is significantly lower than others quoted which have on average been around 20%.[47,57] Of interest, in an analysis of breast cancer histology and age, Wicks et al.[58] found the highest incidence of tubular carcinomas in the age group corresponding to the screened population (50-69 years).[58] Anderson et al.[47] found a difference in proportion of special and variant tumours compared to 'no special type' (or not otherwise specified [NOS]) in prevalence versus incidence screens, and surmised that this might reflect a natural progression of lesions to less well differentiated forms. In their analysis of the Swedish two-county study, Duffy et al.[35] noted a much lower proportion of high grade (III) tumours amongst smaller screen-detected lesions. By comparing size and malignancy grade in the control and 'unbiased' screen-detected groups, the expected distribution corresponded with the observed, demonstrating that any differences in malignancy grade distribution were attributable to size only, an effect therefore independent of length bias. These authors concluded that malignancy grade evolves i.e. worsens as a tumour enlarges. Malignancy grade was considered to represent an underlying variable which faithfully reflected 'malignant potential'. However, grade is a surrogate marker for the latter which ideally should be measured by some biological index relating directly to proliferative activity.

The concept of phenotypic progression is supported by the known heterogeneity of tumours. Thus different cell populations within a single tumour would have variable biological behaviour and growth characteristics. Up to one-third of breast cancers have foci of more than one histological type.[59] Variation in nuclear grade and degrees of pleiomorphism are frequently observed within the same tumour. Furthermore, *in vitro* studies with thymidine labelling have revealed wide variation in indices of proliferative potential between cells derived from a single tumour.[60] Curiously, Ponten et al.[61] carried out extensive DNA ploidy studies on incidence screen detected cancers and reported no differences in ploidy profiles between screen detected and clinical cancers. However, DNA ploidy has been reported to display less intra-tumoral variation than these other proliferative indices.[62]

Hakama et al. (1995)[36] analysed the aggressiveness of cancers amongst a screened population using DNA index (ploidy) and S-phase fraction. On these criteria of proliferative indices alone (and not inclusive of histological data), cancers detected in the prevalence round were of lower malignant potential. However, in subsequent incident rounds, the level of proliferation was similar in control and screened groups, suggesting that "biological aggressiveness" did not increase during the pre-clinical phase of tumour development. By contrast, screen-detected lesions in this study were of smaller size and more favourable stage than controls, this being predictive of a future reduction in mortality from population screening.[36]

Prospects for further reductions of mortality from breast cancer screening

The concept of malignant progression during the pre-clinical phase when lesions are impalpable yet detectable mammographically is attractive, and offers a further explanation for the potential efficacy of Breast Screening Programmes in reducing mortality. To some extent, this phenomenon is related to the issue of pre-clinical dissemination; tumours with greater malignant potential are more likely to metastasise. The proportion of cells within a tumour with the capacity to invade blood vessels, travel in the circulation and establish viable micrometastases will increase with progression to a more malignant phenotype. The latter may be manifest by enhanced activity at several steps in the process of invasion and metastasis. Therefore screening could improve prognosis by detecting lesions of smaller size which are better differentiated, of lower metastatic potential and less likely to have already disseminated. Such lesions could be cured by appropriate loco-regional treatment, and systemic therapy would not be indicated as micrometastases would theoretically be non-existent.

The issue of whether a sub-group of patients with truly localized breast cancer exists is controversial. Moreover, if such a sub-group does exist, it may only represent a small proportion of all screen detected lesions and therefore have little impact overall on the screened population as a whole. In view of the apparent efficacy of screening programmes to date, it might be argued that screening detects not only those lesions which are pre-dissemination, but some which have already metastasised with a minimal micro-metastatic load. The latter could be successfully eliminated with appropriate adjuvant therapy. Results of adjuvant trials reveal that absolute benefits from such therapies are relatively modest – of the order of 5-10%. However, in a pre-clinical setting with a small primary tumour, adjuvant therapies may be much more effective against a lighter micro-metastatic load and complete elimination of all active foci of disease may be possible.

As mentioned above, screening is inherently biased towards slow growing, less aggressive tumours. These have a longer 'sojourn period' and hence are less likely to grow to clinically detectable size prior to screen detection. Evidence suggests that overall, interval cancers do not have a worse prognosis than controls,[56] though not all studies concur with this

view.[63] This group will be composed of a significant number of fast growing tumours which have arisen *de novo* since the last screen. These cancers would be expected to be more aggressive and fatal than screen detected lesions, and their failure to be detected at an earlier stage by screening could undermine the potential for screening programmes to reduce mortality. Increased frequency of screening could increase the proportion of screen-detected cancers and possibly reduce the numbers of fast growing interval cancers, though of necessity those fastest will be the last to be detected as the screening interval is reduced. Moreover, prognosis of these most rapidly growing tumours is probably more dependent upon innate biological parameters than earlier detection at a smaller size. Many of these tumours may indeed be aggressive from the outset, and not as a consequence of any phenotypic drift. More frequent screening would also reduce the average size of screen detected tumours, and thus in turn increase the chances of detecting lesions prior to both systemic dissemination and any progression to a more aggressive phenotype. Further clinical trials are required to resolve these important issues and to maximise the efficacy of screening programmes.

Carcinoma *in situ*

Discussion has deliberately been restricted to invasive forms of breast cancer as these are responsible for mortality. However, with the advent of screening, *in situ* disease has acquired increasing prominence with *in situ* change alone, or in association with micro-invasion, now representing approximately 20-25% of all screen detected cancer.[64] By contrast, prior to screening, only 2-5% of clinical (symptomatic) cancers were exclusively ductal carcinoma *in situ* (DCIS). Though screening is effective at detecting DCIS on account of commonly associated micro calcification, it is currently unknown to what extent this will translate into a reduction of mortality. Not all DCIS will progress to invasive disease, and estimates for this proportion range from 25-50%. It is clear from the reported incidence of DCIS at routine autopsy (up to 15%)[65] that some *in situ* lesions which are detected mammographically and subsequently excised (sometimes entailing mastectomy) would have been of no clinical consequence to the patient during their lifetime. One is therefore faced with the uncertainties of 'non-obligate progression'[66] which poses problems both in terms of the biological behaviour of *in situ* disease and clinical management. Conversely, not all invasive cancers arise from lesions which are recognised histologically as carcinoma *in situ,* though a phase involving some form of increased epithelial proliferation is likely to precede an invasive cancer. Evidence to date suggests that screening programmes have not encouraged over-diagnosis when analysis is confined to invasive tumours. However, until more is learnt about carcinoma *in situ* and its relationship to the natural history of breast cancer, this claim cannot be extended to *in situ* disease. As DCIS may constitute up to a quarter of all screen detected lesions, this justifies some concern regarding both over-diagnosis and 'excessive' treatment.

Conclusion

This chapter has discussed the scientific rationale for breast screening in the context of proposed paradigms of breast cancer biology. Ironically, the philosophy of screening is something of an anathema to the contemporary paradigm of biological pre-determinism according to its strictly orthodox dictates. A screening programme cannot be applied to a disease which is invariably systemic at the outset.

If it is accepted that screening is effective in reducing mortality in certain age groups, then there must be a finite growth period for breast cancers during which disease is localized to the breast with no haematogenous dissemination. A corollary of this is that development of micrometastases can occur between the time of screen-detection and clinical presentation of a cancer.

Analysis of survival curves for breast cancer patients over prolonged periods of follow-up has revealed no evidence for a 'cure' in any sub-group according to statistical criteria. However, just as adjuvant treatment can extend life for patients with clinical breast cancer, so too may early detection by screening achieve a 'personal cure' whereby disease-free survival is prolonged to a point at which a patient dies of a concomitant condition unrelated to breast cancer. Even if cure is not achieved in the statistical sense, this would be of no consequence to individual patients under these circumstances.

The capacity of any screening modality to reduce mortality is dependent upon the frequency of screening. A crucial consideration with breast cancer screening programmes is the potential for improving prognosis as the screening interval is contracted. Clearly increased frequency of screening will reduce the average size of tumours, but it is difficult to predict how this will be reflected by further reductions in mortality consequent on removal of a lesion in anticipation of microscopic dissemination and phenotypic progression. Furthermore, any increased clinical benefits must be balanced against increased costs so as to retain a cost-effective screening programme for a population as a whole. However cogent are theories which offer a biological rationale for screening, the case for indefinite mass screening for breast cancer in terms of clinical efficacy relative to cost remains unproven.[67-69]

References

1. Wilson and Junger WHO, 1968
2. Shapiro S., Venet W., Strax P., Venet L., Roeser R.: Ten to fourteen-year effect of screening on breast cancer mortality. J. Natl. Cancerinist, 1982; 69: 349
3. Tabar L. Fagerberg C.J.G., Gad A. *et al.*: Reduction in mortality from breast cancer after mass screening with mammography. Lancet, 1985; I: 829
4. Holmberg L., Ekbom A., Zack M.: Do screen-detected invasive breast cancers have a natural history of their own? Eu. J. Cancer, 1992; 28A, 4/5 920-923
5. Virchow R.: Cellular Pathology. Philadelphia, Lippincott, , 1863
6. Virchow R.: Die Krankhaften Geschwulste, Berlin, A. Hirschwald, 1863-1873; Vol.I, 26-27
7. Halsted W.S.: The radical operation for the cure of carcinoma of the breast. Johns Hopkins Hospital Reports, 1894; 28: 557
8. Halsted W.S.: The results of operations for the cure of cancer of the breast performed at The Johns Hopkins Hospital from June, 1889 to January, 1894. Johns Hopkins Hospital Reports, 1894-5; 4: 297-350
9. Baum M.: The history of breast cancer. In: Forbes J.F. (Ed.) *Breast Disease*, Edinburgh, Churchill Livingston, 1986; 95-105
10. Brinkley D., Haybittle J.L.: The curability of breast cancer. Lancet, 1973; 2: 95-9
11. Fisher B.: Laboratory and Clinical Research in Breast Cancer - A Personal Adventure: The David A. Karnofsky Memorial Lecture. Cancer Research, 1980; 40: 3863-3874
12. Fisher B., Fisher E.R.: Transmigration of lymph nodes by tumour cells. Science, 1966; 152: 1397-1398
13. Fisher B., Fisher E.R.: Barrier function of lymph node to tumour cells and erythrocytes I. Normal nodes. Cancer, 1967; 20: 1907-1913
14. Fisher B., Fisher E.R.: Barrier function of lymph node to tumour cells and erythrocytes II. Effect of X-ray, inflammation, sensitisation and tumour growth. Cancer, 1967; 20: 1914-1919
15. Atkins H., Hayward J.L., Klugman D.J., Wayte A.B.: Treatment of early breast cancer: A report after 10 years of a clinical trial. Br. Med. J., 1972; 2: 423- 429
16. Fisher B., Redmond C., Poisson R., *et al.*: Eight year results of a randomised clinical trial comparing total mastectomy and lumpectomy with or without irradiation in the treatment of breast cancer. N. Eng. J. Med., 1989; 320: 822-827
17. Veronesi U., Saccozzi R., Del Vecchio M. *et al.*: Comparing radical mastectomy with quadrantectomy, axillary dissection and radiotherapy in patients with small cancers of the breast. N. Eng. J. Med., 1981; 305: 6-11
18. Sarrazin D., Dewar J.A., Arriagada R. *et al.*: Conservative management of breast cancer. Br. J. Surg., 1986; 73: 604 - 606
19. Fisher B, Slack N., Katrych D. *et al.*: Ten year follow up results of patients with carcinoma of the breast in a cooperative clinical trial evaluating surgical adjuvant chemotherapy. Surg. Gynaecol. Obstet., 1975; 140: 528 - 534
20. Early Breast Cancer Trialists Collaborative Group: Systemic treatment of early breast cancer by hormonal, cytotoxic or immune therapy. 133 randomised trials involving 31,000 recurrences and 24,000 deaths among 75,000 women. Lancet, 1992; 339: 1-15 and 7 1-75
21. Haybittle J.L.: Curability of breast cancer. Brit. Med. Bulletin, 1990; 47: 319-323
22. Berkson J., Harrington S.W., Clagett O.T., Kirklin J.W., Dockerty M.B. and McDonald J.R.: Mortality and Survival in surgi-

cally treated breast cancer: A statistical summary of some experience of the Mayo Clinic. Proc. Staff Meetings Mayo Clinic, 1957; 32: 645

23. Brinkley D., Haybitde J.L.: Long-term survival of women with breast cancer. Lancet, 1984; I: 1118 and II: 353

24. Le M.G., Hill C., Rezvani A., Sarrazin D., Contesso G., Lacour J.: Long-term survival of women with breast cancer. Lancet, 1984; II: 922

25. Langlands A.O., Pocock S.J., Keit G.R., Gore S.M.: Long-term survival of patients with breast cancer: A study of the curability of the disease. Br. Med. J., 1979; 2: 1247

26. Adair F., Berg J., Lourdes J., Robbins G.F. Long-term follow up of breast cancer patients: The 30-year report. Cancer, 1974; 33: 1145

27. Hayward J.: Controversies in breast cancer management. 8th International Congress on Senology, Rio de Janiero, Brasil (May, 1994)

28. Todd J.H., Dowle C., Williams M.R. et al.: Confirmation of a prognostic index in primary breast cancer. Br. J. Cancer 1987; 56: 489-492

29. Sigurdsson H., Baldetorp B., Borg A. et al.: Indicators of prognosis in node-negative breast cancer. N. Eng. J. Med., 1990; 322: 1045-1053

30. Folkman J.: What is the evidence that tumours are angiogenesis dependent? J. Natl. Cancer Institute, 1990; 82: 4-6

31. Pickren J.W.: Significance of occult metastases. Cancer, 1961; 14: 1266-1271

32. Fisher E.R., Swamidoss S., Lee C.H. et al.: Detection and significance of occult axillary node metastases in patients with invasive breast cancer. Cancer, 1978; 45: 2025-2031

33. Weidner N., Semple J.P., Welch W.R., Folkman J.: Tumour angiogenesis and metastasis - correlation in invasive breast carcinoma. N. Eng. J. Med., 1991, 324: 1-8

34. Liotta L., Kleinerman J., Saidel G.: Quantitative relationships of intravascular tumour cells, tumour vessels and pulmonary metastases following tumor implantation. Cancer Res., 1974; 34: 997-1004

35. Duffy S.W., Tabar L., Fagerberg G., Gad A., Grontoft O., South M.C., Day N.E.: Breast screening, prognostic factors and survival – results from the Swedish two-county study. Br. J. Cancer, 1991; 64: 1133-1138

36. Hakama M., Holli K., Isola J., Kallioniemi O.P., et al.: Aggressiveness of screen-detected breast cancer. Lancet, 1995; 345: 221-224

37. Fagerberg C.J.G., Baldetorp L., Grontoft O. et al.: Effects of repeated mammographic screening on breast cancer stage distribution. Acta Radiol. (Oncol), 1985; 24: 465

38. Tabar L., Duffy S.W., Krusemo U.B.: Detection method, tumour size and node metastases in breast cancers diagnosed during a trial of breast cancer screening. Eur. J. Cancer, 1987; 23: 959

39. Fisher B. et al.: Surgical adjuvant chemotherapy in cancer of the breast. Results of a decade of co-operative investigation. Ann. Surg., 1968; 168: 337-356

40. Salvadori B. et al.: Prognostic factors in operable breast cancer. Tumori, 1983; 69: 477-484

41. Fisher B., Slack N.H., Bross I.D.J. et al.: Cancer of the breast: size of neoplasm and prognosis. Cancer, 1969; 24: 1071-1080

42. Haagensen C.D.: Diseases of the breast. 3rd Edition. Philadelphia, Saunders, 1986; 659

43. Nemoto T., Vanna J., Bedwani R.N. et al.: Management and survival of female breast cancer: results of a national survey by the American College of Surgeons. Cancer, 1984, 45: 2917-2924

44. Tabar L., Duffy S.W., Krusemo U.B.: Detection method, tumour size and node metastases in breast cancers diagnosed during a trial of breast cancer screening. Eur. J. Cancer Clin. Oncol., 1987; 23: 959-962

45. Tabar L., Fagerberg C.J.G., South M.C., Duffy S.W., Day N.E.: The Swedish Two County Trial of mammographic screening for breast cancer: recent results on mortality and tumour characteristics. In: Miller A.B. Chamberlain J., Day N.E., Hakama

M., Prorok P. (Eds.) Screening for Cancer. Bern, Hans Huber, 1991

46. Hatschek T., Fagerberg G., Olle S. et al.: Cytometric characterisation and clinical course of breast cancer diagnosed in a population-based screening program. Cancer, 1989; 64: 1074-1081

47. Anderson T.J., Lamb J., Donnan P., Alexander F.E., Huggins A., Muir B.B., et al.: Comparative pathology of breast cancer in a randomised trial of screening. Br. J. Cancer, 1991; 64: 108-113

48. Cole P. and Morrison A.S.: Basic issues in population screening for cancer. J. Natl. Cancer Inst., 1980; 65: 1263

49. Klemi P.J., Joensuu H., Toikkanen J., Tuominen J. et al.: Aggressiveness of breast cancers found with and without screening. Brit. Med. J., 1992; 304: 467-469

50. Crisp W.J., Higgs M.J., Cowan W.K., Cunliffe W.K. et al.: Screening for breast cancer detects tumours at an earlier biological stage. Br. J. Surg., 1993; 80: 863-865

51. Abernathy C.M., Hedegaard H. and Weger N.: Screening for breast cancer detects tumours at an earlier biological stage (letter). Lancet 1994; 81: 922

52. Bull A., Mountney L. and Sanderson H. Stage distribution of breast cancer: a basis for the evaluation of Breast Screening Programmes. Br. J. Radiol 1991; 64: 516-519

53. Boyd N.F., Jensen H.M., Cooke G. Lee Han H.: Relationship between mammographic and histological risk factors for breast cancer. J. Natl. Cancer Inst, 1992; 1170- 1179

54. Bennet I.C. McCaffrey J.F., Baker C.A., Burke M.F. et al.: Changing patterns in the presentation of breast cancer over 25 years. Aust. NZ. J. Surg., 1990; 60: 665 - 671

55. Rajakariar R., Walker R.A.: The biological nature of screen-detected invasive breast cancer (meeting abstract) J. Path., 1993; 170: (Supp.) 387A

56. Day N.E.: Screening for breast cancer. Brit. Med. Bull. 1991; 47: 400-415

57. Nicholson S., Webb A.J., Coghlan B., Farndon J.R. et al.: Will screening for breast cancer reduce mortality? Evidence from the first year of screening in Avon. Ann. Roy Coll. Surg., 1993; 75: 8-12

58. Wicks K., Fisher C.J., Fentimen I.S., Millis R.R.: Breast cancer histology and age (meeting abstract). J. Path., 1992; 167: (Supp) 139A

59. Fisher B., Saffer E., Fisher E.R.: Studies concerning the regional nodes in cancer IV. Tumour inhibition by regional lymph node cells. Cancer, 1974; 33: 631-636

60. Fisher B., Saffer E., Fisher E.R.: Studies concerning the regional nodes in cancer VII. Thymidine uptake by cells from nodes of breast cancer patients. Cancer, l974; 33: 271 - 279

61. Ponten J., Holmberg L., Trichopoulos D.: Biology and natural history of breast cancer. Int. J. Cancer, 1990; 5: 1-21

62. Meyer J.S., Witliff J.L.: Regional heterogeneity in breast carcinoma: thymidine labelling index, steroid hormone receptors, DNA ploidy. Int. J. Cancer, 1991; 47: 213

63. Andersson I., Aspegren K., Janzon L. et al.: Effect of mammographic screening on breast cancer mortality in an urban population in Sweden. Results from the Malmo mammographic screening trial (MMST). Brit. Med. J. 1988; 297: 943-948

64. Roberts M.M., Alexander F.E., Anderson T.J. et al.: Edinburgh trial of screening for breast cancer: mortality at seven years. Lancet 1990; i: 241 - 246

65. Anderson J., Nielsen M., Christensen L.: New aspects of the natural history of in situ and invasive carcinoma in the female breast: results from autopsy investigations. Verh. Dtsch. Ges. Pathol. 1985; 69: 88-95

66. Anderson T.J.: Genesis and source of breast cancer. Brit. Med. Bull. 1991; 47: 30s-318

67. Wright C.J., Muller C.B.: Screening mammography and public health policy: the need for perspective. Lancet, 1995; 346: 29-32

68. Baum M.: Screening for breast cancer, time to think – and stop? Lancet 1995; 346: 436

69. Querci della Rovere G., Benson J.R., Warren R.: Screening for breast cancer, time to think – and stop? Lancet 1995; 346: 437

The organisation of breast cancer screening

E.J. Roebuck

The organisation of a Breast Screening Programme will be considered under the following headings:

1. Programme Design
2. The Screening Process
3. Essential Support Services
4. Manpower Considerations
5. Equipment Requirements
6. Implementation
7. Co-ordination

Introduction

Before commencing to consider the organisation of a breast cancer screening programme, it is virtually mandatory to have studied the Forrest report.[1] This report was published in 1986 and the conclusions of the Forrest Working Group were therefore, of necessity, based upon work published prior to that date. The UK experience gained in implementing and running a screening programme has found little at fault with the proposals made in Forrest, and certainly no fundamental principles which need to be revised. Indeed, it has been proven that, starting from what was overall an extremely low level of expertise, it is possible within a short time scale (3 years) to implement a programme which produces results equal to those achieved in trials in specialist centres.[2,3] There are however some details which, in the light of experience, could with benefit be incorporated into any new proposals for breast cancer screening. These will be discussed below.

In the design of breast screening organisation, the detail of the act of basic screening by mammography should come last; major preliminary decisions are an essential prerequisite.

Before a screening programme can be designed a thorough investigation of the epidemiology of the population which it is proposed to screen must be carried out. The organisers of the programme must ensure that the appropriate women in the population are targeted. If the peak age incidence is, say, 45-50 years of age (as seems to occur in some genetic pools)[4] then it is clearly inappropriate to design a programme starting with women at the age of 50 years.

A screening programme will not succeed unless it is designed with the existing health care delivery system in mind, and unless it integrates as smoothly as is possible with that system (or systems), exploiting the strengths of the public and/or private sectors as is appropriate.

Above all there must be the political will to run a programme. It follows that the whole programme will have to be costed in order to ensure that the envisaged design is cost-effective, since it is upon cost-effective (not risk-benefit) considerations that political decisions are made.

1. Programme design

The target population

It is of importance to appreciate that all the published studies of population screening for breast cancer have been undertaken in populations which are predominantly Caucasian, and that these results are not necessarily appropriate for non-Caucasian populations comprised of differing genetic pools and having differing breast cancer incidence profiles.

An epidemiological study of the population will identify the age group most at risk. It is these women who must be targeted, never forgetting that the incidence of a cancer is traditionally regarded as the time at which it becomes clinically apparent. The object of screening is to detect cancers at an earlier stage, and so screening should ideally commence two or so years before a woman enters the peak incidence age group as defined by the criterion of clinical presentation. It is known that, in terms of the risk/benefit ratio for an individual woman, screening using modern techniques is beneficial down to the age of about 35 years.[5] However, the case incidence is so low at this age that population screening is not cost-effective. The studies completed to date (1995) do not provide hard evidence to indicate if population screening below the age of 50 years is or is not worthwhile. The ongoing multi-centre UK trial, which has recently been expanded to include other countries, should produce statistical evidence to enable a judgement to be made as to the age at which population screening should commence.

The frequency of screening

The Forrest Working Group recommended a three-year interval as a starting point for a UK programme, considering that this might well need to be revised following further research. A three-year interval now appears to be too long, and a multi-centre research trial is due to report soon, following which definitive guidance should be available. Published work suggests that, for optimal efficiency, the interval between screening episodes might have to be varied according to age.[6] An approximation for a population might be that younger women (< 55 years) would benefit from annual screening, with an interval of eighteen months for women between 55 and 64 years of age, and two-yearly screening for women over 65.

Women at higher risk

Women considered to be at a higher than average risk of developing breast cancer should have their individual degree of risk accurately assessed and should receive expert genetic counselling. There are no data to indicate the efficiency of screening women at higher risk at more frequent intervals than the usual for that age. It seems reasonable to suggest that women with a significantly higher risk, say 10X, might benefit from more frequent screening, but for women with a 2X or 3X risk this does not appear justified.

2. The screening process

Screening is a sequential three part process which leads to a fourth. First there is the basic screening examination, which, in the case of breast cancer, is a mammographic examination. This is followed by the assessment of any abnormalities detected by the basic screening test. Tissue diagnosis follows, and should really be regarded as an extension of assess-

ment. Finally, in cases where this proves necessary, there is definitive treatment which is not within the scope of the screening programme. However, it is a responsibility of the programme to have an established mechanism to ensure that women found to have a problem are referred for appropriate treatment. Great advantages accrue both to the patient and to the staff if management is determined by the same expert team as is involved in assessment.[3,11]

The invitation to be screened

In order to identify those women for whom screening has been deemed appropriate by the epidemiological study, it is necessary to have an accurate population register. Such registers are not always readily available. In the UK the most accurate register of the population is probably the electoral role, but legally this cannot be used for health service purposes.

Instead reliance had to be upon the General Practitioner-maintained register of patients, which, although now much improved, proved to be far from accurate in the early stages of the NHS screening programme.

To achieve the highest response to invitations to be screened the invitation should be personalised, and preferably appear to be initiated by someone known to the woman, such as her General Practitioner. The invitation should give a firm appointment time, but should also offer the facility to change this, should it prove inconvenient.

Women have the right to refuse an invitation should they so wish. For this reason the number of reminder letters sent, and the energy expended on "chasing" women who do not respond to an initial invitation should be limited. However, to ensure that the woman's refusal is based upon accurate information, a second, reminder, invitation should compare the risks and benefits of screening and clearly identify the risks of not being screened.

Basic screening

The initial examination for all women should be a two-view technique using the mediolateral oblique and the craniocaudal projections.[7,8]

For subsequent screening episodes a woman may only need an oblique projection, but, at the time of reporting the first mammograms, a radiologist should have the facility to request two views at subsequent examinations.

The two-view technique inevitably increases the cost of the basic screening process but the throughput of a basic screening clinic is scarcely altered. The film reading rate increases and the number of cases recalled for assessment decreases when a two-view technique is employed.

These two factors more than offset the increase in costs of the extra film.

There is no doubt that double reading of mammograms improves the sensitivity of the screening process.[9] Inevitably this is at the cost of some decrease in specificity, but it is at the assessment stage that the specificity of a screening programme is achieved.

Double reading may be undertaken by two radiologists or by one radiologist and a fully trained mammographic reader to whom the radiologist can properly delegate this task. Should a delegation system be introduced, it must be appreciated that it is the trained radiologist who has the responsibility for the referral of women for assessment.

There is a risk that double reading can result in an increased rate of recall for assessment. This can be minimised if there are regular full discussions by all radiologist members of the team of every case which has been referred for assessment, this discussion to take place in the light of knowledge of the outcome of assessment. A recall rate of under 3% (a measure of specificity) has been achieved in Nottingham with no reduction in the cancer detection rate (a measure of sensitivity) using this strategy.[10]

Assessment

Assessment is the process by which screen detected abnormalities are further investigated to determine their cause. It is best undertaken in a "one stop" multidisciplinary clinic using triple assessment techniques with clearly defined protocols.[11]

Some centres divide the process so that there is an initial sorting by further radiological investigation before it is determined which women, if any, are referred to a surgeon. This system has disadvantages. The surgeon will have to examine a woman who, because she has been selected for a surgical opinion whereas the other women recalled for assessment have not, has been led to believe that she has a significant problem. This might not be the case, but in this circumstance reassurance is much more difficult.

Some centres even progress to the stage of percutaneous tissue diagnosis prior to surgical referral, and in this circumstance the surgeon has to examine the woman's breasts which may well contain haematoma in the region of the abnormality.

The "one stop" organisation is preferred by the majority of women and has proved so successful that the same organisation is being increasingly adopted for the assessment of symptomatic problems. The preferable organisation is for the same expert team to hold a series of assessment clinics, some designated for symptomatic women and others for screen detected abnormalities.

3. Essential support services

There are services which it is essential must be established before and maintained throughout the duration of a screening programme. It is beyond the scope of this chapter to deal with these in detail, but the importance of these aspects is such that some reference must be made to them.

Education

The population needs to be well and accurately informed regarding the real benefits and potential hazards of the screening procedures to be adopted.[1] The targeted women will need to be given this information in greater detail. In this regard the risks of not being screened should be made quite clear, and comparisons with the risks and benefits of screening made explicit.

The medical profession, particularly family doctors, and also the various non-medical professionals to whom the women to be screened relate, will need specific education. They need to be informed of details which they will require in order to have fully informed consultations regarding screening with women and their families.

Training

Initially all staff who will be working within the screening programme should be fully trained in those aspects of the service which they will be required to undertake. In addition it is of major benefit for each professional group to have a knowledge of the activities of all the others.[12] In this way they will be better able to appreciate their own place in the multidisciplinary team which is responsible for the success of the programme.

Update training will be necessary both to introduce new techniques and protocols, and also to rectify any deficiencies which regular Quality Assurance Audit procedures might identify.

Personal assessment is a vital aspect of quality assurance, which may be accomplished by external methods or by self-assessment.[13] In either case any individual's weaknesses which are identified will need to be addressed by the training programme.

Quality assurance

The foundation of a successful screening programme is an integrated Quality Assurance (Q.A.)

programme.[14,15,16] Not only must all the equipment used within the service be subject to regular Quality Control, but also each professional group will need to establish its own professional Q.A. system. To ensure that these two aspects may both be accomplished is one reason for having an efficient, user-friendly computer system operating before the screening programme is implemented.

Equipment Q.A. is a four-stage process, with a desirable fifth.[17,18,19,20] First, accurate specifications must be agreed for all items.[21] The specifications should evolve from multi-disciplinary discussions involving engineers, physicists, radiographers and radiologists. Secondly, purchase of the equipment. This should be under central control by a group who should be fully aware of the professional needs, and in a position to influence financial aspects such as tendering.[22] Thirdly, acceptance testing at local level by fully trained engineers and physicists is necessary to ensure that the equipment delivered is up to the specified standard. Finally, throughout the operative life of the equipment, regular testing needs to be undertaken according to agreed schedules. Typically, radiographers will undertake daily, weekly and monthly tests, and physicists more complex tests according to quarterly, six-monthly and annual schedules. An additional stage of equipment Q.A. is desirable, namely field trials, undertaken in approved expert centres, of any new items of equipment produced by manufacturers. A dialogue between the manufacturers, the testing centre, and the specification body during the field trial stage is an extremely valuable exercise and should not be inhibited or curtailed.

A fully-integrated Professional Quality Assurance system is the basis of the success of the UK Breast Screening Programme.[23] Each professional group has a central committee, with representatives from each of the health regions, some 18-20 members in total. It is these central committees which, in consultation with the appropriate College, draw up the quality assurance programme for each profession.[13,24,25,26]

Guidelines are issued wherein Objectives are stated, and Criteria devised whereby the achievement of these objectives might be measured. Standards are then agreed, and audit procedures designed to ensure that all members of the professional group are involved in the Q.A. process. Liaison between the central professional committees is achieved by a co-ordinating Q.A. group comprised of the chairmen of the professional groups. Each health region has a Q.A. committee under the chairmanship of a Q.A. Manager. The membership of the Regional Committees is the representative of each professional group together with co-opted members having a specific expertise and officers to undertake any actions determined by the Committee.

4. Manpower considerations

The manpower requirements for each involved professional group need to be assessed with accuracy. This can be achieved conveniently, and relatively simply, by using as a base the number of women who can be screened using one basic screening mammographic apparatus operated by two radiographers. Forrest[1] calculated that about 10,000 women could be screened annually using one machine. Thus, with a 75% acceptance rate and a three-year interval, a target population of some 40,000 women requires one basic screening mammographic unit, and two radiographers to operate it. A total population of 471,000 has within it 40,000 women aged between 50 and 64 years of age. These figures can be regarded as a quantum of population, and extrapolations made from calculations done on them. Thus it can be seen that for a town of a million inhabitants, two basic mammographic machines will be required. In addition to the radiographers to operate these units, there is a requirement for administrative and clerical staff to organise the call and recall system, and to run the screening clinics. Similarly, there are radiologists needed to report the films. Having calculated the requirements for basic screening, the staffing requirements for the assessment of screen detected abnormalities, and all the other activities associated with screening can be assessed using similar logic.

Two important points need to be borne in mind when considering manpower levels:
1. *Part time staff.* The calculations outlined above will indicate the numbers of whole time staff required, but in practice part time staff are extensively employed. This increases the costs, and importantly the training facilities required.
2. *Replacement staff.* In addition to the recruitment of staff required to implement the programme, it is essential to train replacements, otherwise there will be a manpower shortage which will inevitably occur and begin to become apparent some 5-10 years after the commencement of the programme. Take for example radiologists.

In the UK programme it was calculated by the Forrest Working Group that 48 additional whole time equivalent radiologists would be required for 120 basic screening units. Funding sufficient to employ this number was allocated. However, the body which regulated the number of doctors commencing radiologist training at the time (JPAC) refused, or was constrained to refuse, a request to increase the number of trainee radiologists to a level which would support this extra number of radiologists.

Since it takes on average six years to train a radiologist, it is only now, 6 years after the commencement of the programme, that a manpower shortage is beginning to become apparent. This deficiency will inevitably increase. Similar shortages are beginning to appear in other specialities.

To achieve and maintain the highest possible standards of performance each individual involved in the programme should be fully integrated into the screening team, and should be made conscious of this fact. It is advantageous, for example, for individuals who have been involved with a woman's investigation to be aware of the outcome. This applies particularly to radiologists who might have been involved in the basic screening but not in assessment and to radiographers who have undertaken examinations. To avoid boredom and the resultant risk of the lowering of standards, it is important for individuals to undertake more than one task. For instance radiographers should rotate between basic screening, assessment and symptomatic mammography, with additional duties in apparatus and professional quality assurance.[24]

5. Equipment requirements

Computer system

The importance of having an operational computer system established before a screening programme commences cannot be over emphasised.[1]

A computer system is an essential tool to accomplish many of the complex tasks which are associated with breast cancer screening.[27] These include the call and recall system, and consequently the basic requirement is for the computer to maintain a register of women in the target age group. Personal identification data - date of birth, address etc. will be required. This will be expanded to keep a personal screening record indicating dates of invitations and screening episodes, together with a record of events during each episode. In addition to these features management data will be needed, and this can be derived from the records of numbers attending etc. Each professional group will have a data schedule which it requires to perform the monitoring and quality assurance tasks which it should undertake.[13,24,25,26]

Efficient, rapid and accurate data collection and manipulation is absolutely essential for a successful programme. To accomplish this, an up-to-date user-friendly computer system is required. It is beyond the scope of this chapter to detail all the requirements, but when the specification of a system is being determined the following are amongst the key points which should be considered:

- There should be no appreciable delay in screen changes, and waiting times for information to be displayed should be virtually negligible.
- There should be a minimal number of paper interfaces; thus a radiologist should be able to input the report on a mammogram directly, using a light pen or some such device. This will eliminate transcription errors.
- The data collected should be that which is of use to administer and monitor the efficiency of the service. Each involved profession will have a schedule of data items which it requires to administer and monitor those aspects of the service with which it is involved.
- There should be sufficient flexibility, in terms of ad hoc enquiry facilities etc., to enable research projects to be undertaken.
- Efficient transfer of data between various sections of the programme, along agreed pathways, should be an integral feature of the system.

Film processing equipment

Film quality is the most important issue in mammography.[28,29] This depends partially upon the patient-positioning skills of the radiographer, and partly on the film processing. An automatic processor should be used, with large chemical tank capacity. The processing parameters should be accurately controlled, but variable in order to accommodate different film types from time to time. It is common for mammographic films to be subjected to a longer developing cycle time at a somewhat higher temperature than is used for normal radiographic purposes.

Mammographic equipment

Basic screening

For basic screening a high quality but simple apparatus is required, with a single focal spot tube without the facility for magnification or sophisticated investigations. This machine may be static in a fixed building, or may be in a mobile van depending on the location of the population to be served.

The location chosen, mobile or static, should be that which enables the maximum number of women to attend with the minimum of personal inconvenience.

Film processing of the basic screening mammograms is ideally undertaken in a static unit rather than on the mobile van, since the mandatory accurate processor control essential for high quality mammograms is thereby more easily achieved.

Assessment clinics

For assessment of screen detected abnormalities a sophisticated mammographic apparatus is essential. There should be facilities for magnification films, and a variety of compression devices. Stereotactic apparatus, which is an add-on facility for modern apparatus, will be required for the elucidation of screen detected abnormalities which are not visible on ultra-sound.

Ultra-sound equipment

Ultra-sound apparatus is now considered to be an essential part of the equipment of an assessment clinic.[30,31] This should have a high resolution transducer, 7.5 MHz at least, and, if it is a sector scanner, a water-path stand off is required. It is not essential, but many radiologists prefer a transducer with a needle guide attachment.

The case for need for Doppler has not yet been made. Certainly by using Doppler one may produce extra evidence suggesting benignity or malignancy as the case may be, but the need for tissue diagnosis cannot be eliminated. There seems little justification for an additional modality which does not eliminate a step in an existing diagnostic pathway of proven efficiency.

6. Implementation

The implementation programme is best accomplished by an over-seeing multidisciplinary group upon which each professional group involved in screening is represented. If a wide geographical area is to be covered, then it may well be appropriate for the area to be divided into a series of convenient sections based upon the population density in a location. In this event a sub-group for each section should oversee the details of implementation according to the central policy. Tight liaison between the central and peripheral groups is essential. In the design of an implementation programme it is important to remember that:
- The crux of a successful Breast Screening Programme is the assessment process.
- The implementation plan should be assessment led.

Assessment requires an expert multidisciplinary team. Such a team is most likely to be found, or created as a viable entity, if the same individuals are involved with the investigation and management of women with breast symptoms. In the UK the trend is towards the establishment of expert cancer centres. It is in such centres that the assessment clinics for a Breast Screening Programme should ideally be situated. One assessment centre can deal with the referrals from a number of basic screening units.

The number of assessment clinics required for a population can be calculated if it is considered that one clinic can deal with about 10-12 cases per clinic session. The basic screening units will refer about 3%-5% of examined cases for assessment, and can be expected to examine in the order of 70% of the target population.

Having determined the site and capacity of the assessment centres, remembering that some if not all centres will be assessing symptomatic women as well as those with screen detected abnormalities, then the number and location of "satellite" basic screening units can be determined. This will depend upon the population density in the area. An important consideration is that the basic screening units should be conveniently located for each population group; women will travel to have a suspected abnormality assessed, but are less likely to accept inconvenience whilst they still regard themselves as well women. Decisions as to the screening of small elements of population such as small villages should be made following consideration of the alternatives of periodic visits to the village by a mobile unit and the transportation of individual women to a more central location.

Once the overall plan is determined, then the implementation group should commence the educational process (see above). Recruitment of key personnel to run the screening service should commence at an early stage. Meetings between the key personnel and General Practitioners and also local women's organisations are of value as a part of the education process. When a team has been recruited and the equipment has been installed in suitable accommodation and its performance tested, then screening should start. Initially it is preferable to screen a few women, say those of appropriate age group on the staff of a local hospital or clinic. Having proved that the apparatus works, the organisation of the work flow pattern should be tested by inviting a full session of women for screening. Inevitably some alteration in details will be required, and there should be adequate time allowed to accomplish these before screening proper is commenced.

7. Co-ordination

It can be seen from the foregoing that the organisation of a Breast Cancer Screening Programme is a complex and complicated exercise. A programme can only succeed if there is an efficient co-ordinating system. This is best accomplished by having a small dedicated team who have the expertise to justify the confidence of all the professionals working in the programme. The leader of this team, the National Co-ordinator, is the key to its success. The team should be headed by an individual with the expertise to manage the team efficiently, together with the personality which facilitates relationships with both the professionals working within the programme, and the political masters and health officials who control the national policies and finance. Access to both groups by the Co-ordinator should not be constrained. The Co-ordinator should control a budget and have the freedom to expend this in any manner perceived to be appropriate. It is the Co-ordinator who, having an overview, can assess relative priorities and develop initiatives to eliminate deficiencies. The Co-ordinator is in a unique position to know those individuals who are the best sources of expert advice on matters related to screening and also those who are most likely to be able to solve any problems which may arise. An important function of the co-ordinating group is to ensure that the public is kept regularly and accurately informed regarding the successes of the programme and also of any problems which might arise.

Given adequate funding and facilities, then the co-ordinating function will succeed, and the whole programme organisation will function more efficiently, and will itself be more likely to succeed.

References

1. Forrest A.P.M. (Chairman, Working Group on Breast Cancer Screening): Report to the Health Ministers of England, Wales, Scotland and Northern Ireland. London, H.M.S.O., 1986
2. NHS Breast Screening Programme: Review 1995. Sheffield, NHSBSP Publications. 1997; 37: 2
3. Roebuck E.J.: A personal view of the approach to breast cancer screening in the UK.; The Breast, 1994; 3: 60-68
4. Roebuck E.J.: Breast cancer screening in non-Caucasians. In: *Proceedings of the Roentgen Centenary Congress*. Birmingham London, Brit. Inst. Radiol. 1995; 1450: 239
5. Law J.: Risk and benefit associated with radiation dose in breast cancer screening programmes - an update. Brit. J. Radiol., 1995; 68: 870-876
6. Tabar L., Fagerberg G., Day N.E., *et al.*: What is the optimal interval between mammographic screening examinations? An analysis based on the latest results of the Swedish two-county breast cancer screening trial. Br. J. Cancer 1987; 66: 547-551
7. Bassett L.W., Bunnell, D., Johanshahi, R. *et al.*: Breast Cancer detection: one versus two views. Radiology, 1987; 165: 95-7
8. Sickles E.A., Weber W.N., Galvin, H.B. et al.: Baseline Screening Mammography: one versus two views per breast. Am. J. Radiol. 1986; 147: 1149-53
9. Warren R.M.L., Duffy S.W.: Comparison of single reading with double reading of mammograms, and change in effectiveness with experience. Brit. J. Radiol., 1995; 68: 958-962
10. Wilson A.R.M.W.: Proceedings of the Royal College of Radiologists breast group. Edinburgh, 1994
11. Ellis I.O., Galea, M.A., Locker, A., *et al.*: Early experience in Breast Cancer Screening: emphasis on development of protocols for triple assessment. The Breast, 1993; 2: 148-153
12. Roebuck E.J., Wilson A.R.M.: Training in Mammographic Screening. In: *Breast Cancer Screening in Europe*, Gad A., Rosselli del Turco M., (Eds.) Heidelberg, Springer Verlag, 1993; 121-130
13. Royal College of Radiologists: Quality Assurance Guidelines for Radiologists. NHSBSP Publications. Oxford, 1990
14. Europe Against Cancer Study Group: European Guidelines for Quality Assurance in Mammography Screening. LRCB/KUN Nijmengen, Netherlands, 1992
15. Gray, J.A.M.: General Principles of Quality Assurance in Breast Cancer Screening. NHSBSP Publications, Oxford, 1990
16. Pritchard J., ed.: Quality Assurance Guidelines for Mammography. Report of a sub-committee of the Radiology Advisory Committee of the Chief Medical Officer. NHSBSP Publications. Oxford, 1989
17. Young K.C., Ramsdale M.L., Horton P.W.: Review of Mammographic Equipment and its Performance. NHSBSP publications, 1992
18. National Council on Radiation Protection and Measurements. Mammography- A User's Guide. N.R.C.P., 1986; Report n. 85, Bethesda
19. Moores B.M., Watkinson S.A., Henshaw E.T., Pearcy B.J.: Practical guide to Quality Assurance in Medical Imaging. Chichester, John Wiley & Sons, 1987
20. Neilson B.: Technical aspects of mammography. Current Opinion in Radiology, 1992; 4: 118-122
21. Department of Health: Guidance Notes for Health Authorities on Mammographic X-Ray Equipment Requirements for Breast Cancer Screening in 1987. DoH Publication, 1987; STD.: 87/34
22. Briggs P.: Organisation of Breast Cancer Screening. Proceedings of: Breast Screening- Its Impact on Your Future. London, Brit. Inst. Radiol., 1995
23. Roebuck E.J.: Clinical Radiology of the Breast, Oxford, Heinemann Medical Books, 1990; 186-201
24. NHSBSP Radiographers Quality Assurance Co-ordination Committee: Quality Assurance Guidelines for Radiographers. Sheffield, NHSBSP Publication 1994
25. National Co-ordinating Group for Surgeons: Quality Assurance Guidelines for Surgeons in Breast Cancer Screening, Sheffield, NHSBSP Publication, 1992
26. Guidelines for Pathologists: The Royal College of Pathologists Working Group. 1990, NHSBSP publications. IBSN 187, 1997; 65: 8
27. Patnick J., Gray: J.A.M.: Guidelines on the Collection and use of Breast Cancer Data. Sheffield, NHSBSP Publication 1993
28. Kirkpatrick A.E.: Quality Control in Mammography. In: *Breast Cancer Screening in Europe*. Gad A., Rosselli del Turco M., (Eds.), Heidelberg, Springer Verlag 1993; 131-141
29. Lee L., Stickland V., Wilson ARM., Roebuck E.J.: Fundamentals of Mammography. London, W.B. Saunders, 1995; 7-11
30. Guyer P.B., & Dewbury, K.C.: Sonomammography – An Atlas of Comparative breast Ultrasound. Chichester, John Wiley, 1987
31. Tohno E., Cosgrove D.O., Sloane, J.P.: Ultrasound diagnosis of breast Diseases. London, Churchill Livingstone, 1993

Clinical aspects of a screening programme

G. Querci della Rovere, D. Lowry, P. Fulton, J. Spencer Knott, Y. Steel, R. Warren

The role of the General Practitioner

D. Lowry

General Practitioners (GPs) are crucial in ensuring that a breast screening service is effective, in identifying suitable women for screening and in offering support to those with abnormal results.

Their role starts by making women feel positive about screening, for breast awareness can be encouraged at family planning sessions and Well-Women Clinics. Direct questioning identifies women who have a family history of breast cancer and can be offered close monitoring after the age of 35 if two or more first degree relatives are affected. Older women can be told about breast screening in the area and the positive aspects can be explained so they will be more likely to attend once invited. Women over the age of 64 can be screened at their request and GPs are in an ideal position to inform this age group when they attend for other reasons.

A notice in the surgery telling women that the service is being offered in their area may help; press releases will also tell women who are not registered with a GP that the service is available.

Women eligible for breast screening are identified from computerised records at the Family Health Services Authority (FHSA). They are chosen by post code and date of birth as some patients live in a different area from their GPs and would be missed if they were identified by GPs in the area alone.

The computer print-out is then sent to the relevant GP to be checked and approved. The most common error is in the addresses which are often wrong because the patient has not told the FHSA she has moved. Other frequent errors are in the dates of birth and in the post codes which are either missing or simply wrong; these mistakes can be picked up and corrected by GP practices with an age/sex register or computer, but it can be time consuming.

It is helpful to the Screening Service if any patients with a history of breast cancer can be identified. Women who have had a bilateral mastectomy do not need to be screened. Those who have had breast cancer treatment in the past are probably being followed-up and offered regular mammography, although follow-up is variable. If the GP is unsure the woman should be screened.

There are various reasons why a GP advises the Screening Centre not to invite a woman: the most obvious is death (there can be quite a delay before the FHSA delete those deceased from their list). Other reasons include terminal illness or private screening recently (usually within 1 year). If the woman is unfit at present but should be well in six months (for example) this can be indicated on the form. Much of the screening is done in a mobile van with steps: disabled women should be screened at the Centre where there is disabled access for them.

A time limit has to be put on the return of the FHSA lists. In West Essex this limit is 3 weeks. As the years have gone by, the FHSA lists have become more accurate and more GP practices are computerised making it easier to pick up omissions and errors. Unfortunately patients still move without telling us.

The corrected list is sent back to the FHSA who pass the information on to the screening office. Appointments are sent out from here together with a letter from the patient's GP (Fig. 1) explaining the importance of the procedure and suggesting that they make contact if they have any concerns. Very few patients ask for further information.

Any invited woman who fails to attend for her appointment is given a second one and in case of failure the GP is informed. We usually mark this on the notes so that we can discuss it when the patient next attends. Usually, it has been a deliberate policy not to attend, but occasionally the appointment was cancelled for a good reason and then forgotten: jogging the patient's memory results in screening.

Breast Screening Service

St.Margaret's Hospital, Epping. CM16 6TN
Telephone: (0378) 560001

Dear

The Breast Screening Service is now once again available in your area. Your General Practitioner, ... and I would like to invite you to attend. The enclosed leaflet explains the service and the importance of regular screening.

For your convenience an appointment has been made for you at the

SITE..
DATE...

If you would like your appointment changed to a more suitable date or time, or, if you have had a mammogram within a year, please contact this office between 10:00 a.m. and 4:00 p.m. Please bring this letter with you when you attend.

Please do not use talcum powder or spray deodorant when you attend, as they affect the quality of the x-ray film. It would not cause any problems if you use a roll-on deodorant. If you wear separates you will find it easier to undress to the waist.

I expect to send you the results of your x-ray within three weeks of your appointment.

Your sincerely

Dr. Ruth Warren
Consultant Radiologist.

West Essex Health Authority Redbridge Health Authority

Fig. 1. Facsimile of the invitation letter sent by Family Health Services Authority with the co-operation of GPs.

Breast Screening Service

St.Margaret's Hospital, Epping. CM16 6TN
Telephone: (0378) 560001

Please return this form, completed, with the corrected FCP lists.

* 1)   Please refer my patients who need a surgical opinion direct to the Breast Clinic at St. Margaret's Hospital.

* 2)   Please refer my patients who need a surgical opinion direct to
...........................at............................

*3)   Please contact me on.................................. before you refer any of my patients to a surgeon.

*4)   Please delete as applicable.

I enclose a signed letter for my patients on my own headed notepaper.

Signed...........................
Name (please print)...........
Address........................
....
....
Date   ....

West Essex Health Authority Redbridge Health Authority

Fig. 2. The facsimile GPs form requiring surgical opinion for patients.

I do not feel it is helpful to make special contact with non-attenders as they can feel pressured and it can affect the doctor-patient relationship.

Women are notified of a normal result by the screening service about 3 weeks after the mammography; the GP is sent a list of normal women soon after this.

Women with abnormal results are called back to the assessment clinic with a couple of days notice (to reduce the period of anxiety). It was decided against informing the GPs at this stage because of the uncertainty of the diagnosis and the consequent limited contribution the GPs could make.

GPs are sent a letter about each individual patient seen in the assessment clinic with the results of further investigations. This enables us to have an informed discussion with the lady if she has any

queries but the service is so good that this is not usually required.

For women who require treatment, it is important to involve both the GP and the patient in the choice of surgeon; unfortunately GPs can be difficult to contact in a hurry so all GPs are sent a letter (Fig. 2). Most patients feel that they wish to remain in the Screening Centre as they have gained confidence in the "system" but some are referred to other NHS or private hospitals.

Breast Screening has generally been well received by our practice population and, while it has involved us in extra work, it has been rewarding. The population is gradually becoming healthier partly because of screening, and GPs play a vital role in this even when the screening procedure is undertaken at the hospital.

The role of the radiographer

P. Fulton

When the Forrest Report[1] was published, it emphasised the need to provide a high quality service to ensure that the benefits of breast screening outweighed any adverse side effects, as screening was being offered to a healthy population who had not sought help but who were being sought out and invited to participate. This necessary high quality of mammography can best be obtained by dedicated Radiographers using dedicated equipment.

Not all radiographers, however well trained, will make good mammographers; they need a very understanding, sympathetic personality and the ability not only to achieve high standards of work but to maintain it under pressure.

The ladies presenting for breast screening are often anxious; the actual invitation to attend will in many cases raise anxiety and this may cause apparent awkwardness and embarrassment. So the radiographer by her sensitivity and caring approach has to ease these feelings to get the lady as relaxed as possible to enable a good mammogram with good compression to be obtained, whilst at the same time gaining the confidence and satisfaction of the lady so she is willing to attend for future screening.

What is a good mammogram?

Mammography has been described as "the science of imaging and the art of positioning", used to demonstrate early clinically occult cancers. Mammography has to be highly sensitive to detect the malignant lesions with variable growth rates and differing radiological appearances. In the National Health Service Breast Screening Programme (NHS-BSP) each lady attending for her prevalent screen has two-view mammography, a cranio-caudal (CC) view and medio-lateral oblique (MLO) view of each breast.

Cranio-caudal view

The cranio-caudal view when correctly positioned should enable all except the very lateral breast tissue to be visualised (Fig. 3). To obtain this view the woman should face the machine, the breast is gently raised and the film positioned at right angles against the chest wall at the level of the inframammary fold. With the nipple in profile and making sure the medial aspect of the breast remains on the film (as this may not be fully shown on the MLO view) the woman can turn her face away from the breast being x-rayed. If a hand is gently placed on the woman's back she can

gently be eased towards the machine; the compression is gradually applied and at the same time the breast eased forward (Fig. 4). This should give optimum coverage of the breast tissue.

Medio-lateral oblique view

When correctly positioned this view will show maximum breast tissue and allow good compres-

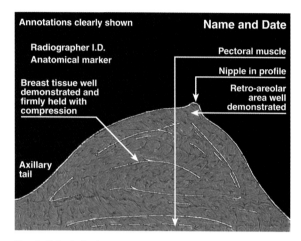

Fig. 3. Criteria for image assessment of cranio-caudal view.

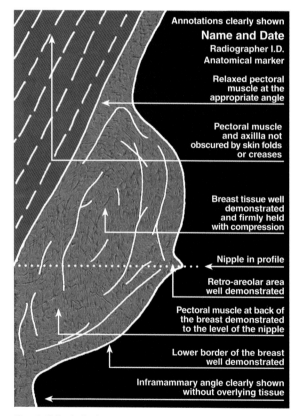

Fig. 4. Criteria for image assessment of medio-lateral oblique view.

sion (Figs. 5-6). The criteria set down by the NHSB-SP for a mediolateral oblique view is that it should show:
a. Nipple in profile.
b. Pectoral muscle visualized at nipple level.
c. Inframammary fold demonstrated.
d. Good compression.
e. Correct exposure and processing.
f. Name, date …

As not all women have the same body build, it is necessary for the radiographers to be experienced enough to be able to adapt the position of the woman and film to demonstrate the breast tissue to the full. It is of importance, when positioning for the MLO view, that the woman is relaxed and the film holder is at the correct height for the woman. If the film is too low, axillary tissue may be missed.

Before compression is applied the breast should be gently raised and eased away from the chest wall. The compression should be even over the whole breast and firm enough to hold the breast in the required position. Not all women find this a comfortable position to be placed in and so a full explanation of the procedure, with an understanding attitude by the radiographer is essential. With good positioning the images of each breast should mirror each other when viewed.

Compression

It is essential for a good diagnostic mammogram that compression is suitably applied. A woman's co-operation must be obtained; an unsympathetic approach by the radiographer can lead to unnecessary discomfort and antagonism by the woman. Good compression will separate superimposed tissue, decrease geometric sharpness and reduce radiation dose; reduction in scatter radiation improves contrast.

Assessment

When an abnormality is suspected on the screening films, further views may be required.
a. Extended craniocaudal, a craniocaudal view with the breast rotated well medially to visualise the axillary tail.
b. True lateral view, either taken from the mediolateral or lateromedial direction. This view will help to visualise areas of asymmetrical density, and is used to localise impalpable lesions.
c. Magnification views are used to demonstrate more clearly the nature of any microcalcifications or masses seen on the original mammogram (Fig. 7). By using a small paddle compression, just the area of interest can be visualised. The localized compression will spread out any superimposed tissue resulting in a sharper and clearer image. Magnification will not only demonstrate the morphology of the microcalcifications but will, at times, demonstrate further calcifications not originally seen, and, in the case of masses, will demonstrate the nature of their borders.

Film processing

However good the positioning of the breast on the film, without good processing and meticulous quality control, cancer will be missed. In a good screening or mammography service only a dedicated processor should be used. This can then be programmed to give optimum performance for the film screen and chemicals combination used and will be as free as possible from artefacts.

Sensitometry tests should be carried out before each screening session and before any batch processing of films; this will ensure the processor is functioning to the required standard and any identified problems can be corrected prior to processing. Mam-

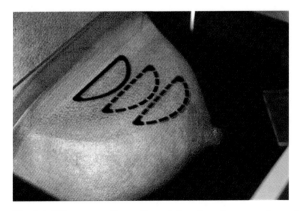
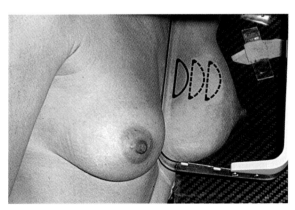

Fig. 5-6. When correctly positioned, the view shows maximum breast tissue and allow good compression.

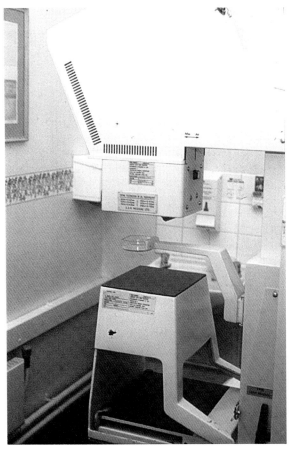

Fig. 7. Mammographic Apparatus for Magnifications view: the distance between the breast and the film is increased.

mography films are particularly sensitive to fluctuations in processing parameters.

If breast cancer is to be detected early, the quality of the mammography and the manner in which it is carried out is of the utmost importance.

The Assessment clinic

G. Querci della Rovere, Y. Steel, R. Warren

In the fourth HM Queen Elizabeth the Queen Mother Fellowship "Breast cancer: the decision to screen" published in 1990,[1] Sir Patrick Forrest estimated that no more than 10% of the women screened would be recalled for further investigations in an assessment clinic. In practice most of the Screening Centres have a lower recall rate of 3 to 6%. This is very important because a recall letter is cause of extreme anxiety to a woman. Two-view mammography has considerably reduced the recall rate but there might be doubts as to its cost-effectiveness.[2]

Staffing

The aim of the assessment clinic is to provide the woman with a definitive answer to the suspicion created by the screening process.

This should be achieved as quickly as possible: ideally the same day for benign cases, whereas for patients with cancer the diagnosis is probably better delivered in two visits.

To achieve this objective the assessment clinic should ideally be staffed by a radiologist, a surgeon, a cytopathologist, radiographers and a Breast Specialist nurse. In reality however it is impractical and not cost-effective to have three Consultants in the same clinic.

A compromise would be to have the assessment clinic run by a single clinician trained in mammography, ultrasonography, cytopathology and treatment of breast diseases.

Investigations

It is imperative that as soon as the woman arrives at the assessment clinic she has explained to her the reason for the recall and is reassured as much as possible. In fact, only a minority of the recalled women will be found to have breast cancer.

During the interview with the patient the clinician should inquire regarding risk factors, previous breast pathology, present breast complaints and the use of drugs, particularly hormone replacement therapy and anticoagulants.

The patient is then examined: often a careful examination aimed at the area of the mammographic abnormality allows the clinician to feel a lesion which could have been missed.

Breast ultrasound should be a routine investigation of the breast, ideally carried out at the same time as the clinical examination. Ultrasound in the context of the assessment clinic is used mainly to differentiate a solid from a cystic lesion; further analysis of a solid lesion is also possible with a doppler study which assesses the degree of vascularization of a lesion (increased vascularity is suspicious of malignancy).

A breast cyst is shown as a circumscribed transechoic lesion with sharply defined margins and strong distal enhancement. Small cysts often appear to contain echoes which may be due to thick viscid content but will still show distal enhancement.

The benign fibroadenoma will present as a solid welldefined round or lobulated mass with an even internal echo pattern. Border definition is sharp and there is normally no distal effect, although occasionally there is central attenuation or accentuation. The mass is mobile and compressible. A small percentage of well defined solid lesions are malignant and in these cases a doppler study could be useful to increase or reduce the level of suspicion. Variation in internal echo pattern or loss of border definition should raise the possibility of malignancy. There are three main features of the malignant lesion which are seen in varying combinations:

1. Mass or nidus with uneven echo pattern (under 1 cm in size the echo pattern is even). The margins often remain fairly sharp in medullary and colloid carcinomas.
2. A surrounding highly reflective zone or halo.
3. A distal central alternating shadow seen in both planes. Edge refractive shadowing is non-specific.

Further radiological views are also useful in trying to clarify the nature of the mammographic suspicious features. Cranio-caudal views are mandatory when only mediolateral oblique views were taken.

Extended craniocaudal views are essential for lesions visible only in the axillary tail of the mediolateral oblique view.

Cone-compressed and magnified views are valuable to assess microcalcifications and other mammographic irregularities, particularly those of low level of suspicion; very often a radiological view with further compression will show that there is in fact no lesion.

At the end of the clinical-radiological assessment, three possible levels of suspicion can be achieved:

R3 probably benign
R4 probably malignant
R5 malignant

If we had to rely only on radiological information, to reduce to a minimum the risk of missing carcinomas, we would have to biopsy all the suspicious lesions (R3, 4, 5); possibly the majority of recalled women.

If on the other hand, we want to minimise the number of biopsies, we could decide to biopsy only R4-5 lesions, with the knowledge however of leaving behind a number of carcinomas and still having a discrete number of benign biopsies.

An alternative to this predicament is to improve the sensitivity and specificity of the assessment by introducing into the diagnostic phase another parameter, FNA cytology.

If a definite lesion has been confirmed at the assessment clinic its nature should be established by fine needle aspiration (FNA) cytology. The investigation can be carried out clinically if there is a palpable lump or under ultrasound or radiological guidance. FNA under radiological guidance can be through a perforated plate (Fig. 8) or with stereotaxis (Fig. 9).

In theory FNA with stereotactic control should be the most accurate and the procedure of choice; however in practice this may not so due to the fact that the breast is not a rigid structure and often the lesion, instead of being transfixed by the needle, is simply pushed downwards, failing to produce a representative specimen.

We compared the accuracy of FNA through a localizing window and with stereotaxis practising on targets; we observed that for lesions up to 2.5 cm from the skin surface the accuracy was 90% both for stereotaxis and the localizing window; however for lesions deeper than 2.5 cm the accuracy (10 mm target) was still 90% with stereotaxis but only 70% with a localizing plate.

If we consider that the average thickness of the compressed breast is 4 cm and that most lesions are in the upper half of the breast we can conclude that most FNAs under X-ray control can be carried

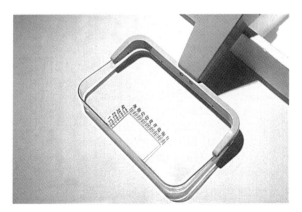

Fig. 8. Fine needle aspiration (FNA) cytology under radiological guidance using a perforated plate.

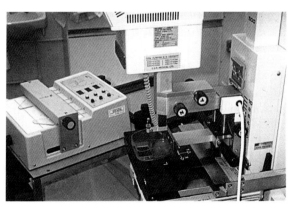

Fig. 9. The same process with stereotaxis.

out reliably through a perforated window. The level of suspicion on cytology is expressed as follows:
CO-1 no cells, inadequate;
C2 benign;
C3 suspicious, probably benign;
C4 suspicious, probably malignant;
C5 malignant.

If we now combine the radiological with the cytological levels of suspicion we can have several possible combinations; these are better expressed in a diagram which also shows our present policy on open biopsies (Fig. 10).

All the C4-5, R3-4-5 combinations are biopsied:
C2, R4-5 and
C3, R4 are biopsied
C2, R3 and C3, R3 are not at present biopsied but reassessed between 6 and 12 months.

This policy helped us to achieve a malignant/benign biopsy rate of 4:1.

We reviewed the combined (cytological-radiological) levels of suspicion of 113 benign biopsies (microcalcifications 40%, circumscribed lesions 17%, asymmetry or distortion 21%, stellate lesions 22%) and found that 48% were C2R3 or C3R3. We feel we could reduce by 48% the number of benign biopsies by adopting a policy of careful follow-up of C2R3 and C3R3 lesions.[3]

By adopting this policy we would also delay the diagnosis of cancer in 0.5% of cases (1DCIS and 1 Tubular ca.).

At the end of the assessment the women with benign breast changes will be reassured and returned to routine screening; the patients with cancer will be told the diagnosis and the treatment options explained. Most screen detected cancers are small and have an excellent prognosis: this fact should be stressed to the patient. It is imperative that the surgeon who will be in charge of the case informs the patient of the diagnosis of breast cancer.

There will be a third group of women who, at the end of the assessment phase, will have lesions of low or high level of suspicion. In these cases we repeat an FNA cytology test either to obtain a definite positive result of malignancy or in the case of benign cytology to reduce to a minimum the chances of sampling error.

Women with highly suspicious lesions undergo a diagnostic biopsy whereas those with lesions which are probably benign are, after full explanation and discussion with the patient, reassessed in 6 to 12 months.

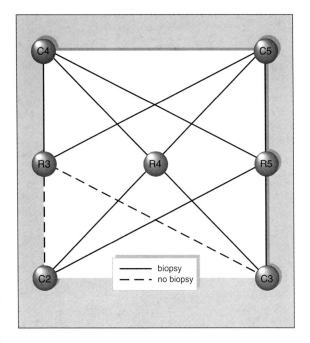

Fig. 10. Present policy on open biopsies.

The role of the breast specialist nurse in breast screening (Figs. 11-21)

J. Spencer Knott

The Breast Care Specialist Nurse provides a supportive and advisory service to women who have or might have breast cancer. Within the field of education she aims to improve the capabilities of others involved, both lay and professional, and to deliver care to this client group.

Within this role it is a great privilege to work with women and their families who are facing one of the greatest traumas of their lives; that of a diagnosis of breast cancer!

With the implementation of the National Breast Screening Programme early breast cancers are diagnosed. We have however invited well women, and their reactions both to the assessment clinic invitation and to the diagnosis can be quite diverse. The 1991 Breast Cancer Screening Report[4] highlights the need to develop the specialist nursing service within the Breast Screening Programme endeavouring to lessen the anxiety in women called for assessment. The nurse is part of the multidisciplinary team. It is vital that we all speak the same language with the same goals and that a climate of openness and honesty exists. The establishment of good communication ensures continuity of appropriate care, information, advice, physical and psychological support.

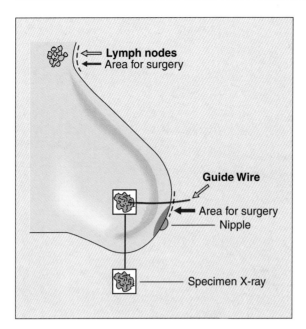

Fig. 11. Diagram showing guidewire localisation.

The assessment clinic

About 3 to 6% of the women screened are recalled to the assessment clinic. An information leaflet is sent out with the recall appointment. This explains the procedures that may occur on this occasion. Research shows that information according to the need can decrease anxiety and enhance one's ability to cope. The nurse introduces herself as part of the team. It is not easy to take in who's who in a strange environment, however hard those in the Clinic try to keep a relaxed atmosphere.

Once a diagnosis of breast cancer is given it is essential that the Breast Care Nursing Service provides:
Time and privacy for confidentiality;
Information and psychological support;
Telephone contact;
Continuity of care.

Information given needs to be tailored to individual needs, stepping stones as opposed to abrupt overload of news. There needs to be time to let the news sink in and explore resulting concerns. Concerns can vary enormously.
"Everyone dies from breast cancer, don't they?"
(a patient)

"It is always in the paper, many patients haven't received the right treatment"
(a patient)

"My mother has Alzheimer's Disease and I really can't leave her to come into hospital for an operation"
(a patient)

Treatment options

There is no consensus of opinion about breast cancer treatment. There is evidence that women who are keen to take part in the process of treatment choice may have less psychological problems later on. Relevant information must be given to assist this process. Demands and expectations have changed in the last few years. Media coverage can contain alarmist messages and can cause confusion particularly if a woman has been diagnosed within days of a TV programme.

"I felt as if an explosion had happened in my body and I was waiting for all the pieces to come down on top of me"
(a patient)

"I fell into a black hole today. I feel I am drowning in the blackness"
(a patient)

Declining treatment

The woman may wish to decline treatment and is quite entitled to support in her decision. It is of paramount importance that communication continues to be open and honest. The woman needs to be aware of the risks she is taking and that the opportunity is there to return and discuss the situation again. The team may find this quite a dilemma and this is when supporting each other is so important. It is important that working within this stressful role the specialist nurse, if she wishes, has access to independent psychological support for herself.

Wide excision and axillary dissection

After diagnosing a breast cancer that is impalpable the pre-operative preparation includes inserting a fine guidewire into the breast to guide the surgeon to find the lesion during the operation. It is of paramount importance that this is fully explained. Around the mixture of feelings of disbelief that something can really be wrong, the information given clarifies the situation thus minimising anxiety.

The majority of screen detected cancers are treated by local excision and axillary dissection. Information is given concerning the length of hospital admission, the recovery time, the use of drains and possible

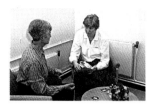 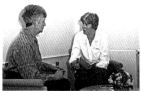 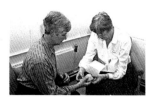 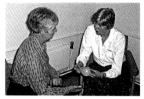

Fig. 12-13. The nurse is counselling the patient, giving information.

Fig. 14-15. As a practical support she is showing a prostheses to the patient.

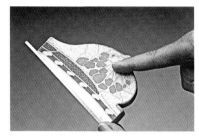 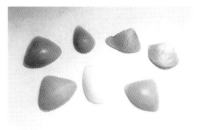 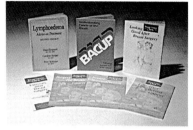

Fig. 16. Cross-section model of a breast.

Fig. 17. Range of prostheses available: temporary, permanent and suitable for swimming

Fig. 18. Breast cancer care; lymphoedema advice.

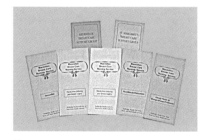 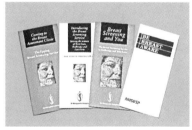 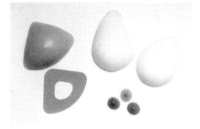

Fig. 19. Handy hints leaflets. In house.

Fig. 20. Breast screening leaflets.

Fig. 21. Adhesive prostheses using skin support, custom made nipples.

complications. Arm exercises are recommended with advice on precautionary measures to reduce the risk of lymphoedema of the arm and hand. It must be stressed that further treatment (radiotherapy, chemotherapy or hormone therapy) may depend on the histology report. It must be stressed how diverse breast cancer can be and that there are different types of this disease. What may be the best treatment for one woman might not be so for another.

Mastectomy

Within the context of early diagnosis multifocal disease presents a dilemma for the woman and her family. Our message is early diagnosis, conservative surgery and better prognosis and therefore few women are prepared to accept a mastectomy for early breast cancer.

Basic diagrams or a cross-section model of the breast enables better understanding.

Mastectomy with or without reconstruction requires increased comprehension.

Photographs, contact with a trained volunteer willing to provide her own experience and being aware of the full range of prostheses are all tailored to the needs of the individual, and help the woman to come to terms with the operation. Awareness of altered body image problems and anxieties about sexuality need to be assessed and monitored. Appropriate intervention or referral to other agencies may be necessary.

Breast care support group

The setting-up of a support group is another way of providing continuing support for any woman who has had treatment for breast cancer. The emphasis is on good health and on looking and feeling better. Providing a network of support with monthly meetings and invited speakers allows experiences to be shared.

One of the positive aspects to come out of our group has been the setting-up of a volunteer tea rota for the Assessment Clinic. The tea is warmly welcomed by the women either attending for tests or by those who are being given a diagnosis: indeed it is served by those who fully understand what the women are experiencing. An open invitation to the group is extended to all the patients and their families or close friends.

We are used to being a reactive Health Service; we must learn to be pro-active within our National Breast Screening Programme and the education of professional and lay people in the diagnosis and treatment of breast cancer must also be pro-active.

The Government's strategy "Health of the Na-tion" has set national targets, one of which is to reduce deaths from breast cancer.

A high quality screening programme has introduced skill and specialist knowledge to symptomatic services, thereby resulting in improved breast services for women.

We have the opportunity for early diagnosis with good acceptance rates in the National Breast Screening Programme. Let us all work together to reduce mortality from breast cancer.

References

1. Forrest P.: Breast Cancer: the decision to screen. The Nuffield Provincial Hospital Trust Pub., 1990
2. Bryan S., Brown J., Warren R.: Mammography screening: an incremental cost effectiveness analysis of two views versus one view procedures in London. J. Epid. Comm. Health 1995; 49, 70-78
3. Querci della Rovere G., Morgan M., Patel A., Steel Y., Warren R.: A way to reduce the number of benign breast biopsies in a screening programme; Joint Meeting of Senology EUSOMA, Florence 1997
4. Vessey M.: Breast cancer screening. Evidence and experience since the Forrest report. NHSBSP Pub., 1991

The Radiology of Breast Cancer

Film reading and recall of patients

R. Warren

Film reporting in symptomatic mammography and screening

The symptomatic mammogram request is like any other radiological referral, an instruction to the radiographer and the radiologist for a radiological examination and a report is required in response to a clinical problem. The report stands alone when the films are not available, and it is normal for the text of the report to respond to the query in quite specific ways. Commonly in Britain the report is a string of descriptive free text describing the appearance of the mammogram, some quasi-pathological description of the stroma, and a description of lesions that may not be of clinical significance. This is followed by, if the report is to be useful at all, some clear comment on whether cancer is present or not. There may be advice on additional tests that may be useful.

Reports of this sort can be quite confusing to those not familiar with the complexities of breast disease, such as the General Practitioner. They may, without intending to do so, generate doubt and the need for additional tests. Kopans[1] has recommended standard mammography reporting to remove the doubts associated with such descriptive communications. In our own centre a standard format has been developed with the breast surgeons by group discussion within the diagnostic team, and all other users receive this format. An initial statement gives the Wolfe pattern[2] and notes implants where relevant. The two breasts are reported separately, and only striking or symptomatic benign features are described. It is understood that the critical judgement is whether cancer is present or absent from each breast. This gives a report much less cluttered with difficult terms, a clear comment on the clinical relevance of benign or malignant lesions described, and advice for further tests (or no action) which helps practitioners advise the patient appropriately.

In the screening situation, an even simpler format is required to avoid the false alarms for which screening has been criticised.[3] The result may be communicated to the woman without the intermediary of her doctor, and so clear cut reassurance must be given for a normal result, or for one containing an innocent benign feature. In the screening situation moreover, the result may well be generated by a computer in the form of a letter that is of standard format. Recalls for additional investigation may well be addressed to the woman herself, and will probably not contain details of why the assessment is needed. The format must be wholly acceptable to women, and designed so that panic is not caused. Good arrangements must be made for any additional tests in a short time course of not more than a few days. In order to produce reports of this sort it is quite common to use computer codes, or even bar code readers which record results directly into the computer.

Method of reading mammograms

In the symptomatic service, or where small numbers of films are read at a time, the films may be viewed on standard radiographic viewing boxes. It is important that the boxes are sufficiently bright, and do not have scratched surfaces. The films should be mounted in a standard format so that errors of side or position of a lesion are not made, and in order to make this easy standard radiographic procedures must be adopted for marking the medial and lateral side and for the position of the identity label. In this way a lesion can be localized at a glance by an experienced radiologist.

The calcifications and other features critical to cancer diagnosis may be very small, approaching the grain size of the film, and so the use of some form of magnification by lenses is almost universal. This can take the form of a large hand lens held close to the film, or a binocular viewer of about 2 diopters strength (Fig. 1). Such a binocular viewer also masks the brightness from extraneous areas of the viewing box. When a hand lens is used it may be useful to mask bright uncovered parts of the viewing box with black card or film. It is usual to read the films initially at a distance for bold features such as contour deformities, and then close, to observe fine detail, and each radiologist develops his own scanning pathways around the films.[4,5]

For screening of large numbers of mammograms, multiviewers have been devised so that the films can be loaded by a technician for the radiologist(s) to read. Such viewers (Fig. 2) can carry the films of a hundred or so examinations in a position designed for the comfort of the reading radiologist. Attempts are being made to devise digital readers for reading mammograms, but are not yet in any way approaching a useful stage of development.

Who should report the films?

Mammography is a traditional radiological technique, and so from the time of its development, the natural person to give a report was the consultant radiologist. With the onset of large screening programmes on a national basis, and the difficulties that ensued in finding sufficient trained radiologists willing to report the endless flow of large numbers of screening films, consideration has been given to whether radiographers, breast physicians, obstetricians or nurses could be trained to read the films. In general any person with adequate training can achieve good results, and the use of non-radiologists has sometimes taken place for second reading of the films.[6]

How many readers should examine each film?

Conventional radiology normally is read by one radiologist only, except in teaching departments where double-checking of trainees may be required. In the clinical setting, the referring clinician may examine the films in addition to the radiologist. In screening mammography, large numbers of repetitive films are read, and it is realised that inattention may result in missed cancers. In some of the trials double reading of the films by radiologists has taken place. This matter has been scientifically examined on several occasions now,[7,8] and the use of double reading by radiologists has given rise to between 9 and 15% more cancers being diagnosed, an extra level of staff input that has a definite cost. It is becoming the norm

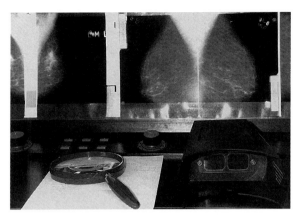

Fig. 1. A hand lens of the type available for reading mammograms and the binocular viewer designed for use in mammography film reading.

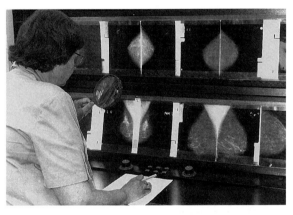

Fig. 2. A radiologist reading films on one format of the multiviewer systems available for reading large numbers of mammograms. The transparent bands holding the films can be moved horizontally, so that the films are rolled up around drums at each end. The slight slope of the lower bank of films places them in the ideal position for film interpretation. Up to 800 films of 24×30 format can be accommodated on the viewer.

in a well run screening service to employ two radiologists for reporting the films to achieve adequate levels of sensitivity, and studies of the cost effectiveness of the second view are becoming available.

When it is not possible to use two trained radiologists, other options arise. Other doctors such as breast physicians, surgeons in breast surgery or obstetrics and gynaecology, nurses or radiographers can all be trained to read mammograms, provided they submit themselves to suitable training programmes, and undertake appropriate follow-up of the cases to gain ongoing experience.

The radiologist has two advantages: firstly he is trained for many years in a speciality where visual acumen is developed in pattern recognition to a sophisticated level; secondly he is familiar with the faults and artefacts that may occur in the complex chain involved in the production of a radiograph, and the use of the equipment features to maximise the technical quality of the film, and will work in a natural way with the technician for constant improvement in technical quality of the film, so critical an issue in mammography.

Training and experience

Mammography is a form of radiology that is specialised, and there is growing recognition of the amount of training needed to achieve good sensitivity and specificity.

A critical feature of a high quality screening programme is in depth training of the personnel, both in film interpretation and in radiopathological correlation of the images.

Knowledge is gained from following the cases through surgery, and following up the interval cases to view with hindsight the features of the small cancers that must be diagnosed for obtaining a good outcome to screening. Learning for both the individual and the team goes on over a much longer period than may be expected.[7]

Methods have been devised for monitoring the performance of radiologists by using test films, and these can be used on sequential occasions to demonstrate improvement.[8] While physical performance of the radiographic chain is critical in achieving good outcomes, the quality of interpretation of the mammogram may be the most important factor in diagnosing the small invasive cancers that ultimately determine the success of screening.

Recall decisions

After the films have been reported, a selected group of women must be recalled for further tests. High quality office procedures must be adopted, particularly when large numbers of women are screened, to ensure that every minor query raised by the radiologist or film reader is acted upon. This has been an issue in cervical cytology where failed recall procedures have given rise to missed cancers.[9]

It is obvious that when only one report is available then it is those queries raised that will give rise to the recalls. More complex is the situation when more than one report is available. A decision must be made whether to recall every query raised, to reach a consensus, or to use the opinion of the most experienced person. This may give rise to very different recall rates, and it is essential that the benefit in

improved sensitivity gained by the second report is accrued.

Recalling the women

When a woman is recalled after a mammogram, whether in a screening programme or after symptomatic mammography, she will automatically jump to the conclusion that cancer has been found. Depending on the recall rate of the particular centre the likelihood of a positive diagnosis may be of the order of one in six to one in twenty.

Therefore this situation is likely to give rise to anxiety which is out of place in a large number of cases. It is therefore important that the timing between notifying a recall and the actual test is as short as practically possible, that the wording of the letter is well thought out and that those conducting the additional tests are sensitive to the anxieties. Honesty of all concerned in the context of recognisable caring is the current style.

A "one-stop clinic" is the ideal situation when all the tests are done with the mammography and a final report is given, particularly for those who are to be reassured. In the case of patients found to have cancer, it is sometimes too heavy an impact emotionally to give all the information at one visit, and some form of phasing (but in a context of honesty) may be helpful. The presence of a nurse counsellor is beneficial. When there is a delay between the mammogram and the additional tests, it is important to communicate the final conclusion as soon and as clearly as possible to the woman.

Reference

1. Kopans D.: Standardised-mammography reporting. Radiol. Clin. N. Amer., 1992; 30; 257
2. Wolfe J., Wilkie R.: Breast pattern classification & observer error. Radiol. 1978; 127: 343-344
3. Devitt J.: The false alarms of breast cancer. Lancet, II, 1989; 334: 1257
4. Noton D., Stark L.: Eye movements and visual perception. Sci Amer., 1971; 224: 35-43
5. Kundel H., Nodine C.: A visual concept shapes image perception. Radiol., 1983; 146: 363-368
6. George W., Sellwood R., Asbury D., Hartley G.: Role of non-medical staff in screening for breast cancer. Brit. Med. J., 1980; 280: 147-149
7. Warren R.: Team learning and breast cancer screening. Lancet, 1991; 338: 51
8. Gale A.G., Wilson A.R.M.: Evaluation of radiologists performance in reading mammograms. Br. J. Radiol., 1991; 64: 476
9. Warren R., Duffy S.: Comparison of single reading with double reading of mammograms, and change in effectiveness with experience. Brit. J. Radiol., 1995; 68: 958-962
10. Brown J., Bryan S., Warren R.: Mammographic screening: an incremental cost-effectiveness analysis of double *versus* single reading of mammograms. B.M.J., 1996; 312: 809-12

Radiology of the normal breast and differential diagnosis of benign breast lesions

S. Ciatto, D. Ambrogetti

The normal breast

The appearance of the normal breast at mammography varies with age and individual characteristics. Before the menopause the parenchyma is well represented and usually occupies about half of the breast volume, being localized in the subareolar and upper outer region (Fig. 1). The amount and distribution of parenchyma is quite variable, especially before the menopause, when changes are possible even in the same subject under special circumstances (*e.g.* pregnancy, lactation).

The opacity of breast parenchyma is a determinant of mammographic sensitivity. The normal parenchyma is opaque enough to mask the limited density of a small carcinoma. So far, this is the most convincing explanation for the failure in reducing mortality in women aged 40-49 years by mammographic screening.

Table I. Relative risk of developing breast cancer according to mammographic parenchymal pattern.

Authors	Cases	Relative risk by mammographic pattern			
		NI	PI	P2	DY
Wolfe	76	1.0	2.6	12.0	30.7
Ciatto	61	1.0	1.0	1.9	1.9
Ciatto	279	1.0	3.7	5.4	8.3
Wilkinson	42	1.0	2.1	2.1	5.8
Hainline	171	1.0	1.5	2.7	7.2
Egan	385	1.0	2.3	2.0	10.0
Krook	67	1.0	2.5	4.0	6.8

Modified from Rosselli Del Turco *et al.*[2]

Epithelial and connective tissues are depicted as densities of variable size, from small nodular (Fig. 2) to large sheet-like homogeneous opacities (Fig. 3). These two dominant patterns have been proposed by Wolfe[1] to classify the normal breast into four categories of increasing density, associated with a progressively increasing risk of subsequent breast cancer. Parenchymal patterns have been studied by several authors, but none of them was able to reproduce Wolfe's original results (Table I). Although there is

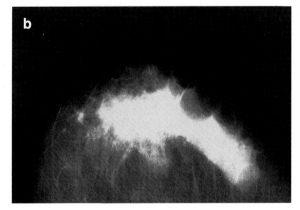

Fig. 1. Normal pre-menopausal breast. Breast parenchyma is depicted as a large opacity occupying about half of the breast volume, localized in the subareolar and upper outer region of the breast. **a**:medio-lateral oblique view; **b**:cranio-caudal view.

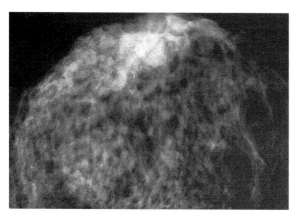

Fig. 2. Normal breast. Breast parenchyma: micronodular opacities (Wolfe's pattern PI or P2).

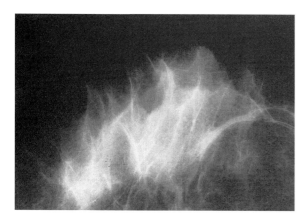

Fig. 3. Normal breast. Breast parenchyma: sheet-like large opacities (Wolfe's pattern DY).

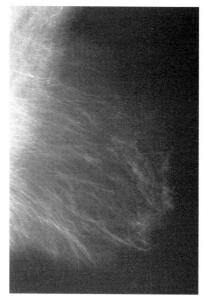

Fig. 4. Normal post-menopausal breast. The parenchymal opacity has regressed completely, and only radiolucent fat tissue is left.

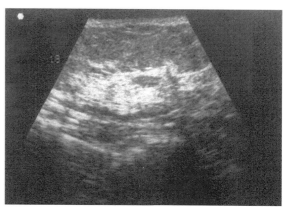

Fig. 5. Normal breast. Ultrasonography (10 MHz): an hyper-echoic island of parenchyma is surrounded by hypo-echoic fat.

general agreement that denser breasts (P2-DY patterns) are associated with a slightly higher risk of breast cancer, it is unclear whether parenchymal patterns are really indicative of an intrinsic increased risk, or denser breasts are simply masking the presence of minimal cancer[3] which will surface during the subsequent follow-up. In fact, parenchymal patterns are not currently used for clinical purposes (e.g. selecting women for different surveillance regimens). After the menopause parenchymal densities gradually disappear, until the breast is essentially made of fat and fibrous tissue (Fig. 4).

This regression is variable in time and extent, depending on individual characteristics (e.g. endogenous extra-ovarian production of oestrogens, hormone replacement therapy), and fibro-adipose or dense breasts will occasionally be seen in young or older women, respectively. The features of the normal breast at sonography are also strictly correlated to the amount and distribution of the epithelial and connective tissue with respect to the surrounding fat. Fat is hypo-echoic and is depicted as a rather homo-

geneous greyish background on which hyper-echoic parenchyma stands out in white granular patches of variable size (Fig. 5). For these characteristics the sensitivity of sonography is not affected, as for mammography, by the presence of parenchyma which, on the contrary, offers the ideal hyper-echoic background for hypo-echoic circumscribed lesions, either benign or malignant (Fig. 6). On the contrary the post-menopausal breast, made essentially of fat and fibrous septa, offers the worst contrast at sonography and some intermediate-hypo-echoic lesions (mostly benign fibroadenomas) may be difficult to differentiate from fat lobules (Fig. 7).

Benign breast disease

The appearance of benign lesions of the breast is often typical, but in some cases the differential diag-

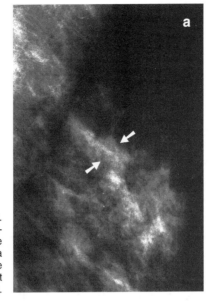
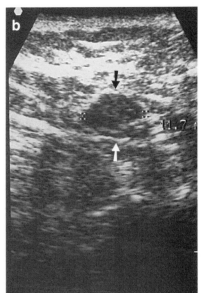

Fig. 6. Pre-menopausal breast. At mammography (**a**) a small fibro-adenoma (arrows) is masked in the radiologically dense parenchyma which, on the contrary, offers the best hyper-echoic contrast at sonography (**b**) (arrows).

Fig. 7. Post-menopausal breast. At mammography (**a**) a fibro-adenoma stands out as a sharp opacity on the radiolucent fat background, whereas it is much less evident at sonography (**b**), being almost iso-echoic to fat.

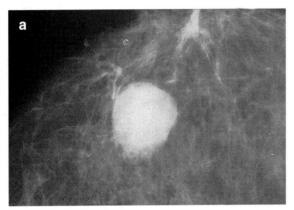
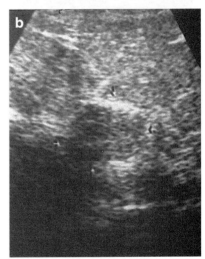

nosis with breast cancer is not easy as they may share the same mammographic/sonographic features. Clinical evidence or patient's age and history may help, but in some cases, fine needle aspiration cytology or even surgical biopsy are necessary to define the exact nature of the lesion.

Listed below are the most common benign lesions and the diagnostic problems which may arise for each of them.

Cysts

Cysts are very common, especially in the 4th-5th decade. When not masked by surrounding parenchymal opacities, a cyst is depicted at mammography as a sharp-bordered round opacity (Fig. 8), (incompletely filled cysts may be oval shaped). Calcifica-

tions of cystic wall are typical (Fig. 9) but infrequent. It is almost impossible to differentiate a cyst from other sharp-bordered non-calcified opacities (e.g. fibroadenoma, medullary carcinoma), although suspicion of cancer should arise only for isolated opacities in older women.

Sonography is the ideal instrumental method to diagnose a cyst as the an-echoic appearance (usually with posterior acoustic enhancement and lateral acoustic shadowing) is typical of this lesion (Fig. 10). Sonography may be particularly useful to diagnose small cysts in elderly women, which may be suspected to be circumscribed carcinomas at mammography (Fig. 11). Aspiration is the simplest, cheapest and fastest method of diagnosing a cyst, and is therapeutic at the same time, as the majority of cysts will not refill after complete aspiration.[4]

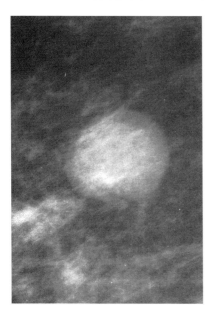

Fig. 8. Cyst: typical appearance at mammography.

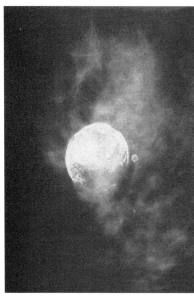

Fig. 9. Cyst: typical calcification of cystic walls.

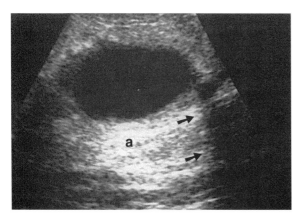

Fig. 10. Cyst: typical appearance at sonography: an-echoic lesion, with posterior acoustic enhancement (a) and lateral acoustic shadowing (arrows).

In the presence of an isolated palpable mass, aspiration is always indicated. If the mass is a cyst, diagnosis and treatment will be achieved at the same time. If the mass is solid, aspiration will provide material for cytological examination which will help the differential diagnosis between cancer and solid benign lesions.

Some clinicians, especially radiologists, are against an extensive use of aspiration, and prefer to confirm the presence of a cyst by sonography. In our experience, a woman will not be fully satisfied with a diagnosis of benign cyst if she has a breast lump. The aspiration of the cyst will by far compensate the minimal discomfort of skin puncture and the woman's anxiety will be fully removed.

Aspiration allows the evaluation of the characteristics of the cyst fluid. Non blood-stained cyst content is associated with a negligible risk of intracystic growth. Even when the cyst fluid is blood-stained, no intracystic lesion is found in the majority of cases and the few intracystic lesions are benign papillomas (see Table II). Intracystic cancer, that is otherwise unapparent cancer growing from the inner face of the cystic wall, is an infrequent event. Most reports of intracystic cancer are dealing with clinically or radiologically evident carcinomas, associated with haemorragic pseudocysts, and are erroneously reported as intracystic.

When the cyst fluid is blood-stained, instrumental evaluation of the cystic wall is important to assess the presence of intracystic growth. Sonography (Fig. 12) is far simpler than pneumocystography (Fig. 13) which is currently no longer used. Cytological examination of the cyst fluid may reveal cells from papilloma or cancer but its sensitivity is low and it should be performed only on blood-stained fluids (Table II). Surgery is justified only when an intracystic growth is suspected.

Fibroadenomas

Fibroadenomas are also very common. They are typical of the 2nd decade, when there is no question of differential diagnosis with cancer, but they may be a common finding also in older age. At mammography, fibroadenomas are depicted as homogeneous intense opacities with sharp margins, virtually indistinguishable from cysts except for their oval rather than rounded shape (Fig. 14). At sonography, fibroadenomas are homogeneously hypo-echoic. In young women sonography is much more reliable as it shows the whole margin of the lesion (Fig. 15), being unaffected by the opacity of surrounding parenchyma, whereas in post-menopausal women fibroadenomas may be difficult to appreciate as they are often iso-echoic to the surrounding fat. After the

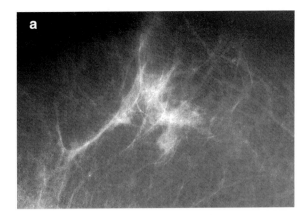
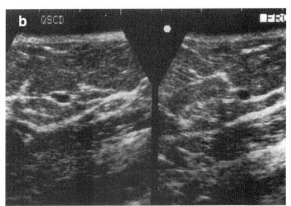

Fig. 11. Circumscribed opacity at mammography (**a**) may suggest medullary carcinoma in an elderly woman, but sonography (**b**) demonstrates a cyst, and no other assessment is necessary.

menopause, typical coarse "wax drop" macrocalcifications may be evident within the fibroadenoma, and may be easily shown either at mammography or sonography (Fig. 16). Unfortunately, there is no possibility of reliable differential diagnosis between small non-calcified fibroadenomas and small carcinomas with regular borders at either mammography or sonography (Fig. 17). Age and history may help, but aspiration cytology is the best criterion to avoid an excess of benign biopsies, which are unnecessary, as fibroadenoma is a benign lesion carrying no risk of progression to cancer.

Benign phyllodes tumour

When the lesion has not reached its typically giant size, the benign variety of phyllodes tumour is indistinguishable from a fibroadenoma, as both mammography and sonography will depict it as an hypoechoic lesion with regular margins (Fig. 18).

The history of rapid growth might suggest the diagnosis of phyllodes tumour but surgical biopsy will always be necessary to confirm its benign or malignant nature.

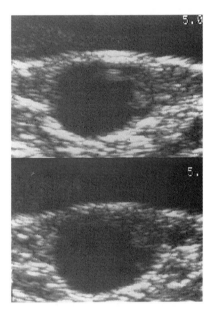

Fig. 12. Intracystic papilloma: evidence of intracystic growth at sonography.

Table II. Probability of intracystic growth according to the appearance of cyst fluid at aspiration.

Intracystic lesion	Total aspirated cysts	Cyst fluid appearance	
		Blood stained	Non-blood stained
Cancer *	1	1	–
Papilloma	5	5	–
None	6776	119	6657

* Accidental finding of *in situ* lobular carcinoma adjacent to the cyst
modified from Ciatto *et al.*[5]

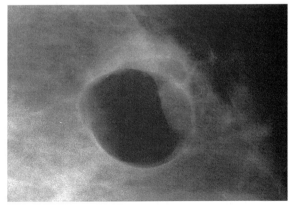

Fig. 13. Intracystic papilloma: evidence of intracystic growth at pneumocystography.

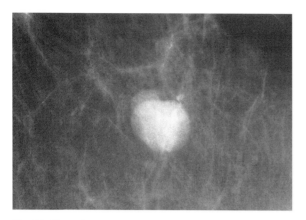

Fig. 14. Fibroadenoma: typical appearance at mammography.

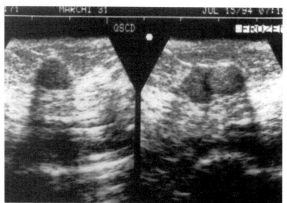

Fig. 15. Fibroadenoma: typical appearance at sonography.

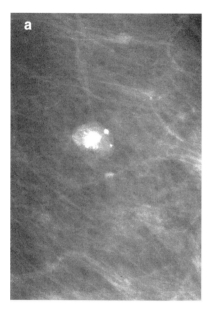

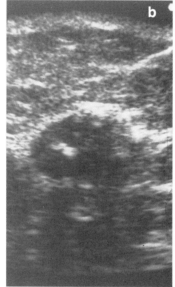

Fig. 16. Fibroadenoma: typical calcifications evidenced at mammography (**a**) or at sonography (**b**).

Lipoma

The mammographic diagnosis is easy as lipoma is radiolucent (Fig. 19). It may be difficult to differentiate a lipoma from the surrounding fat either at mammography or sonography, but this has almost no clinical relevance as the diagnosis of lipoma is generally already evident at physical examination, and no further diagnostic procedure is necessary.

Nipple discharge and papilloma

Nipple discharge is a frequent cause of self-referral to a breast clinic for consultation. Although in most cases it has no clinical relevance, in a few cases nipple discharge may be the only sign of cancer. The prevalence of cancer is significantly associated with the type of discharge, being irrelevant for milky or coloured discharge, and high for blood stained discharge and for serous discharge in elderly women (Table III).

As a practical rule, isolated milky or coloured discharges and even serous discharges in pre-menopausal women are not worth further assessment, which should be limited to blood stained discharges or serous discharges in post-menopausal women. Multiduct and bilateral discharges are also associated with irrelevant risk, as cancer is almost invariably associated with uniduct and unilateral discharge.

Mammography and sonography are of no use unless for a few cases of large papilloma, usually subareolar, which may present coarse calcifications (Fig. 20). Thus assessment should be based on cytological examination and on galactography. Cytology may reveal cancer and papilloma cells in the discharge but although it is highly specific, it is not very sensitive (Table IV), and thus a negative or inadequate cytologic report is not fully reliable.

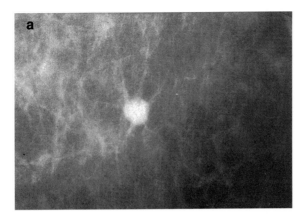
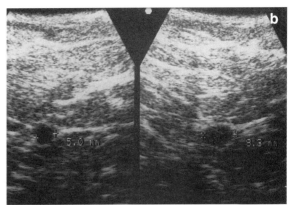

Fig. 17. Medullary carcinoma: The lesion has sharp margins at mammography (**a**), and at sonography (**b**). A false benign report is common in these cases.

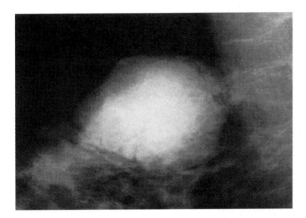
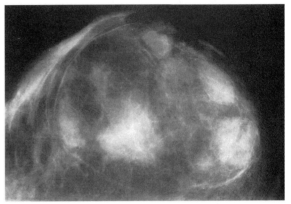

Fig. 18. Benign phyllodes tumour: the appearance at mammography is the same as that of a fibro-adenoma.

Fig. 19. Lipoma: typical radiolucent appearance at mammography.

At galactography papillomas are usually depicted as small spherical masses (Fig. 21), but multiple defects may be due to multiple papillomas as well as to intraductal carcinoma (Fig. 22). Even a sharp stop or a rupture of the injected duct, which usually suggests the presence of cancer, may be associated with a large papilloma. The majority of blood stained discharges are not associated with papilloma or cancer and routine resection of major subareolar ducts represents an over-treatment in most cases, and moreover it may miss peripherally located lesions.

Galactography is fundamental to assess the presence and the site of intraductal growth, and allows guided limited resection. When no lesion is shown at galactography and malignant cells are evident at cytologic examination, the whole injected ductal tree should be resected.

Mastitis

Acute mastitis is relatively frequent also in non-pregnant non-lactating women. Mammography and sonography will confirm the presence of skin and breast oedema but they will allow no reliable differential diagnosis with inflammatory carcinoma. The latter is currently based on the typical signs of benign mastitis (acute onset, pain, skin circumscribed reddening, fever) and on aspiration cytology.[8]

When an abscess is present it may be revealed at mammography as a circumscribed opacity with ir-

Table III. Prevalence (%) of otherwise unapparent breast cancer associated with nipple discharge, according to the type of discharge - 5,305 consecutive cases.

Type of discharge	Age			Total
	<40	40-59	>59	
Serous	0.00	0.16	2.70	0.16
Milky	0.09	0.18	0.00	0.13
Purulent	0.00	0.44	28.60 *	0.83
Blood stained	2.61	2.89	8.82	3.96

* 2 of 7 cases
Modified from Ciatto *et al.*[6]

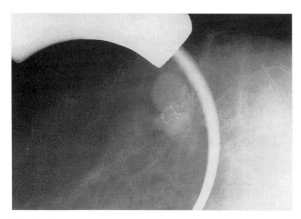

Fig. 20. Subareolar gross intraductal papilloma identifiable for the presence of coarse calcifications.

Table IV. Frequency of suspicious findings at different diagnostic procedures in 18 cancer cases associated with nipple discharge.

Procedure	Intraductal carcinoma	Invasive carcinoma	Total cancers
Palpation	3/8	6/10	9/18
Mammography	1/8	5/10	6/18
Discharge cytology	2/8	5/10	7/18
Galactography	2/8	5/10	7/18
All above	5/8 *	8/10 **	13/18

* 3 cases of intraductal carcinoma underwent surgery with a diagnosis of multiple papilloma at galactography.
** 2 cases of invasive carcinoma underwent surgery for persistent blood stained discharge with no other evidence.
Modified from Ciatto et al.[7]

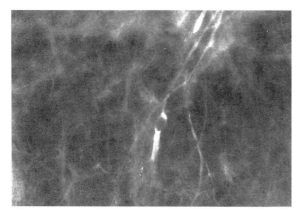

Fig. 21. Galactography: a filling defect due to an isolated papilloma is evident in the injected duct.

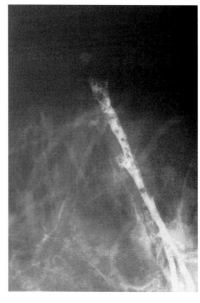

Fig. 22. Galactography: multiple filling defects due to papillomas are evident in the injected duct.

regular, poorly-defined margins (Fig. 23), which may suggest the presence of carcinoma. At sonography differential diagnosis may also be difficult but the central part of the abscess is often an-echoic with scattered hyper-echoic foci due to necrotic fragments (Fig. 24). Aspiration is the simplest and fastest method to achieve a reliable diagnosis when purulent material is aspirated.

Chronic mastitis may be associated with breast lump and skin dimpling, and cancer may be suspected. At mammography the diagnosis of chronic mastitis may be easy if typical linear periductal calcifications, usually bilateral, are evident (Fig. 25).

Surgical outcomes

Previous surgery may cause diagnostic problems at breast imaging, due to the presence of the scar causing star-like opacities or parenchymal distortion. The presence of circumscribed areas of liponecrosis (oil cysts) (Fig. 26) or of gross coarse calcifications (Fig. 27) is typical of a surgical outcome, but when these features are absent the differential diagnosis with cancer may be difficult and tissue diagnosis may be necessary. This is one of the reasons for reducing the frequency of unnecessary surgical biopsies as much as possible.

Benign microcalcifications

Microcalcifications are often present in the normal breast. For some of them no diagnostic problems arise, as they are diffuse, bilateral, and have a typical benign morphology: tea-cup (Fig. 28), punctate (Fig. 29), anular/circular (Fig. 30).

In some other cases benign microcalcifications may be unilateral and clustered and have a crystalline granular morphology (Fig. 31). In these cases differential diagnosis may be very difficult at mammogra-

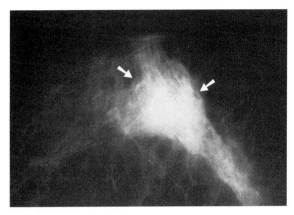

Fig. 23. Acute mastitis: an abscess is visualized at mammography as a pseudonodular area of increased density (arrows).

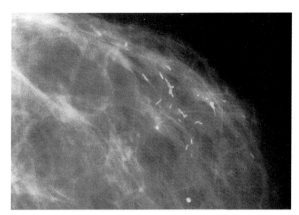

Fig. 25. Chronic mastitis: typical periductal linear calcifications.

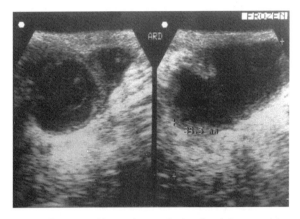

Fig. 24. Acute mastitis: an abscess is visualized at sonography as an irregular mass with predominant an-echoic component, and scattered hyper-echoic foci and septa.

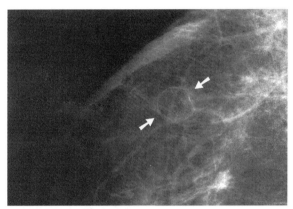

Fig. 26. Surgical outcome: radiolucent circumscribed area due to fat necrosis (oil cyst arrows).

phy and a high frequency of unnecessary biopsies are caused by such lesions.[9]

Sonography is of no help in these cases[10] and stereotaxic cytology is the only test which may be employed to reduce the number of unnecessary biopsies.[11]

Cancer-like lesions

Some benign lesions, which are neither pre-cancerous nor associated with increased risk of cancer, may simulate breast cancer at mammography. This occurs with sclerosing adenosis (Fig. 32) or radial scar (Fig. 33), which have a star-like distorted appearance which may often justify a false positive mammographic report. Although some characteristics (radiolucent central area, absence of palpable mass, visualization on a single view only) may suggest the right diagnosis, they are not sufficiently specific[12] and most cases are sent for surgical biopsy

due to the high predictive value associated with this mammographic pattern.[9] Even at microscopic examination these lesions may create problems of differential diagnosis with scirrhous or tubular carcinoma. This diagnostic difficulty might explain those few reports claiming an association of radial scar with cancer.[13]

Reporting benign lesions in clinical or screening practice

The criteria for reporting the presence of benign lesions may be different in clinical and screening practice. In clinical practice radiologists are usually requested to define the nature of a suspicious palpable lesion, and they should report typical benign signs (e.g. calcifications of fibroadenoma, cysts or periductal mastitis at mammography, cystic appearance at sonography) to confirm a benign diagnosis, reassure the clinician, and avoid unnecessary surgi-

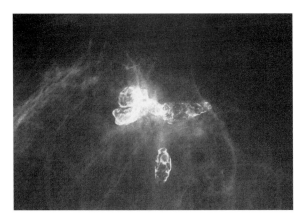

Fig. 27. Surgical outcome: typical gross calcifications within the surgical scar.

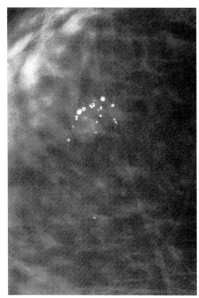

Fig. 30. Anular/
circular benign
micro-
calcifications.

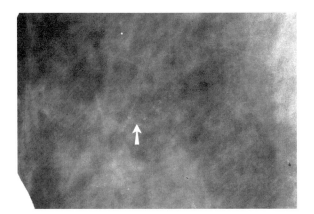

Fig. 28. Tea-cup like benign microcalcifications (arrow).

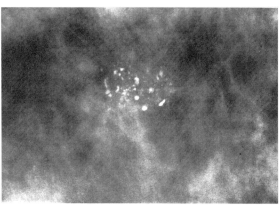

Fig. 31. Cluster of benign cristalline granular microcalcifications which may be misinterpreted as malignant and thus cause unnecessary surgical biopsy.

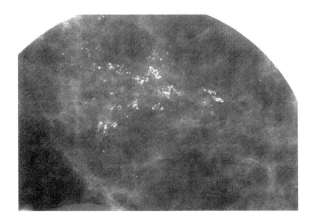

Fig. 29. Punctate benign microcalcifications.

cal biopsy. In screening practice the situation is quite different: we are dealing with healthy asymptomatic women, and the aim of screening is to detect early cancer, not to report the presence of benign abnor-

malities which carry no risk of cancer. Reporting a benign lesion would only possibly cause the woman anxiety and unnecessary assessment or even biopsy. Thus, it is a common policy for screening radiologists not to describe any typically benign lesion detected at screening, the report being limited to a "negative" or to an "absence of suspicious findings" formula. This policy should be extended also to typically benign lesions detected at clinical mammography in breast regions other than the site of the palpable or symptomatic lesion for which the woman is referred.

What you can ask of imaging

Some clinicians expect that breast imaging should

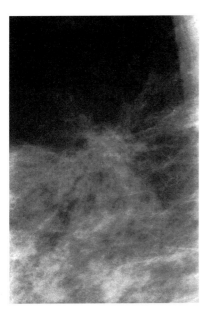

Fig. 32. Sclerosing adenosis: an irregular opacity with infiltrating-like margins simulating cancer.

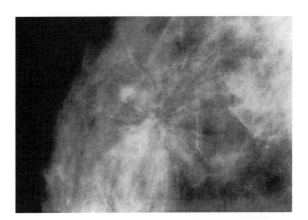

Fig. 33. Radial scar: mammography. Typical appearance with gross distortion, radiating spicules and radiolucent central core.

classify women according to their relative risk of developing breast cancer, either by applying some classification based on mammographic pattern, such as Wolfe's, or simply by identifying the presence of "dysplasia", or "fibrocystic disease", often assumed as consistent with "dense breast".

It should be clear that breast imaging has no such power. Mammographic parenchymal patterns scored well only in Wolfe's hands, and nobody has been able to confirm his results. In the literature the average relative risk associated with high risk patterns (P2-DY) is around 2:1, a figure which does not justify any special surveillance. Breast imaging does not recognize the presence of "dysplasia", atypical ductal or lobular hyperplasia is unapparent at mammography or sonography, and the presence of a radiologically dense breast is not a synonym of fibrocystic disease, which may be diagnosed only when cysts are visible at sonography. Moreover, even fibrocystic disease is associated with a negligible increase in the risk of developing breast cancer, and justifies no special action or surveillance. The evidence of a radiologically dense breast should only alert the clinician about the reliability of a negative mammographic report. Thus, breast imaging allows no reliable prediction of breast cancer risk in the current practice, and should not be used as an excuse to justify excessively frequent clinical or instrumental controls of selected patients.

References

1. Wolfe J.N.: Breast patterns as an index of risk for developing breast cancer. AJR 1976; 126: 1130-1139
2. Rosselli Del Turco M., Ciatto S., Mezzalira L.P., Camargo J.R., Petracco A.: The role of mammographic patterns in the selection of women for periodical mass screening. Int. J. Breast Mammary Pathol.-Senologia 1983; 2: 75-78
3. Egan R.L., Mosteller R.C.: Breast cancer mammographic patterns. Cancer 1977; 40: 2087-2090
4. Ciatto S., Rosselli Del Turco M., Cariaggi P.: Diagnostic and therapeutic role of breast pneumocystography. Int. J. Breast Mammary Pathol.-Senologia 1983; 2: 27-29
5. Ciatto S., Cariaggi P, Bulgaresi P.: The value of routine cytologic examination of breast cyst fluids. Acta Cytol. 1987; 31: 301-304
6. Ciatto S, Bravetti P, Cariaggi P. Significance of nipple discharge clinical patterns in the selection of cases for cytologic examination. Acta Cytol 1986; 30: 17-20
7. Ciatto S., Bravetti P., Berni D., Catarzi S., Bianchi S.: The role of galactography in the detection of breast cancer. Tumori 1988; 74:, 177-181
8. Cardona G., Ciatto S.: Criteria of clinical and radiological diagnosis in nonpuerperal acute phlogistic-like processes of the breast: considerations on 97 consecutive cases. Tumori 1981; 67: 31-34
9. Ciatto S., Cataliotti L., Distante V.: Nonpalpable lesions detected with mammography: review of 512 consecutive cases. Radiology 1987; 165: 99-102
10. Ciatto S., Catarzi S., Morrone D., Rosselli Del Turco M.: Fine needle aspiration cytology of nonpalpable breast lesions: US V8 stereotaxic guidance. Radiology 1993; 188: 195-198
11. Ciatto S., Rosselli Del Turco M, Bravetti P.: Nonpalpable breast lesions: stereotaxic fine needle aspiration cytology. Radiology 1989; 173: 57-59
12. Ciatto S., Morrone D., Catarzi S., Rosselli Del Turco M., Bianchi S., Ambrogetti D., Cariddi A.: Radial scars of the breast: review of 38 consecutive mammographic diagnoses. Radiology 1993; 187:757-760
13. Fisher E.R., Palekar A.S., Kotwal N.: A non-encapsulated sclerosing lesion of the breast. Am. J. Clin. Pathol. 1979; 71: 240-246

The radial scar (Stellate lesions)

N. Perry, I. Morrison

The radial scar/complex sclerosing lesion is a proliferative and benign condition demonstrating architectural distortion as its major radiological feature. There may be an associated soft tissue element, but whether there is centralised soft tissue thickening, or the presence or absence of a tumour nidus, the predominant feature is that of deformity of the breast architecture with variable retraction of the surrounding soft tissues.

These so-called stellate lesions may be easy to detect mammographically, but if small they can be extremely difficult to identify within a dense fibroglandular breast (Fig. 1). Providing there has been no trauma or previous surgical intervention to the area the important differential diagnosis of a stellate abnormality lies between the radial scar/complex sclerosing lesion and invasive malignancy. The two of course may co-exist, likewise a radial scar may be present with an *in situ* malignancy.

Pathology

Radial scar[5-6] is a benign pathological entity characterized by central fibro-elastosis, surrounded by radiating parenchymal and epithelial structures. Previous and alternative terms include sclerosing adenosis with pseudo-infiltration,[7] infiltrating epitheliosis,[2] non-encapsulated sclerosing lesion[4] and indurative mastopathy.[9] Andersen and Gram[1] report a high incidence of associated papillomatosis, epithelial hyperplasia and microcalculus formation.

The Royal College of Pathologists working group[8] has set down guidelines that a radial scar be defined as a lesion 10 mm or less in maximum diameter with a dense and poorly cellular fibro-elastotic centre with radiating epithelial structures in a stellate formation. A complex sclerosing lesion (Fig. 2) has similar features but, measures more than 10 mm in maximum diameter and generally has more complex and extensive benign changes peripherally, *e.g.* sclerosing adenosis.

Risk of malignancy

Attention has been re-focused in recent years on the presence and significance of stellate lesions due to the flourishing use of screening mammography. The National Breast Screening Programme in the

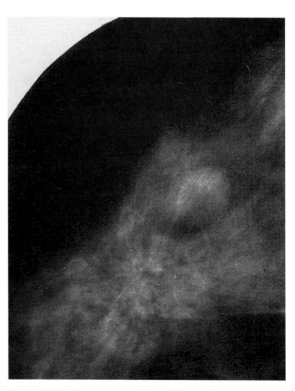

Fig. 1. A typical appearance of a radial scar with quite marked architectural distortion but little in the way of a central mass. The size of this may be judged in comparison to a 7mm cyst which was incidentally present just anteriorly.

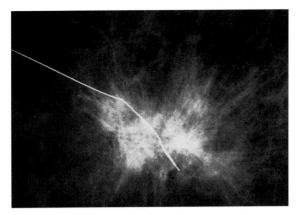

Fig. 2. A complex sclerosing lesion. This is also more complex in its radiological appearance. It is larger and denser than a typical radial scar although there is not so much a central mass as central thickening and the predominant feature is once again that of distortion. The pre-operative wire marking film demonstrates the fact that this fairly obvious abnormality was in fact impalpable.

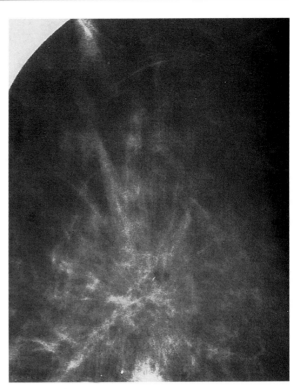

Fig. 3. Another classical radial scar appearance, demonstrating spicule bunching.

United Kingdom screens over 1 million women a year mammographically and, as image quality and production continues to improve, a breast assessment centre may expect to deal with a significant number of these lesions. Tabar and Dean[11] report a screening incidence of 0.9 per 1,000 women screened.

The radiological appearance of a stellate lesion carries a significant risk of malignancy of approximately 40-50%. Differentiation however needs to be made between this radiological appearance and the spiculate mass where there is a central mass with spiculate margination. The positive predictive value for malignancy here is much higher and in the region of 90-95%.

There has in the past been much controversy over whether a radial scar is a completely benign entity or whether it carries a pre-malignant association. Notable proponents of a totally benign character include Fenoglio and Lattes,[3] Tremblay,[12] Azzopardi[2] and Rickert.[9] Eminent supporters of the pre-malignant theory include Fisher,[10] Linell[6] and Sloane.[10]

The Breast Unit at St. Bartholomew's Hospital retrospectively reviewed the recorded cases of radial scar since computerised records were commenced in 1989, due to the observed frequent incidence of atypical hyperplasia or carcinoma in association with radial scars. 45 patients with radial scar were analysed - 40 of these being screen detected. 16 (35%) had associated malignancy and a further 8 cases (18%) showed atypical hyperplasia (Table I).

On the basis of these figures in conjunction with other published data, this unit would support the pre-malignant theory. Many major breast units now believe that there is sufficient circumstantial evidence to admit the possibility that radial scars/complex sclerosing lesions may be associated with the development of malignancy and that this fact should be taken into account when considering their appearance and management.

Further analysis was done to determine features that could prove helpful to the radiologist in immediate diagnostic management. Most cases will be found through screening as a radial scar presenting through the symptomatic service and will in most cases have been discovered as a chance finding rather than a palpable mass. The decision to biopsy here is usually standard. In screening however the importance lies with what management the radiologist should pursue. Is it a reasonable policy to leave these abnormalities on the basis that the typical appearance of a radial scar is most likely to be benign, or should they all be referred for surgery? Indeed can radiological appearances reliably predict the presence of a radial scar without significant associated pathology?

Table I. Analysis of associated pathology in 45 radial scars.

	Number
Uncomplicated radial scar	21
Associated atypical hyperplasia	8
Associated invasive malignancy	7
Associated in situ malignancy	9

Radiological features

Classical radial scar features are those of architectural distortion with typical lack of a central tumour nidus. Various radiologists refer to black stars or white stars which is likely in many cases to reflect no more than their personal visual subjective biases. The black star theory holds that the multiple lucent linear markings are due to elastosis causing distortion of fat. A 'wheat sheaf' or clumping appearance of spicule branching is certainly seen (Fig. 3) and this correlates to the common finding of the appearance of a radial scar varying according to the radiographic projection. Certainly it is quite typical to be able to visualise this lesion mammographically with ease in one projection but have extreme difficulty visualising it in the orthogonal projection. This may lead to complications during wire localisation. Sonographically, there may be a hypo-echoic area with dense acoustic shadowing. However, these features are not reliable and cannot reliably be differentiated from malignancy or previous surgical scarring.

Radiological prediction of malignancy

A widely held view is that, if palpable, this mammographic lesion is most likely to represent malignancy. However, most aspirators will bear testament to the toughness of a radial scar at fine needle aspiration. Some have experienced the bending of a needle whilst attempting to traverse or aspirate such pathology. Another classically described feature is that the spicules of a radial scar will not traverse the subcutaneous tissue and tether the skin whereas malignancy may do this. Change in the shape or size of lesion over time is not a reliable predictive factor for malignancy or benignity. Both radial scars and many grade 1 invasive tumours with a high desmoplastic reaction, also tubular malignancies, may remain relatively static over many years. In a series of 126 radial scar/complex sclerosing lesions, Sloane and Mayers[10] found a relationship between size of the lesion and the presence of malignancy. 38 out of 50 lesions that were 7 millimeters or more in size had associated malignancy or atypical hyperplasia as opposed to only 6 out of 76 that were 6 mm or less in size. These same authors also report an association with age, 37 out of 66 lesions studied where the woman was over 50 years old had associated malignancy or atypical hyperplasia as opposed to only 7 out of 56 up to the age of 50.

The presence of microcalcification in our series was found to be of some help in predicting associated pathology although again not entirely reliable. Retrospective analysis of the 21 screen detected cases where distortion was the predominant mammographic feature showed microcalcification associated with 8 out of 11 cases where there was associated significant pathology as opposed to 3 out of 10 uncomplicated radial scars (Table II).

Certainly on these grounds microcalcification appeared to be much more likely to indicate a significant associated pathology. We further analysed 14 screening cases which had typical appearances mammographically of a radial scar and of these 6 out of 6 cases where there was associated pathology showed microcalcification as opposed to 1 out of 8 uncomplicated radial scars (Table III).

In all cases the microcalcification was scattered and punctate, often being fairly scanty in appearance. What is undoubtedly true is that no attempt can be made to categorise such a mammographic abnormality without high image quality and specialised assessment techniques to include coned compression and paddle micro-focus magnification facilities.

Certainly therefore we did not consider radiological differentiation reliable. Does cytology help? We analysed the cytological findings on the 14 cases with typical appearances of radial scar (Table IV). One of the atypical hyperplasia cases had an inade-

Table II. Analysis of 21 radial scars where distortion was the predominant feature mammographically with regard to microcalcification content.

	Number	Micro-calcification
Uncomplicated radial scar	10	3
Associated atypical hyperplasia	6	4
Associated carcinoma	5	4

Table III. Analysis of the importance of microcalcification in 14 cases having typical radiological features of a radial scar.

	Number	Micro-calcification
Uncomplicated radial scar	8	1
Associated atypical hyperplasia	3	3
Associated carcinoma	3	3

Table IV. Cytological findings with 14 cases having a typical appearance of radial scar mammographically.

	Number	C1	C2	C3	C4	C5
Uncomplicated radial scar	8	4	0	3	1	0
Associated atypical hyperplasia	3	1	0	1	1	0
Associated carcinoma	3	0	1	0	2	0

quate cytology and one of the carcinomas had a benign cytology. Not only is this a difficult lesion to analyse cytologically, it is also a difficult lesion to sample from the radiologist's point-of-view. Five out of 14 lesions (36%) had inadequate cytology whereas the unit's inadequate rate from all lesions runs at approximately 7-9%. Fenestrated plate cytology with its advantage of variable angle and depth of sampling from different puncture sites may be preferable in this particular lesion to stereotactic approach.

In conclusion, it is not reliable or safe to attempt to differentiate, on radiological grounds, a benign or malignant cause for a stellate lesion on a mammogram.

Summary

The experience of the St. Bartholomew's Hospital unit indicates a high incidence of hyperplasia and carcinoma in association with radial scars lending support to the pre-malignant theory. Lesions which were radiologically classical for radial scars were frequently associated with significant pathology.

Micro-calcification, if present, in our series, was a good predictor of associated pathology. Is it safe to leave such a lesion even in retrospect, if it is possible to identify it on a previous mammographic study? It would not seem advisable, certainly not without the woman's informed consent. There are several recorded cases of malignant "radial scars" where there had been no radiological change over several years, the decision to biopsy being prompted by a change of policy to excise all such lesions. The removal of a suspected radial scar is strongly advised even in the presence of negative cytology.

References

1. Andersen J.A., Gram J.B.: Radial scar in the female breast. Cancer, 1984; 53: 2557-2560
2. Azzopardi J.G.: Problems in Breast Pathology. Philadelphia, Saunders, 1979; 174 -187
3. Fenoglio C., Lattes R.: Sclerosing Papillary Proliferations in the female breast. A benign lesion often mistaken for carcinoma. Cancer, 1974; 33: 691-700
4. Fisher E.R., Palekar A.S., Kotwal N., Lipana N.: A non encapsulated sclerosing lesion of the breast. Am. J. Clin. Pathol., 1979; 71: 239-246
5. Hamperl H.: Strahlige Narben und Obliterierende Mastopathie: Beitrage Zur Pathologischen Histologie der Mamma. XI. Virchows Arch (Pathol anat), 1975; 369, 55-68
6. Linell F., Ljungberg O., Andersson I.: Breast Carcinoma. Aspects of early stages, progression and related problems. Acta Pathol. Microbiol. Scand (A) (suppl), 1980; 272: 1-233
7. McDivitt R.W., Stewart F.W., Berg J.W.: Tumors of the Breast. Atlas of tumor pathology Fasc. 2. Washington, 1968
8. Pathology Reporting in Breast Cancer Screening (2nd edition), NHSBSP Publication, 1995
9. Rickert R.R., Kalisher L., Hutter R.V.P: Indurative mastopathy: A benign sclerosing lesion of breast with elastosis which may simulate carcinoma. Cancer, 1981; 47: 561-571
10. Sloane P.B., Mayers M.M.: Carcinoma and atypical hyperplasia in radial scars and complex sclerosing lesions: Importance of lesion size and patient age. Histopathology. 1993; 23(3): 225-31
11. Tabar L., Dean P.B.: Teaching atlas of mammography. New York, Thieme Stratton, 1985
12. Tremblay G., Buell R.H., Seemayer T.A.: Elastosis in benign sclerosing ductal proliferation of the female breast. Am. J. Surg Pathol., 1977, 1: 155-158

Circumscribed breast masses

A.R.M. Wilson

Introduction

A circumscribed mass demonstrated on mammography can be defined as a localized rounded lesion of predominantly homogeneous density with convex margins; this is in distinction to an asymmetric density, which is made up of tissue of mixed density and has predominantly concave margins, and a spiculate mass, which is associated with surrounding radial architectural distortion.[1]

Circumscribed masses in the breast demonstrated on mammography account for between 15% to 20% of breast carcinomas detected at screening. Review of interval screening breast cancers has shown that up to 25% of false negative cases are represented on the previous screening mammogram as circumscribed masses, many of these occurring in the "review areas" (the retro-areolar area and behind, inferior and medial to the breast disc).[2,3]

Screening radiologists should pay particular attention to these areas. Similarly, review of incident screen detected cancers has shown that a significant proportion are demonstrated on the previous screening mammograms as subtle small circumscribed masses. However, the vast majority of circumscribed masses seen on mammography are benign.[4,5] Distinguishing benign from malignant circumscribed masses on their mammographic features alone is not usually a problem but these lesions require careful evaluation at the time of screen reading.

Further assessment of those that do not fulfil the radiological criteria of benignity should include further imaging, including mammography and ultrasound, clinical examination and needle biopsy (fine needle aspiration (FNA), for cytology and/or needle core biopsy) where indicated (Triple assessment).[6-9] Only by so doing can unnecessary open surgical procedures be avoided for what prove to be benign abnormalities. This approach to assessment also has the advantage of providing a definitive pre-operative diagnosis of malignancy allowing the breast team to plan treatment and the patient to make informed decisions about treatment options supported by the breast care nurse.

Detecting and distinguishing significant circumscribed masses demonstrated on mammography

There is a large number of both normal and abnormal processes that can appear as circumscribed masses on mammography; a comprehensive list of causes is shown in Table I. Features that are helpful in differentiating benign from malignant masses include their:
– number;
– size;
– density;
– composition;
– position;
– character of their margins;
– contour;
– any associated features;
– the age of the patient.

Each of these is described separately but it is stressed that all features should be considered together when weighing up the probabilities of a mass representing malignancy and no single characteristic should be regarded as diagnostic.

Single or multiple masses

The differential diagnoses of single and multiple circumscribed masses are shown in Table I; malignancy is more likely with a solitary than multiple lesions. However, before dismissing multiple masses as benign they must all be seen to have similar features and a careful search made for a mass with

Table I. Round masses on mammography.

Multiple Round Masses

- *Cysts*
- *Fibroadenomas*
- *Papillomas*
- *Multifocal carcinoma*
- *Galactocoele*
- *Metastases*
  - Carcinoma
  - Melanoma
- *Lymphoma*

Solitary Round Masses

- *Normal structures*
  - Nipple
  - Normal breast lobule
  - Intramammary lymph node
  - Vascular structures
  - Skin lesion (mole, sebaceous cyst, naevus)

- *Common causes*
  - Cyst
  - Fibro-adenoma
  - Carcinoma
  - Abscess
  - Haematoma
  - Galactocoele
  - Papilloma

- *Uncommon causes*
  - Phyllodes tumour
  - Hamartoma
  - Metastasis (contralateral breast, melanoma, lung, ovary)
  - Adenoma

- *Rare causes*
  - Sarcoma
  - Fibromatosis
  - Tuberculosis
  - Sarcoid
  - Haemangioma
  - Neurofibroma
  - Leiomyoma
  - Granular cell tumour

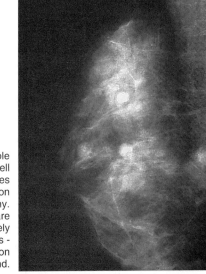

Fig. 1. Multiple small well defined masses demonstrated on mammography. Simple cysts are the most likely diagnosis - confirmed on ultrasound.

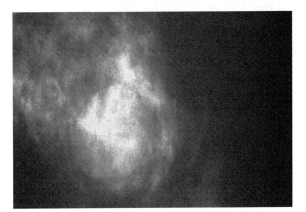

Fig. 2. A solitary 2.5 cm diameter well defined mass as shown on mammography. A surrounding halo is clearly demonstrated. This appearance is strongly in favour of a benign lesion; a cyst is the most likely diagnosis.

significantly different characteristics that may warrant further assessment. Figure 1 shows the typical mammographic features of multiple benign circumscribed masses.

Size

On its own the size of an abnormality is not of particular importance as malignant tumours may be identified at any stage in their development.[5] However, as a general rule a well circumscribed mass that is less than 1 cm in diameter is unlikely to be malignant while any circumscribed mass over 2 cm in diameter warrants further assessment (Fig. 2). An ill-defined mass of any size requires further investigation.

Density and composition

Density and composition are important in assessing the nature of a mass found on mammography.[10] Masses of reduced density compared to normal adjacent tissue (radiolucent) are very likely to be benign (Fig. 3). The commonest causes of a radiolucent mass are oil cyst, lipoma and galactocoele; these rarely cause much diagnostic difficulty.

Masses of mixed density containing tissue of fat density are also highly likely to be benign (Fig. 4). The differential diagnosis includes normal lymph nodes, (Figs. 5a-b) fibro-adenoma (Fig. 6), galactocoele and haematoma.

Masses showing increased density are deserving of careful evaluation as most malignant circumscribed malignant lesions are radio-opaque (Fig. 7).

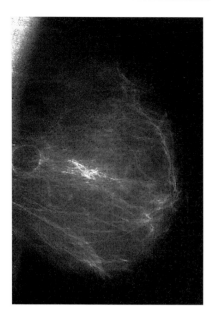

Fig. 3. A well defined reduced density mass demonstrated in mammography - the typical appearances of an oil cyst .

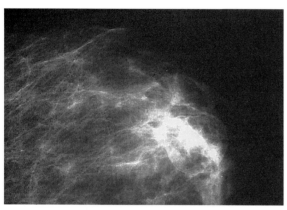

Fig. 4. A mammogram demonstrating a mixed density mass behind the nipple.

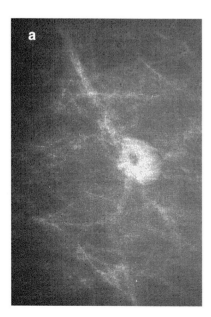

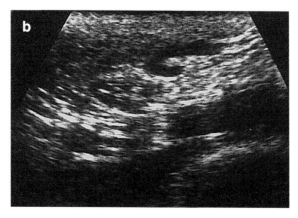

However, increased density is a non-specific feature with many benign lesions, such as cysts and fibroadenomas, often showing significantly increased density when compared to the adjacent normal breast tissue.[11]

Position

A circumscribed mass can occur in any part of the breast. However, masses demonstrated in certain areas are deserving of special attention. These areas are often referred to as the "review areas" and include the retro-areolar area, the retroglandular space on the mediolateral oblique projection (Figs. 8 a-b), the medial aspect of the breast and the infra mammary angle (Figs. 9 and 10 a-b). The majority of circumscribed masses in the axillary tail of the breast are normal lymph glands but all such masses should be carefully reviewed and further assessment arranged if there is any doubt about their nature.

Margin

The characteristic of the margin of a circumscribed mass are probably the most important single feature in deciding the need for further assessment. A well defined mass with clearly circumscribed margins, where differentiation of tumour edge from normal breast tissue is sharply defined, is unlikely to represent malignant disease (Fig. 11); the risk of malignancy in a solitary well defined mass is reported to be between 2 and 0.5%. Benign circumscribed masses often show a surrounding halo (Figs. 2 and 11) (either partial or complete), a feature that is very rarely seen in malignant lesions.

However, if the margins of the circumscribed lesion are ill defined, such that there is no clear distinction between the margin of the mass and adjacent normal breast tissue (Fig. 12), then the risk of malignancy is significant; all poorly defined cir-

Fig. 5. The mammographic (a) and ultrasound (b) appearances of a normal intramammary lymph node. (a) The lucent central area represents fat in the lymph node hilum. (b) The morphology correlates with that shown on mammography.

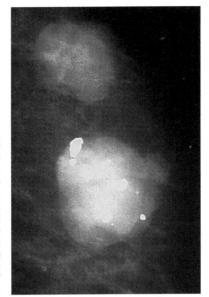

Fig. 6. Mammography showing the typical appearances of two fibro-adenomas, one shown as a simple lobulated mass and the other containing characteristic course "popcorn" calcification.

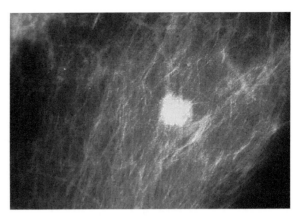

Fig. 7. A small circumscribed malignant mass on mammography showing markedly increased density compared to the adjacent normal breast tissue and ill-defined margins - compare to figure 6.

cumscribed masses require further assessment. Virtually all circumscribed masses that represent invasive carcinoma will have ill defined margins; only a few benign lesions will show this feature. Circumscribed masses with margins that are mostly well defined but with a portion that is ill defined (Fig. 13) should be managed in the same way as other ill-defined masses. Most of these will prove to be benign, the ill defined portion of their margin being caused by overlying normal breast parenchyma, but the risk of malignancy is such that at least further imaging is required.

Contour

Benign circumscribed masses are almost always circular or oval and often show lobulation (Fig. 6). The exceptions are haematoma and infection (abscess), but the history usually points to the diagnosis in these cases.

Most malignant lesions show some degree of irregularity to their contour; some circumscribed malignancies also show lobulation, particularly papillary and medullary carcinoma (Figs. 14a-b).

Palpability

Another feature, of less importance, is whether or not the abnormality is palpable. A circumscribed lesion that is palpable at small size on imaging (approximately 1 cm or less in diameter) is more likely to be malignant than one that is not.

This is true because the desmoplastic reaction

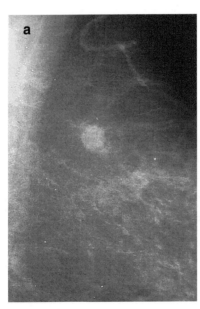

Fig. 8. A small invasive carcinoma represented by the ill defined mass lying behind the breast disk on this mediolateral oblique mammogram (**a**) and the ultrasound of the same lesion showing an ill defined hypoechoic mass with distal acoustic shadowing (**b**).

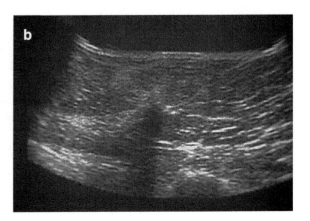

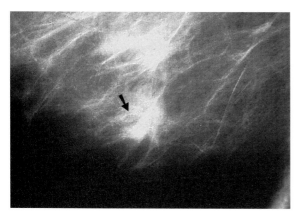

Fig. 9. A small circumscribed carcinoma lying in the infra-mammary angle as shown on a medio-lateral oblique mammogram.

excited in the surrounding breast tissue is often palpable around the tumour mass, exaggerating the true size of the lesion.

However, this is not a reliable means of differen-tiation between benign and malignant lesions; small benign inflammatory lesions may be easily palpable while small invasive carcinomas very often are not.

Associated features

The presence of calcification in and around a circumscribed breast lesion is often a helpful fea-ture in deciding its nature. Macrocalcification within a mass can be characteristic of fibroadeno-ma which has undergone partial hyaline degener-ation (Fig. 6).

This appearance is diagnostic and needle biopsy is unnecessary; malignant change within a fibro-adenoma is extremely rare.

Pleomorphic calcifications, on the other hand, in or around a circumscribed lesion are of much more significance and should suggest the diagnosis of ductal carcinoma *in situ* (Fig. 14a); the soft tissue mass in these circumstances does not necessarily indicate the presence of invasive malignant disease

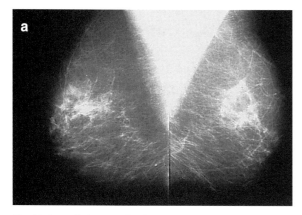
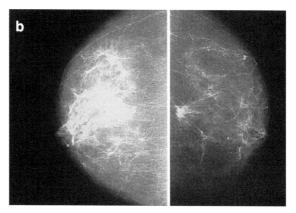

Fig. 10. A small circumscribed carcinoma with associated disturbance of architecture is clearly demonstrated medially in the breast on a craniocaudal mammogram (**b**); the lesion is very difficult to identify on the mediolateral projection (**a**).

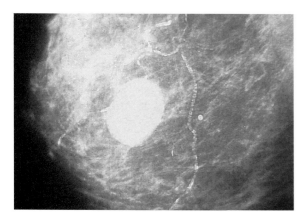
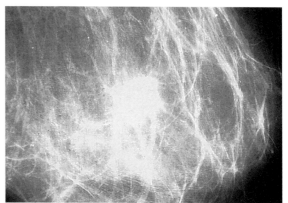

Fig. 11. Mammography showing the typical well circumscribed margins, with a clearly visible surrounding "halo", of a benign mass.

Fig. 12. An example of a poorly defined mass demonstrated on mammography compared to figure 11 the distinction between probably benign and probably malignant masses on the basis of their margin is clearly demonstrated.

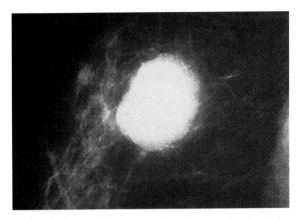

Fig. 13 A circumscribed mass with a clearly defined anterior border but poorly defined posterior border.

as, not infrequently, the mass represents a localized non-malignant inflammatory response to the *in situ* disease.

Age

The differential diagnosis of circumscribed masses is influenced by the age of the woman. Those presenting in women under 35 years are very likely to be benign, fibro-adenoma being the most likely diagnosis. Between 35 and 45, cysts are common but after 35 all circumscribed masses should be fully assessed if they do not show definitively benign features on imaging.[4,5]

Histological correlation

Circumscribed breast carcinomas without evidence of adjacent desmoplastic reaction to produce architectural distortion are said to be more likely to

be of high histological grade, the tumour growing rapidly without stimulation of a response from the adjacent breast tissue. The most likely diagnosis of a poorly defined circumscribed mass in the breast which is malignant is ductal carcinoma of no specific type. However the full range of breast tumours can give this appearance, including lobular carcinoma. Mucinous carcinoma and medullary carcinoma typically produce circumscribed mass in the breast as opposed to a stellate lesion or a spiculate mass.

Assessment of circumscribed breast lesions

If there is any doubt in the mind of the mammogram film reader about the nature of a circumscribed lesion then further imaging and clinical assessment should be mandatory. The assessment process for circumscribed masses is straightforward. The single most useful imaging tool is ultrasound. Ultrasound, using frequencies of at least 7.5 MHz, should be the routine initial imaging investigation for circumscribed masses detected on mammography. It will demonstrate the vast majority of masses and facilitate image guided biopsy, should this be indicated. Ultrasound will usually easily differentiate solid from cystic lesions (Figs. 15 -16); where there is doubt needle aspiration should be attempted. All solid lesions deemed worthy of further assessment should undergo fine needle aspiration for cytology and/or needle histology.

If a circumscribed lesion is not visible on ultrasound further mammography is indicated. It should not be assumed that a mass that is not seen on ultrasound either does not exist as a true mass or is benign. Paddle compression is particularly useful in confirming the presence of a circumscribed mass and will often give more information about the contour and mar-

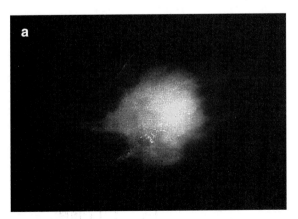
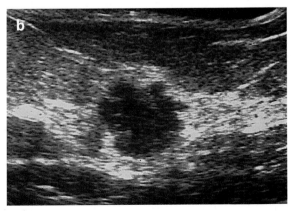

Fig. 14. Mammogram showing a mass with a lobulated contour with associated pleomorphic microcalcification representing DCIS both within the mass and in the surrounding tissues (**a**), and the ultrasound of the same malignant mass clearly demonstrating the lobulated irregular contour (**b**).

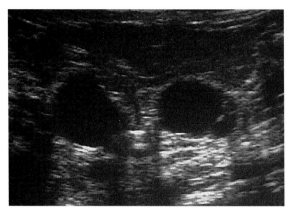

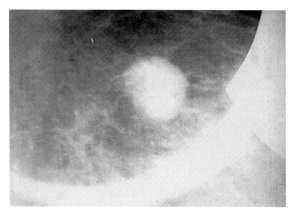

Fig. 15. Ultrasound showing the characteristic features of a simple cyst - an an-echoic mass with crisp well defined margins, posterior wall bright-up, and distal acoustic enhancement.

Fig. 17. A paddle compression mammogram clearly showing the ill defined nature of the contour of a circumscribed malignant mass.

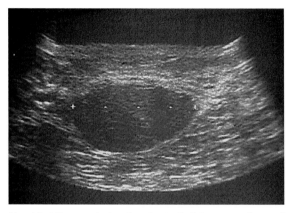

Fig. 16. Ultrasound showing the typical features of a well defined solid lesion (compare to figure 15) - all solid circumscribed lesions identified at assessment require FNA or core biopsy regardless of their imaging features.

gins (Fig. 17).[12,13] X-ray guided FNA or core biopsy should be performed if the mass is not clearly benign.

Summary

Circumscribed masses are common findings on screening mammography and most are benign. Differentiation of definitively benign from possibly malignant circumscribed masses is usually straightforward, with mass margin and density being the most important mammographic features. Ultrasound is the most useful imaging tool for further assessment.

References

1. Kopans D.B., Swann C.A, White G.W., *et al.*: Asymmetric Breast Tissue. Radiology, 1989; 171: 639-643
2. Bird R., Wallace T., Yankaskas B.: Analysis of cancers missed at screening mammography. Radiology 1992; 184: 613-617
3. Burrell H., Sibbering D., Wilson A.R.M., *et al.*: The mammographic features of interval cancers and prognosis compared with screen detected symptomatic breast cancers. Radiology 1996; 811-817
4. Stomper P., Leibowich S., Meyer J.: The prevalence and distribution of well circumscribed nodules on screening mammography: analysis of 1500 mammograms. Breast Disease 1991; 4: 197-203
5. Sickles E.: Nonpalpable, circumscribed, noncalcified, solid breast masses: likelihood of malignancy based on lesion size and age of patient. Radiology 1994; 192: 439-442
6. Feig S.: Breast masses: mammographic and sonographic evaluation. Radiological Clinics of North America 1992; 30: 67-92
7. Ellis I., Galea M., Locker A., *et al.*: Early experience in breast cancer screening: emphasis on development of protocols for triple assessment. The Breast 1993; 2: 148153
8. Sickles E., Parker S.: Appropriate role of core breast biopsy in the management of probably benign lesions. Radiology 1993; 188: 315
9. Sickles E., Parker S.: Appropriate role of core biopsy in the management of probably benign lesions (editorial). Radiology 1993; 188: 315
10. Tabar L., Dean P.: Teaching Atlas of Mammography. Stuttgart, Georg Thieme Verlag, 1985
11. Jackson V., Dines K., Bassett L., Gold R., Reynolds H.: Diagnostic importance of the radiographic density of noncalcified breast masses: analysis of 91 lesions. AJR 1991; 157: 25-28
12. Berkowitz J.E., Gatewood O.M.B., Gayler B.W.: Equivocal mammographic findings: evaluation with spot compression. Radiology 1989; 171: 369-371
13. Sickles E.A.: Breast masses: mammographic evaluation. Radiology 1989; 173: 297-303

Microcalcifications

R. Given-Wilson

Introduction

Microcalcifications are common. They are seen in approximately a third of all mammograms. The great majority are benign but in a small percentage arc a marker of malignancy.

In a typical screening population malignancy will be detected in 0.5-0.8% of women. 20% of this is due to ductal carcinoma *in situ* (DCIS). This is usually detected by the presence of calcification.[1] In the remaining 80% of malignancies, half will have microcalcification accompanied by other signs such as a mass or distortion.

Thus, although malignant microcalcification is seen in up to 0.5% of all mammograms, it accounts for only one sixtieth of all cases of microcalcifications visualised. Over 98% of microcalcifications are due to benign processes. It is therefore essential to be able to distinguish benign from malignant microcalcifications both to detect malignancy and reduce unnecessary biopsies.

It is important to have an understanding of the pathological processes producing calcifications and the anatomical structures within which they arise. These determine their shape, density and distribution, the features that allow differential diagnosis. Malignant calcifications are typically pleomorphic (variable in shape and size), clustered (>5 calcifications in a small area), linear and branching.

Calcifications occur in many structures in the breast. Of importance to the radiologist are those arising in ducts and lobules, which commonly represent or simulate malignancy. Knowledge of the natural history of conditions associated with calcifications facilitates determination of a management strategy.

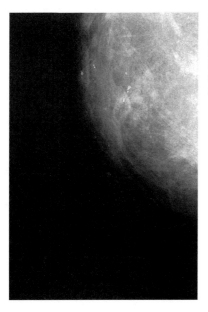

Fig. 1. Multiple small ring calcifications, some of which are seen on this tangential view to lie intradermally, represent sebaceous gland calcification.

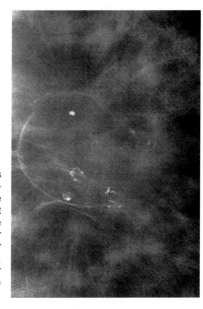

Fig. 2. Fat necrosis. Areas of liponecrosis microcystica calcificans are associated with an oil cyst following surgery. There are also some smaller more amorphous linear calcifications in this area, presumably an earlier stage of the same process.

Calcifications classified by structure of origin

Calcifications outside ducts and lobules

These are benign and rarely cause diagnostic difficulty. They are characteristically ring, tubular or curvilinear. All are benign shapes.

Vascular calcification

This is very common. This produces curvilinear and tubular calcifications and may be widespread throughout the breast. It may rarely cause diagnostic difficulties if there is only a small area and typical parallel lines and curves cannot be seen. It is commoner in patients with diabetes, renal failure and those undergoing dialysis.[2]

Sebaceous gland calcification

This is distinguished by its intradermal location and can be clearly demonstrated by tangential views if necessary. This consists of small clusters of 2-6 calcifications individually measuring about 1 mm in diameter within sebaceous glands. These tend to be concentrated in the inframammary fold, the areola and the axilla, but may be occasionally scattered over the breasts (Fig. 1). They are likely to be due to inflammation such as chronic folliculitis. Skin calcification and ossification can also be seen in Albright's hereditary osteodystrophy and osteoma cutis.[3]

Fat necrosis

Liponecrosis microcystica calcificans is well defined ring calcification, 1-4 mm in diameter which occurs around small areas of fat necrosis. These are more common in association with trauma such as surgery or with plasma cell mastitis, but are often scattered in the breast with no obvious underlying cause. Larger areas of fat necrosis up to several centimetres across can follow trauma and may have a striking appearance with a dense rim or sheets of calcification. Occasionally in the early stages of development, rim calcification around fat necrosis or sheet calcification may simulate malignant calcification, as may irregular calcification in diffuse, saponified fat (Fig. 2). In addition fat necrosis can cause stellate distortion leading to confusion.

Foreign bodies

Calcification can occur in reaction to any foreign body. Its shape will depend on that of the structure it is responding to. Surgical sutures lead to curvilinear and tubular calcification around a scar, similar to vascular calcification shapes. Calcification of suture material commonly occurs following irradiation, but is rarely seen in the non-irradiated breast.[4] Parasitic worms, not surprisingly, cause small worm-shaped calcifications (Fig. 3). They are rare but commoner in women of African origin. Schistosomiasis is also rare but has been reported to cause breast calcifications indistinguishable from malignancy[5] and Trichinella can cause pectoral muscle calcification. Implants may cause sheets of fat necrosis-type calcification around them. Direct injection into the breast has been practiced for augmentation. Silicon injection has been carried out in North America and paraffin has been used in a similar fashion in the Far East. This results in multiple ring calcifications of varying sizes around subsequent granulomas (Fig. 4).

Stromal calcifications

Occasionally calcification of unknown aetiology

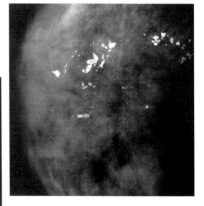

Fig. 5. Bizarrely-shaped and variable calcifications are seen throughout the upper right breast in this asymptomatic woman. They were due to stromal calcification of unknown aetiology.

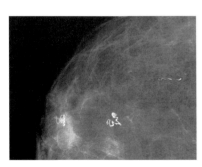

Fig. 3. Curvilinear calcification within parasitic worms is occasionally an incidental finding.

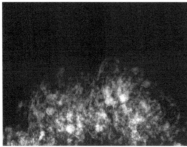

Fig. 4. Multiple ring calcifications are the result of direct injection of augmentation material into the breast many years previously.

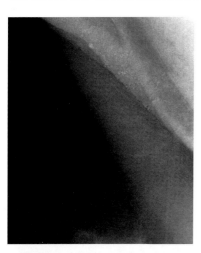

Fig. 6. Cream in the axilla has rolled into little rods simulating DCIS. In this case the dermal location is clearly seen.

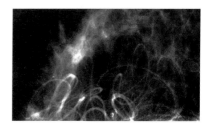

Fig. 8. Hair artefacts producing typical curvilinear densities overlying the back of the cc view.

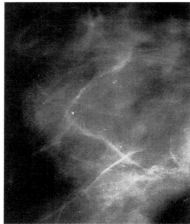

Fig. 9. Widely scattered pearl-like calcifications in adenosis. These were unchanged on a subsequent screening mammogram three years later. Curvilinear and tubular vascular calcification is also seen.

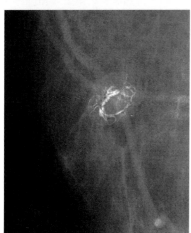

Fig. 7. A calcified wart.

occurs in the fibrous breast stroma. This may be variable and quite bizarre in shape with punctate well defined calcifications mixed with large linear and sheet-like shapes (Fig. 5). This can occasionally simulate malignancy but is usually more extensive and bilateral.

Artefacts simulating calcification

These can arise from a variety of sources. Talcum powder, deodorants and creams in the axilla or inframammary fold may become aggregated into small rods and balls. This can simulate malignant calcification but its distribution should allow distinction (Fig. 6). Intradermal densities can be caused by tattoos and warts (Fig. 7). A careful record by the radiographer of any visible skin lesions should avoid confusion. Also, the patient's scalp hair should be pulled well back during mammography to avoid it being projected on the film where it can cause blurred curvilinear densities usually seen on the back of the craniocaudal view (Fig. 8).

Dirt on the screens, film scratches or pick off during processing all produce small white artefacts which should be distinguishable from calcification by their brightness on careful inspection of the films. Fingerprints on the film should be recognisable by their whorled patterns.

Calcification in the lobule

Lobules are the commonest site of breast calcifications. The majority are markers of benign breast disease (fibrocystic changes). Those that are malignant represent lobular carcinoma *in situ* (LCIS) and cannot be distinguished from benign lobular calcifications. This diagnosis cannot be made radiologically. Adenosis, sclerosing adenosis and microcystic disease are variants of fibrocystic benign breast disease.

Adenosis

Overgrowth of the epithelium lining the terminal duct lobular unit can lead to calcium deposits within distended lobules. These concretions are rounded pearl-like calcifications, of uniform density and size and arranged in tiny round clusters (likened to little raspberries or dogs paw prints) or in ones or twos (like diplococci) (Fig. 9). They are often scattered throughout both breasts wherever there is glandular tissue and frequently associated with a spectrum of benign breast disease. When localised they may cause diagnostic difficulties. Following fatty involution scattered lobular calcifications may remain within adipose tissue with no visible surrounding glandular tissue.

Sclerosing adenosis

In this variant there is a greater degree of stromal fibrosis associated with epithelial hyperplasia within the lobules. This results in distortion of normal lobular architecture and can produce calcifications which show variations in density, shape and size (Fig. 10).

There may also be architectural distortion of breast stroma visible on a mammogram. These appearances simulate malignancy. Alternatively amorphous, powdery calcification within tiny cysts may produce softer, less dense, lobular calcifications giving a cumulus cloud effect on mammography (Fig. 11).

Microcystic disease

Again, part of the spectrum of benign breast disease and often seen in association with the conditions above and with macrocystic disease, the calcifications may be scattered or clustered. The lobules enlarge to form tiny cysts 1-5 mm in diameter. The epithelium secretes fluid containing calcium salts which precipitate within the cysts producing a layer of sludge at the bottom which has been likened to tea leaves in a tea cup.

These have a characteristic mammographic appearance. When viewed from the side on a true lateral horizontal ray film, crescents of calcium are seen lying horizontally. When viewed from above on a cranio-caudal film the calcifications are seen as rounded lower density splodges. It is worthwhile searching for this appearance with a true lateral and cranio caudal magnification view as it represents a definite benign disease process (Figs.12 and 13).

Lobular carcinoma *in situ* (LCIS)

Lobular carcinoma *in situ* is not a direct precursor of malignancy but a marker of increased risk, thus some authors prefer the term lobular neoplasia. It denotes a risk of 1% per year of developing invasive cancer, either ductal or lobular type, in either breast (7 x increased risk above the general population). Neoplastic cells replace the normal epithelium of acini and intralobular ductules. The abnormal cells cause expansion of individual acini as well as enlargement of the entire lobule. It is commonly multifocal and bilateral. It can rarely lead to the formation of calcifications which are indistinguishable from lobular calcifications seen in adenosis or sclerosing adenosis. These conditions are much commoner than LCIS. For all practical purposes therefore, LCIS is

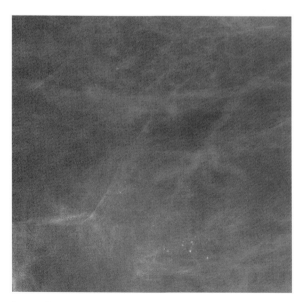

Fig. 10. Two small clusters of fine granular calcifications. The shape of each cluster is triangular and appearances simulate two small foci of DCIS. Histology of both groups showed sclerosing adenosis.

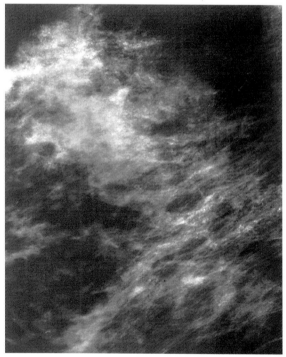

Fig. 11. Extensive soft cumulus cloud type calcification in sclerosing adenosis. This was unchanged at repeat screening mammography at three years.

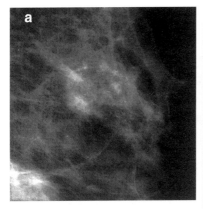 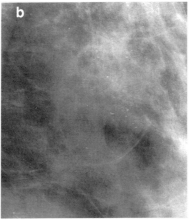 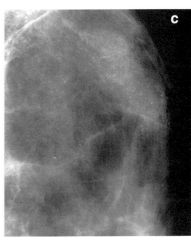

Fig. 12. **a.** On the original screening mammogram some fine indeterminate calcifications are seen in the upper part of the left breast on the oblique view. A magnified true lateral view of the area; **b.** shows characteristic linear crescentic calcifications lying horizontally on the cc view; **c.** confirms the presence of lower density rounded calcifications. The appearances are characteristic of microcystic disease and were unchanged on a repeat screening mammogram after three years.

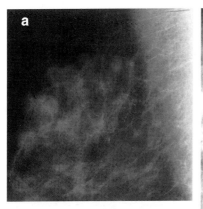 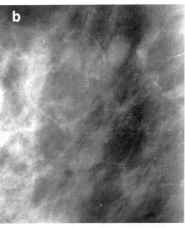 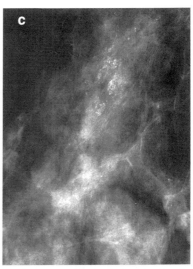

Fig. 13. **a.** Fine indeterminate calcifications are again seen lying in a linear segmental distribution in the upper part of the right breast on the screening mammogram; **b.** A magnified true lateral view of the area confirms the presence of multiple small round clusters of rounded calcifications interspersed with linear crescents characteristic of microcystic disease; **c.** The cc view confirms the presence of rounded benign appearing calcifications. Larger rounded masses which represent macrocystic disease are seen in the breast and these were confirmed on ultrasound. Cytology from the area was benign and the calcifications are unchanged on a repeat screening mammogram at three years.

not a diagnosis which is made mammographically. It is usually an incidental finding in breast biopsies and the best management is uncertain. Commonly an expectant watch policy is adopted.

Calcification in ducts

The majority of breast cancer arises from ductal epithelium, of which a proportion arises from DCIS. DCIS appears to be a direct precurser of invasive tumour, evolving into invasive cancer in up to 50% of cases.[6] It is a diagnosis most commonly made mammographically, accounting for up to 20% of screen detected malignancy and about 5% of symptomatic cancers. Benign ductal calcifications also occur in plasma cell mastitis (PCM) and atypical ductal hyperplasia (ADH). PCM should be easily distinguishable from DCIS radiologically. ADH is more difficult to identify.

Plasma cell mastitis

In this benign condition also known as mammary duct ectasia, enlarged ectatic ducts are filled with

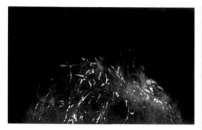

Fig. 14. Florid plasma cell mastitis.

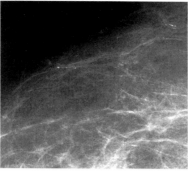

Fig. 15. Extensive fine linear calcifications were widely distributed throughout both breasts. In addition vascular calcification is seen. The individual calcifications have a ductal distribution. Some of them do not have entirely smooth margins so that they simulate DCIS. Their widespread location however favours plasma cell mastitis and they were unchanged on further screening mammography three years on confirming a benign diagnosis.

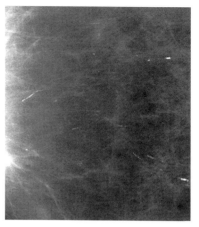

Fig. 16. Linear calcifications lie in a ductal distribution within one quadrant of the breast. There is virtually no associated soft tissue density. The irregular granular margins of the individual calcifications are suspicious. Histological examination confirmed the presence of comedo DCIS.

inspissated eosinophilic material, lipid containing histiocytes and desquamated duct epithelium. Sometimes ovoid crystalline bodies and cholesterol crystals are present. These may calcify within the ducts giving rods or needles of dense well circumscribed round ended calcium of up to a centimetre long and 1-3 mm thick. They are frequently distributed throughout both breasts in a ductal pattern converging on the nipple though they may only occupy one segment. They are commonest in the subareolar area. Duct inflammation is invariably present and rupture may also occur and lead to oval, lucent-centred, ductally distributed calcifications interspersed with the rods (Fig. 14). Rings of fat necrosis may also be associated. Plasma cell mastitis calcification tends to be widely spaced within the breast. This and the smooth well defined borders of individual calcifications usually allows differentiation from DCIS (Fig. 15).

In a fatty breast enlarged ducts in this conditon may be visible as soft tissue linear structures especially beneath the areola and in a dense breast sometimes the duct contents will be distinguishable as lines of greater lucency up to 5 mm thick converging on the nipple. There is often long-standing slit-like nipple inversion. Although women may present with pain or nipple discharge, the majority of these women are asymptomatic.

Ductal carcinoma *in situ* (DCIS)

In DCIS malignant cells are confined within the basement membrane of the ducts. It can be extensive within a duct system and may involve adjacent lobules (cancerisation of the lobules). Tiny foci of invasion (up to 1 mm diameter) may also be present and are

defined as micro-invasion. It can be multifocal (more than one lesion, single quadrant) or multicentric (more than one quadrant involved) and in these cases breast conserving surgery may be inappropriate.

DCIS is characterized pathologically into high and low grade by the growth pattern (comedo, solid, cribriform, or micropapillary), cell size (large or small), presence or absence of necrosis, and nuclear morphology. Large cell size, necrosis, comedo growth pattern and more abnormal nuclear morphology are associated with high grade DCIS. These features determine the mammographic appearance and likelihood of detection. DCIS may occur in pure form or more often in combination with different types of DCIS occurring in a single lesion.

Comedo DCIS produces radiologically visible calcification in 94% of cases.[7] It accounts for the majority of screen detected DCIS. Large malignant cells fill and expand involved ducts. They undergo central necrosis and the necrotic tissue calcifies producing casts of the ducts with linear and irregular shaped calcifications.[8] These are very variable in shape and size but may be up to several millimetres long. Although these are the hallmark of comedo DCIS there is often extensive granular and punctate calcification in addition (Fig. 16). Presumably these represent calcifications in necrotic debris that have not yet coalesced to form casts. 14% have granular calcification alone. Casting calcifications may branch and form X or Y shapes. There is marked variation in density both within and between calcifications and they have very irregular borders. They follow a ductal distribution and cluster shapes are thus typi-

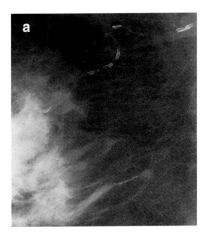 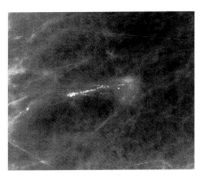

Fig. 17. **a.** There is striking tubular vascular calcification in the upper part of this breast. Further similar linear calcification is seen inferiorly but is associated with a small asymmetric soft tissue density;
b. A magnification view shows that the inferior linear calcification has an irregular border and is variable in density. The small associated mass remains irregular on a magnification paddle view. The appearances are suspicious of DCIS with an invasive lesion. Histology confirmed the presence of comedo DCIS with a 5 mm invasive ductal carcinoma grade I.

cally linear or triangular with convergence on the nipple (Fig. 17).

The calcifications that are visible in comedo DCIS are likely to be representative of the extent of disease. In cases of pure comedo DCIS 88% show less than 20 mm discrepancy between mammographic and histological measurements of the extent of disease. Comedo DCIS however has a relatively high recurrence rate following local treatment as it corresponds to high grade DCIS.

In cribriform and micropapillary DCIS involved ducts are expanded by malignant cells but these grow in a regular fashion with sieve-like spaces between arches of malignant cells or small papillary projec-tions with intervening clefts. Crystalline calcifications are produced from active secretion into these spaces. Necrosis is not a major feature.

It appears that only half of cribriform/micropapillary DCIS (53%) produces radiologically visible calcifications. It is more likely to be mammographically occult than comedo type and may present symptomatically.[7] When calcification is visible it is likely that the disease extends well beyond the area of calcification and thus mammography underestimates the histological extent of disease by more than 20 mm in 44% of cases of pure micropapillary/cribriform type DCIS. The calcifications in this condition tend to be small (less than 0.5 mm diameter) and granular leading to confusion with benign lobular calcification. However they show greater variability in density, shape and size than in benign conditions and their distribution is ductal, linear and segmental (Figs. 18-19).

These features should give rise to suspicion. In addition there is overlap with 22% of calcified small

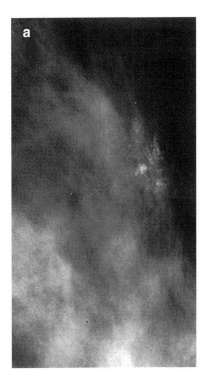 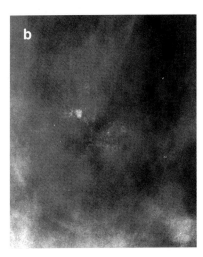

Fig. 18. **a.** Lateral and
b. cranio-caudal views of a small cluster of small calcifications found on screening mammography. The cluster shape is rounded. The individual calcifications are mainly rounded but there are some polyhedral shapes and a little variability in size and density. Some of the calcifications also appear to line up in rows.
The appearance is indeterminate but sterotactic fine needle aspiration cytology yielded suspicious cells.
Histology confirmed the presence of cribriform and solid DCIS.

cell DCIS showing linear calcification similar to comedo DCIS.[8] Other forms of DCIS, clinging and solid, may also produce calcifications of variable but often punctate shape and a high index of suspicion is needed to diagnose them. These patterns are associated with low grade DCIS.

Two factors influence the recurrence rate after local excision of DCIS, the size of the lesion (> 2.5 cm is associated with a higher recurrence rate) and a high pathological grading.[1] High grade (large cell) DCIS has a higher recurrence rate than low grade (small cell) type.

Although screen detected DCIS is usually diagnosed on the basis of microcalcifications it can have a variety of less common manifestations without calcification. For instance it may produce a stellate lesion, duct thickening, asymmetry or a circumscribed or ill defined mass.[9]

Atypical ductal hyperplasia

In this condition there is an intraductal epithelial proliferation with cells which show architectural and/or cytological atypia. However the degree of atypia is insufficient quantitatively or qualitatively to allow a diagnosis of DCIS. It is a risk marker for malignancy and carries a 4 to 5 times risk of subsequently developing invasive malignancy.[10] It is commonly found on biopsy in combination with a spectrum of benign breast disease.

It is present in up to 31% of biopsies undertaken for benign microcalcifications.[11] The calcifications it produces are usually in secretions in the lumen of affected ducts with irregular punctate and linear forms. Because of its ductal origin, the calcifications tend to show a segmental linear distribution and may simulate DCIS or benign breast disease such as sclerosing adenosis (Fig. 20).

Calcifications associated with masses

Most types of breast masses can have associated calcifications. The form of these may aid diagnosis of the mass. They may be benign or malignant.

Carcinoma

Many invasive cancers show associated DCIS type calcification either within the mass or surrounding it. This may indicate the extent of associated DCIS and aid in planning surgery (Fig. 21). Invasive carcinoma also often shows coarser dystrophic calcifications usually within areas of necrotic tumour. When extensive DCIS is seen in association with invasive tumour there is an increased risk of recurrence after local treatment.

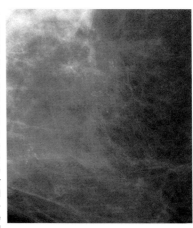

Fig. 19. Magnification view of three small clusters of calcification found on screening mammography. Again fine polyhedral calcifications show some variability in shape and size and tend to line up in rows. The appearances are suspicious for DCIS and histology confirmed the presence of mixed papillary and cribriform DCIS.

Lymph nodes

Rarely, nodes containing metastases from breast carcinoma will calcify.[12] This can be typical DCIS-type calcification within ductal structures formed by a well differentiated tumour (Fig. 22). Alternatively, as in primary tumours, more amorphous calcifications will occur in necrotic areas and can be up to several millimetres across. More commonly, however, nodes show calcification of benign aetiology, usually inflammatory. Popcorn-type calcification is common following TB (Fig. 23). Also punctate nodal calcification can occur following gold therapy for rheumatoid arthritis.

Radial scars

These often show calcifications. They are highly proliferative epithelial lesions and the majority of calcifications represent a spectrum of benign breast disease within and around the main lesion.[13] In up to

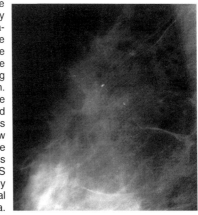

Fig. 20. A large cluster of variably shaped calcifications is seen in the upper part of the breast on the screening mammogram. There are some granular and rounded shapes and also a few linear ones. The appearance is suspicious of DCIS but histology showed atypical ductal hyperplasia.

30% of screen detected radial scars however there is associated malignancy and typical DCIS type calcifications associated with the radial scar may suggest this[14] (Fig. 24).

Fibro-adenomas and papillomas

These are common in the screening population. Their nature is usually obvious, particularly if a benign appearing mass is accompanied by typical dense clumps of popcorn-type calcification within its fibrous stroma or eggshell-like rim calcification (Fig. 25). Often the original fibroadenoma has hyalinized and just the calcification is still visible. Again this should cause no diagnostic difficulty. Calcifications in fibro-adenomas, however, are also common within the epithelium-lined clefts which curve within the tumour. This calcification is then linear and branching. It is generally well defined and often the branches have characteristic clubbed ends formed by the blunt ends of the cleft. It should form a rounded or oval cluster and the circumscribed border of the soft tissue mass may be visible around it. These features, when present, will allow differentiation from malignant causes of calcification but this is not always possible (Fig. 26).

Calcifications within a papilloma may be very similar. These masses tend to be near the nipple and aligned within the ducts. Single papillomas are benign but multiple papillomatosis is a risk marker for malignancy indicating an increase risk of 4 to 5 times.

Fibroadenolipomas

These have such a characteristic radiological appearance that they should not cause confusion. However they contain the elements of normal breast tissue and these can undergo benign breast disease.

We have seen plasma cell mastitis producing linear calcification within a fibroadenolipoma. Malignancy within a fibroadenolipoma has not been described.

Galactocoele

These can contain clumpy thick calcification but will rarely be seen in the screening population.

Haemangiomas

These may contain thick, clumpy or variable bizarre-shaped calcification.

Warts

These may also show irregular calcifications but should be clinically obvious.

Changing calcification

Calcifications of benign aetiology obviously start at some point in time and must change and develop after this. However, change is a feature of malignancy and therefore any change in breast calcification should be regarded with suspicion. The commonest change in malignant calcification is increase in number and extent with time (Fig. 27). The amount of time taken for this to happen is variable, but if no change has occurred in three years malignancy is unlikely. Alternatively calcification may decrease and resolve with time; this can also be a marker of malignancy as it indicates an active disease process. It leads to problems with management as disappearing calcifications are more difficult to biopsy (Fig. 28).

Management

The majority of calcifications seen on screening mammograms will appear clearly benign and no recall is necessary (Fig. 29).

When there are clustered calcifications which

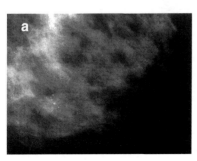

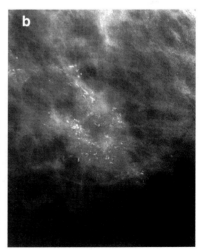

Fig. 21. **a.** A screening mammogram shows a small cluster of round calcifications inferiorly in the breast. These were felt to be benign and were not assessed.
b. Three years later there has been marked change within the area. Typical casting comedo type DCIS calcifications are seen associated with a dense spiculated mass. Histology confirmed the presence of a 9 mm invasive ductal carcinoma (grade III) with associated comedo DCIS.

raise any suspicion on screening films, it is reasonable firstly to obtain any previous mammograms. If the calcifications have a benign appearance and have been present and unchanged for over three years no further action is needed.

Women with suspicious or new clustered microcalcifications will need recall for further assessment which will include a history and a clinical examination as well as true lateral and cranio-caudal magnification views of the calcifications. When these show a definite benign appearance such as microcystic disease or vascular calcification, the woman can be reassured and discharged to routine screening.

If the appearance is suspicious of malignancy, the woman should be referred for surgical biopsy. Prior to excision, discussion and counselling, fine needle aspiration cytology and staging will be needed. Fine needle aspiration cytology may be guided by palpation, ultrasound or mammography (usually stereotaxis) according to the clinical and imaging findings. Guided core biopsy may also be used as histology and may help in planning surgical management, particularly if invasive malignancy is shown.

The more difficult situation arises for the radiologist when magnification views show indeterminate calcification. The majority of women with indeterminate calcification will have benign disease and excision biopsy should be avoided in them. Guided cytology or wide core needle histology should be obtained from the area of calcifications, preferably with stereotaxis in order to give the most accuracy. When this is atypical or malignant, referral for excision is indicated. When the cytology or histology is benign it is reasonable to adopt a watch policy with repeat mammograms and assessment at one year.

Assuming that these show no change, a screening mammogram can then be performed at two years giving a total of three years follow up.[15]

Any change with either increase or decrease in the number of the calcifications during this period should prompt a reassessment with repeat cytology and careful consideration again of the need for excision biopsy. Management will always be tempered by consideration of the woman's wishes. Most women will, having received full explanation, tolerate a policy of follow up well, but a few cannot tolerate any uncertainty and will prefer to have excision biopsy.

It is more difficult to obtain adequate cytological samples from microcalcifications than other breast lesions.[16] Lofgren et al found a 29% inadequate sample rate from calcifications versus 26% overall for impalpable lesions on fine needle aspiration cytology. On those occasions when the cytology is insufficiently cellular for diagnosis, it should ideally be repeated after an interval. Diagnostic cytology results are more likely to be obtained if a cytopathologist or cytotechnologist is present at the time of aspiration so that adequacy can be assessed immediately. Further passes can then be made if the sample is insufficient.

Policy will vary locally with regard to action over atypical cytology. Screening radiologists need to be aware of the positive predictive value (PPV) of cytological grades from their own cytopathologist. The PPV for atypical cytology may vary from 10% to over 50% in different centres. Thus the local rate will determine whether atypia is considered as an indication for excision or whether it prompts careful follow up and repeat cytology to try to obtain a definite benign or malignant result.

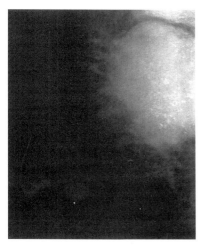

Fig. 22. Pathological nodes within the axilla containing metastatic invasive ductal carcinoma forming casting DCIS-type calcifications.

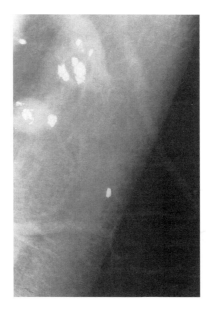

Fig. 23. Well circumscribed popcorntype calcification is visible within several normal sized axillary nodes in this asymptomatic woman of Indian origin. These are presumably due to old TB.

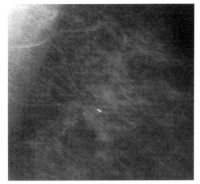

Fig. 24. A radial lesion which was impalpable and detected on routine screening. Spicules are relatively long and there is little soft central soft tissue mass compared to the size of the lesion suggesting that it may be a radial scar. There is associated linear and round calcification within the area. Histology confirmed the presence of a radial scar with associated papillary DCIS and atypical ductal hyperplasia containing calcifications.

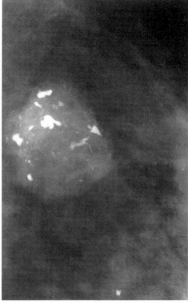

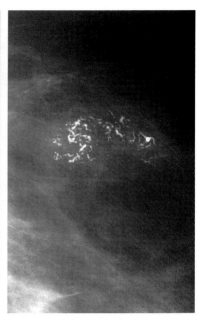

Fig. 25. A lobulated well circumscribed soft tissue mass is associated with popcorn shaped calcifications. Some of these show linear projections with clubbed ends. The appearances are characteristic of a fibroadenoma.

Fig. 26. There is an ill defined soft tissue density associated with multiple linear and comma shaped calcification which shows considerable variability in size and a little irregularity and beading of the margins in places. The appearance is unusual. The differential lies between comedo DCIS and a hyalinized fibroadenoma. Histology confirmed the presence of hyalinized fibroadenoma with no evidence of malignancy.

Post-operative changes

Benign histology

In a proportion of cases when surgical biopsy has been recommended by the radiologist because of suspicious mammographic findings, benign histology will be found. When the calcifications have been completely excised no further follow up is necessary. In some of these however, usually when the calcifications are extensive, only an incisional biopsy will have been performed and there will be residual

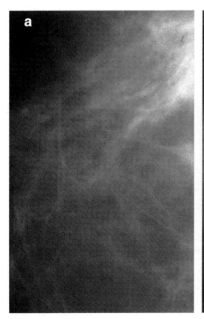

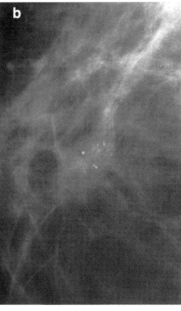

Fig. 27. **a.** A single small linear calcification.
b. Same area on a subsequent screening mammogram three years later. There is now a tiny cluster of linear calcifications with a single benign appearing rounded calcification. This cluster is associated with a small asymmetric soft tissue density which has appeared since the previous mammogram. The appearances are suspicious of malignancy and histology confirmed the presence of invasive ductal carcinoma (grade II) 4 mm in diameter and containing DCIS.

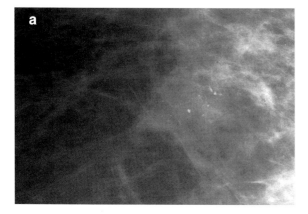

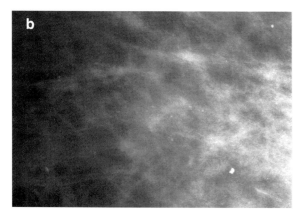

Fig. 28. **a.** There is a small linear shaped cluster of fine variable polyhedral and linear calcifications. The appearances are indeterminate and stereotactic fine needle cytology was benign.
b. On early recall a year later the calcifications are disappearing. This change is suspicious. Excision biopsy was subsequently undertaken and confirmed the presence of comedo DCIS and a focus of invasive ductal carcinoma (grade III).

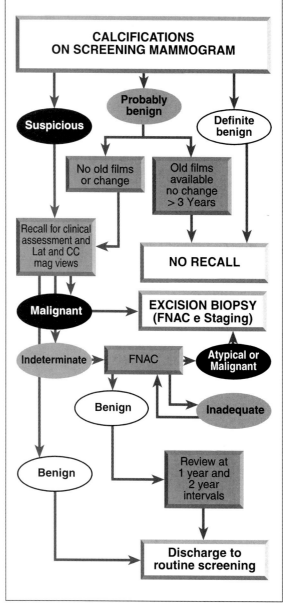

Fig. 29. Management.

calcifications. Assuming that the specimen contains representative calcification it appears safe to follow a policy of mammographic follow up rather than repeat excision. In 39 such cases followed for an average of 32 months Homer found no cases of malignancy developing.[17]

Malignancy

When malignancy is found on surgical biopsies performed for microcalcification, in up to 40% incomplete excision may be suspected because the tumour was close to the margins of the surgical specimen (within 5 mm). This may happen when the original biopsy was planned for diagnosis rather than therapy or because of the difficulty of identifying the extent of calcifications intra-operatively. Post-operative mammography can be used to help guide re-excision if breast conserving surgery is planned. It should be delayed at least a month after surgery to allow wound healing. When more than five residual calcifications are seen in women with DCIS the mammogram is a good predictor of residual disease.[18]

After breast conserving surgery regular mammographic follow up is advisable to allow early detection of recurrence. It should initially be carried out annually, then on a tapering protocol.

Post-radiation

Unexcised residual calcifications may or may not disappear post-radiation therapy. If they persist this

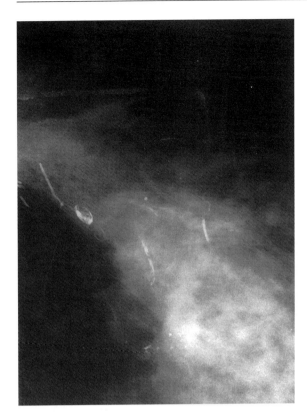

Table I. Diagnostic features of calcifications.

	Benign	Malignant
Distribution	Single or Diffuse	Clustered (>5 in a small area)
Cluster shapes	Round	Linear, triangular, rhomboid
Form	Round, popcorn rings, needles, parallel lines	Casting, (linear & branching) granular, pleomorphic
Size	Uniform	Variable
Density	Uniform	Variable – within and between calcification

The presence of typical benign calcifications does not exclude co-existent malignancy and each area of calcification within a breast should be judged separately (Figs. 31).

Fig. 30. Five years following wide local excision and radiotherapy for invasive ductal carcinoma. Fat necrosis and associated tubular sutural calcification is seen at the site of previous surgery. Some vascular calcification is noted more lateral to this in the breast. Medially in the breast however there is a new cluster of fine granular and linear calcifications with a little asymmetric soft tissue density. Histology confirmed recurrent malignancy with further foci of comedo DCIS and invasive ductal carcinoma.

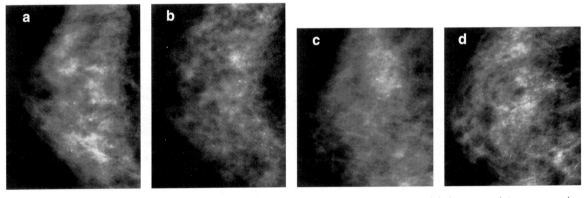

Fig. 31. **a.** and **b.** show extensive benign microcystic calcifications within the right breast. **c.** and **d.** three years later on screening mammography, the benign calcifications are still present but in addition there is a cluster in the medial aspect of the breast of fine irregular and linear calcifications. Histology confirmed the presence of extensive comedo DCIS in this area with widespread microcystic changes within the breast.

does not necessarily indicate viable tumour but careful follow up is necessary to ensure stability. New calcifications are suspicious of malignancy.[19]

43% of mammographically detected recurrences are manifested by calcifications.[20] The distribution and appearance of these calcifications are similar to those of malignant appearing calcifications in the pre-treated breast (Fig. 30). 20-25%, of irradiated breasts however, develop benign calcifications within fat necrosis, sutures or duct ectasia. It is important to recognise these and avoid unnecessary biopsy.[21]

Composition of microcalcifications

Microcalcifications detected radiologically may not be easily visualised by the pathologist. Larger calcifications may be fragmented and lost during the preparation and cutting of slices for histological examination. Finer calcifications fall into 2 main categories:

Type I

Calcium oxalate dihydrate (wedelellite). This forms small polyhedral shapes which may be difficult to see on mammograms. It is usually associated with benign or borderline lesions. The crystals are birefringent and may also be difficult to visualise on microscopy except with the use of polarized light.

Type II

Amorphous calcium phosphate or hydroxyapatite. This is non-crystalline, it is associated with both benign and malignant conditions. It stains readily with haematoxylin and is more readily visualised microscopically.[22]

The pathologist examining breast lesions needs to be aware if microcalcifications were present on the mammogram so that a specific search can be made to confirm their presence in the histological specimen. Otherwise they may be missed (Table I) (Figs. 31a,b,c,d).

References

1. Bassett L.W.: Mammographic analysis of calcifications. Radiol. Clin. N. A., 1992; 30, 1: 93-105

2. Evans A.J., Cohen M.E.L, Cohen G.F.: Patterns of breast calcification in patients on Renal Dialysis. Clin. Rad., 1992; 45: 343-344

3. Kopans D.B., Meyer J.E., Homer M.J., Grabbe J.: Dermal deposits mistaken for breast calcifications. Radiology, 1983; 149: 592-594

4. Stacey-Clear A., McCarthy K.A., Hall D.A., Pile-Spellman E.R., Mrose H.E, White G., Cardenosa G., Sawicka J., Mahoney E., Kopans D.B.: Calcified suture material in the breast after radiation therapy. Radiology, 1992; 183: 201-208

5. Gorman J.D., Champaign J.L., Sumida F.K., Canavan L.: Schistosomiasis involving the breast. Radiology 1992 185: 423-424

6. Rosen P.P., Braun D.W. Jr., Kinne D.W.: The clinical significance of pre-invasive breast carcinoma. Cancer, 1980; 46: 919-25

7. Holland R., Hendriks J.H.C.L., Verbeek A.L.M, Mravunac M., Schuurmans Stekhoven J.H.: Extent, distribution, and mammographic/histological correlations of breast ductal carcinoma *in situ*. Lancet, 1990; 335: 519-22

8. Stomper P.C., Connolly J.L.: Ductal carcinoma *in situ* of the breast: Correlation between mammographic calcification and tumour subtype. AJR, 1992; 159: 483-485

9. Ikeda D.M., Anderson I.: Ductal carcinoma *in situ*: atypical mammographic appearances. Radiology 1989; 172: 661-666

10. Dupont W.D., Page D.L.: Risk factors for breast cancer in women with proliferative breast disease. N. Engl. J. Med. 1985; 312: 146-151

11. Stomper P.C., Cholewinski S.P., Penetrante R.B., Harios J.P., Tsangaris T.N.: Atypical hyperplasia: frequency mammographic and pathological relationships in excisional biopsies guided with mammography and clinical examination. Radiology 1993; 189: 667-671

12. Helvie M.A., Rebner M., Sickles E.A., Oberman H.A.: Calcifications in metastatic breast carcinoma in axillary lymph nodes. AJR, 1988; 151: 921-922

13. Greenstein Orel S, Evers K., I-Tien Yeh, Troupin R.H.: Radial scar with microcalcifications: Radiologic, pathologic correlation. Radiology, 1992; 183: 479-482

14. Sloane J.P., Mayers M.M.: Carcinoma and atypical hyperplasia in radial scars and complex sclerosing lesions: importance of lesion size and patient age. Histopathology 1993; 23: 225-231

15. Sickles E.A.: Breast calcifications: Mammographic evaluation. Radiology, 1986; 160: 280-293

16. Lofgren M., Andersson I., Lindholm K.: Stereotactic needle aspiration for cytologic diagnosis of non palpable breast lesions. AJR 1990; 154: 1191-1195

17. Homer M.J.: Nonpalpable breast microcalcifications: Frequency, management and results of incisional biopsy. Radiology, 1992; 185: 411-413

18. Gluck B.S., Dershaw D.D., Liberman L., Deutch B.M.: Microcalcifications on postoperative mammograms as an indicator of adequacy of tumor excision. Radiology, 1993; 188: 469-472

19. Greenstein Orel S., Troupin R.H., Patterson E.A, Fowble B.L.: Breast cancer recurrence after lumpectomy and irradiation: Role of mammography in detection. Radiology, 1992; 183: 201-206

20. Stomper P.C., Recht A., Berenberg A.L., Et al.: Mammographic detection of recurrent cancer in the irradiated breast. AJR, 1987; 148: 39-43

21. Mendelson E.B.: Radiation changes in the breast. Seminars in Roentgenology 1993. Vol. XXVIII No.4 p. 344-362

22. Frouge C., Meunier M., Guinebretiere J.M., Gilles R., Vanel D., Contesso G., Di Paola R., Blery M.: Polyhedral microcalcifications at mammography: Histologic correlation with calcium oxalate. Radiology, 1993; 186: 681-684

Further reading

Lanyi M.: Diagnosis and Differential diagnosis of breast calcifications. New York, Springer Verlag, 1988

Tabar L., Dean P.B.: Teaching atlas of mammography. Stuttgart Georg Thieme Verlag, 1985

Distortion of architecture and asymmetry

C. Kissin

Distortion of breast parenchyma is a very worrying mammographic finding and, if previous trauma and surgery can be excluded, there is a high likelihood that it is due to malignancy. Even the benign radial scar has been found to contain foci of carcinoma in up to 19% of cases[1] and the overlap between the mammographic features of benign and malignant radial lesions is so great that carcinoma cannot be excluded without surgery. However, if the breast is known to be, or is likely to be, scarred from previous injury, accurate assessment of mammographic and ultrasound features can be very difficult. The detection of breast cancer may therefore be compromised in the 11% of women in the screening age group (50-64 years) who report having had previous breast surgery (88% for benign disease) and in those who have experienced significant injuries from seat belts and newel posts.

Some degree of asymmetry in the breast tissue is a common mammographic finding[2] and statistically is usually benign. However, such asymmetry may hide an underlying mass lesion or may contain parenchymal distortion or microcalcification which is not initially evident. The presence of any of these features would greatly increase the risk of malignancy. An area of asymmetrical breast tissue therefore warrants full and thorough assessment although the rate of detection of malignancy may be relatively low.

Assessment

All mammograms showing parenchymal distortion need full assessment unless there is a clear history of significant assault to the breast. Without a history of injury or surgery the cause of distortion must be pursued thoroughly, even if relative mammographic stability has been documented, and core biopsy may be necessary if a definite answer is not otherwise obtained.

Similarly, most areas of asymmetry present in two views (or in one view if only one projection is available) need to be recalled for assessment and further evaluation. However, if the mammographic appearances of this asymmetry have been stable over a period of time, malignancy is much less likely and recall may not be necessary.

At assessment, clinical evaluation is vital and ultrasound may be very helpful in identifying a focal lesion or architectural disturbance in the relevant quadrant of the breast. However, ultrasound is undoubtedly less reliable in the fatty breast and has been found to have relatively low sensitivity in the detection of invasive lobular carcinoma (ILC) (68% compared with over 90% for invasive ductal carcinoma).[3,4] ILC presents not infrequently as a diffuse area of asymmetry with or without parenchymal distortion and thus the absence of a sonographic lesion cannot be regarded as a completely reassuring finding when investigating such mammographic features.

Specialist mammographic views using focal compression and magnification over the area of suspi-

Table I. The value of focal compression views in the mammographic assessment of architectural distortion and of asymmetry.

In asymmetry	In suspected distortion
To reveal underlying distortion	To confirm presence of distortion (Fig. 1)
To identify underlying mass lesion (Fig. 2)	To assess presence and density of tumour core
To identify microcalcification (Fig. 3)	To identify microcalcification
To assess skin changes	To assess length and lucency of spicules

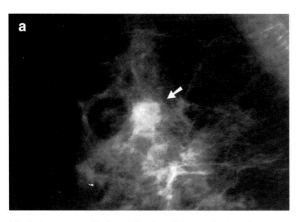 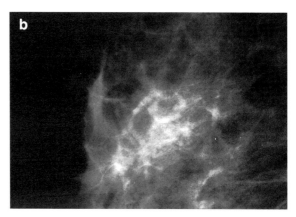

Fig 1. An unmagnified paddle view (**b**) reveals that the apparent focal asymmetry (**a**) is merely a positional shadow.

cion, will provide considerable additional diagnostic information. Such 'paddle views' can increase the internal pressures within the breast by up to 60% compared with those pressures experienced during routine mammography.[5] The value of these specialist views is shown in Table I.

These assessment techniques will usually be supplemented with cytological sampling in order to provide accurate triple assessment.

Features at assessment

I. Asymmetry only

a. Generalised

Radiotherapy

The irradiated breast typically shows a generalised diffuse increase in density, marked trabecular thickening and skin thickening. The diffuse density

is due to oedema of the breast tissue which occurs maximally 6 months after starting radiotherapy and then starts to resolve in the subsequent 3-6 months.[6] The associated phenomenon of collagen bundle oedema causes the distinctive trabecular thickening which resolves more slowly than the diffuse density, possibly due to the development of associated fibrosis. Generalised skin thickening is usually obvious at 6 months after radiotherapy and it contributes to the increased density of the treated breast. In 35% of cases this has resolved by 3 years[7] but local or periareolar thickening may persist for long periods due to induced fibrosis and surgical interference with normal lymph drainage. Coarse, rounded, benign-type calcifications can be seen in approximately 25% of irradiated breasts[7] and these are felt to be a direct

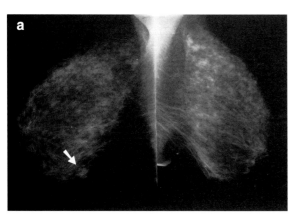 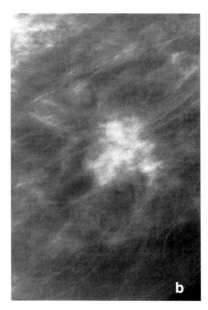

Fig. 2. **a**. A small area of asymmetry is noted in the lower part of the right breast. **b**. A paddle magnification view over this reveals an underlying irregular mass lesion, associated parenchymal distortion and some adjacent suspicious microcalcification. This proved to be a 13mm grade 3 IDC with adjacent comedo DCIS.

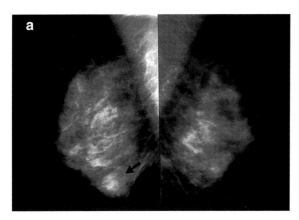 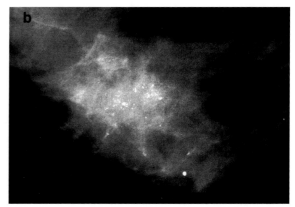

Fig. 3. **a**. There is a relatively large area of localized asymmetry in the lower part of the right breast. **b**. A magnified focal compression view over this reveals extensive suspicious microcalcification within the asymmetry. Histology showed a 14mm grade 2 IDC.

result of the radiation. These develop up to 6 years after radiotherapy.

Inflammatory carcinoma

Inflammatory carcinoma of the breast, where there is infiltration of the subdermal lymphatic plexus by tumour and often metastases in the axillary lymph nodes also, causes a very similar appearance to that seen after radiotherapy with diffuse density, trabecular thickening, skin thickening and distension of the lymphatics in the subcutaneous tissues (Fig. 4). A similar picture is seen in acute mastitis and where there is obstruction to the lymphatic or venous drainage of the breast.

Hypoplasia of the opposite breast

It is usually readily apparent that there is underdevelopment of the breast parenchyma on one side

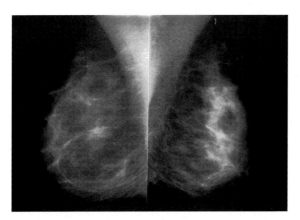

Fig. 4. The left breast shows a generalised diffuse increase in density, marked trabecular thickening and widespread skin thickening due to an extensive inflammatory carcinoma.

rather than a generalised increased density on the other. Such unilateral hypoplasia of breast tissue may be an isolated finding or it may be associated with absence of the pectoralis major muscle on that side and abnormalities of the ipsilateral forearm (Poland's syndrome).

b. Localised

Accessory breast tissue

Accessory breast tissue is a localised area of tissue which is most commonly seen in the axillary tail of the breast but may lie anywhere along the milk line which extends from the axilla to the groin. The accessory tissue may drain into the duct system of the main breast or it may have its own duct system or indeed its own nipple. Accessory breast tissue is palpable as a smooth, soft, otherwise normal area of breast tissue. There is no detectable ultrasound abnormality and no evidence of distortion on paddle views.

Patchy involution

Uneven involution of breast parenchyma after the menopause may temporarily leave a residual island of otherwise normal breast tissue which can create diagnostic confusion. Again there is no evidence of mammographic distortion in association, no microcalcification and no associated ultrasound abnormality. Cytology will reveal normal breast tissue only and the diagnosis therefore is largely one of exclusion.

Hormone replacement therapy

Hormone replacement therapy (HRT) causes demonstrable mammographic changes in the breast

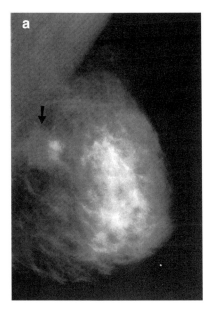

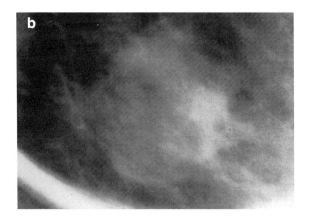

Fig 5. **a**. A 20mm diameter Grade 3 IDC seen as a localised asymmetrical opacity in the oblique projection. **b**. Paddle magnification view shows no spiculation or distortion, thus suggesting rapid growth.

parenchyma in up to 24% of women.[8] 58% of these show bilateral diffuse generalised increase in density but the rest show more patchy changes with the development of multifocal asymmetrical parenchymal densities in 17% and cysts in 25%.

Carcinoma

Whilst an asymmetrical opacity is a recognised appearance of invasive lobular carcinoma (ILC) this can also be seen with invasive ductal carcinoma (IDC) and ductal carcinoma *in situ* (DCIS).

ILC is seen as an asymmetrical opacity only, with no evidence of a central tumour nidus, in 7-27% of cases,[9,10] and up to 85% are of a density no greater than that of the surrounding normal breast tissue. This therefore can make the mammographic manifestations subtle and detection can be difficult.

Up to 4% of IDCs present as an asymmetrical mammographic opacity only, with no evidence of spiculation or parenchymal distortion.[9] These are found to be largely aggressive grade 3 tumours which are growing too fast to allow a desmoplastic response within the surrounding breast tissue (Fig. 5).

DCIS is most commonly seen as suspicious clustered microcalcifications (62%) but up to 15% may

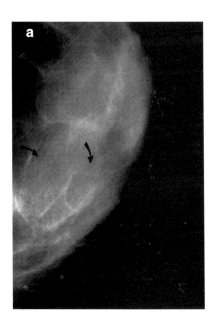

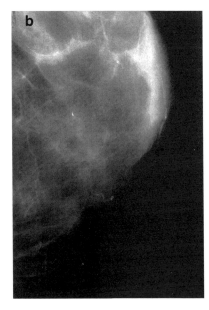

Fig. 6. **a**. CC view of left breast where diffuse increased parenchymal density is present medially at the site of a vigorous FNAB performed one hour previously.
b. Six weeks later appearances have returned to normal.

Table II. Causes of inflammation of the breast.

Breast inflammation	
Infective	**Non-infective**
Lactational mastitis	Acute periductal mastitis
Secondary infection of: – periductal mastitis – haematoma – cyst – penetrating injury	Inflammatory carcinoma Acute fat necrosis

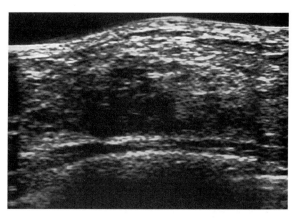

Fig. 7. 41 year-old woman presented with sudden onset of pain in the right breast. A palpable lump and reddening of the overlying skin quickly appeared. Ultrasound examination revealed an ill defined irregular hypo-echoic lesion consistent with infection.

be identified only as a nodular or more diffuse mammographic density with or without architectural distortion.[11]

Minor trauma

Injury to the breast, either as a result of accidental trauma, fine needle aspiration biopsy or core biopsy, can cause local oedema and haemorrhage resulting in an ill defined parenchymal density with no distortion and possibly some thickening of the overlying skin (Fig. 6). After fine needle aspiration biopsy these mammographic features can be noted immediately and have usually resolved two weeks later.[12]

Mammographic changes after the use of a 14-gauge core-biopsy gun include poorly defined increased density, due to haemorrhage, in 51% and air at the biopsy site in 42%.[13] Greater injury to the breast may lead to mammographic changes of fat necrosis (architectural distortion, asymmetrical density and lipid cysts).

Inflammation

Inflammation of the breast can be infective or non-infective (Table II) and, of course, the latter may progress to the former. The diagnosis is usually clinically obvious but mammographically there may be no more than an ill defined area of increased parenchymal density, due to inflammatory infiltrate and oedema, with overlying skin thickening. Ultrasound will show skin thickening and a diffuse increase in the subcutaneous fat echoes with some irregular areas of posterior attenuation within the parenchyma. When this progresses to abscess formation an irregular heterogeneous mass with some posterior enhancement will be identified (Fig. 7).

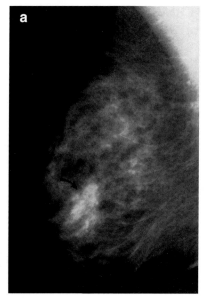 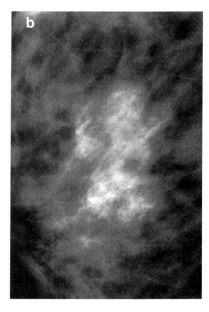

Fig. 8. **a**. + **b**. Focal compression over the area of asymmetry revealed an underlying irregular mass which proved to be a 14mm grade 2 IDC.

Clearly this may closely resemble an inflammatory carcinoma.

Previous surgery on the opposite breast

The excision of breast tissue from one breast can give the impression of localised asymmetrical increase in density on the opposite side. Evidence of parenchymal scarring and skin thickening or deformity may be seen on the treated side.

II. Asymmetry with an underlying mass lesion

Well defined mass

Focal compression views may reveal a well defined mass within an area of asymmetry. In a lady in the screening age group this is likely to be a simple cyst. The differential diagnosis includes an intramammary lymph node, a long-standing fibro-adenoma and a phyllodes tumour. If the lesion is found to be solid it requires cytological sampling to clarify the diagnosis.

Simple breast cysts are commonly seen both in perimenopausal women and in those taking HRT. The typical smooth, sharp, rounded mammographic margins may be obscured by the generalised or patchy increased density in both breasts which often also accompanies the HRT, but the true nature of the lesion should be readily identifiable with ultrasound.

Irregular mass

An irregular or spiculate mass within an area of asymmetry is likely to be a carcinoma (Fig. 8) but this appearance can be seen with fat necrosis. Secondary features of malignancy may be identified in addition, such as thickening of the overlying skin, adjacent distortion and microcalcifications.

III. Asymmetry with distortion

a. Benign

Fat necrosis

In a significant number of patients with fat necrosis there is no definite history of trauma (40%) but in many there has been recent injury, such as from a seat belt, or surgery. There is a wide spectrum of mammographic appearances ranging from well defined oil cysts with rim calcification (Fig. 9) through irregular, nodular or spiculate masses to irregular parenchymal distortion and suspicious-looking microcalcifications.[14]

Radial scar

Focal compression over an area of asymmetry may reveal an underlying radial distortion. A benign radial scar is composed of a central zone of fibroelastosis from which epithelial structures radiate out. It is therefore classically seen to have a relatively lucent central core and long lucent spicules in association (Fig. 10). Relatively few (8%) contain microcalcification but up to 25% have a clinically palpable

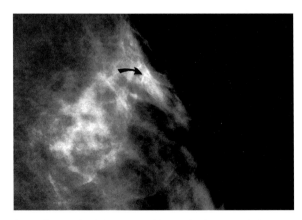

Fig. 9. Severe bruising to the left breast had occurred after seat belt injury. 4 months later calcified oil cysts are seen confirming fat necrosis.

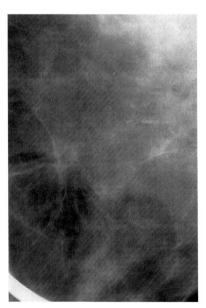

Fig. 10. Paddle magnification view revealing the typical features of a radial scar.

abnormality and up to 55% demonstrate ultrasound features commonly associated with malignancy.[15] Thus, a benign radial scar and a low grade tubular carcinoma can mimic each other very closely. In addition, up to 19% of histological radial scars have been shown to have a focus of malignancy associated, usually located around the periphery of the lesion. This is found more commonly in lesions greater than 7 mm in diameter and in women over the age of 50.[1] Clearly therefore, even if benign cytology is obtained at sampling, all radial distortions within the breast should be excised.

b. Malignant

Invasive lobular carcinoma

Both IDC and DCIS can be seen mammographically as a diffuse area of asymmetry with some architectural distortion (13.5% and 15%)[9,11] but more often these features suggest the diagnosis of invasive lobular carcinoma.

ILC often presents problems in mammographic perception.[16] It accounts for approximately 10% of breast cancers detected at screening and yet 16% of those presenting as interval cancers. It characteristically spreads by diffuse infiltration of single rows (or "Indian files") of cancer cells into the surrounding parenchyma in a manner that does not destroy the glandular anatomy nor generate substantial connective tissue reaction. This contributes to the frequent absence of a well defined tumour nidus and to the relatively low radiographic opacity of the lesion (52-85% are of a density less than or equal to that of the surrounding parenchyma, compared with only 17% of IDCs).[9,10] Indeed between 8 and 16% are reported to be mammographically occult and in others the radiographic definition can vary markedly with pro-

jection (up to 32% being seen in one projection only).[9]

The rarity of microcalcifications within ILCs (between 0 and 28%)[9,16,17] further contributes to the difficulty of diagnosis and ultrasound is estimated to have only 68% sensitivity (there is a high false negative rate, especially if the lesion is small or if it is seen mammographically as distortion and asymmetry only).[4]

ILCs may present as spiculate mass lesions (16-69%),[9,17] but 27-57% are seen as a diffuse ill defined area of parenchymal asymmetry with subtle architectural distortion or distortion only visible on focal compression (Fig. 11).[9] In these circumstances a core biopsy may be more likely to give a definitive diagnosis than cytological sampling (up to 48% of fine needle aspiration biopsies of ILCs may be negative for malignancy or yield an inadequate sample).[18]

Tumour recurrence

In a patient who has had previous surgery for malignancy, comparison with old films is invaluable to assess whether the degree of distortion or asymmetry is increasing, or if a new mass or new microcalcification is developing in association. These features and the development of a clinical abnormality would suggest the development of local recurrence (Fig. 12). Breast-conserving surgery, particularly where there has been haematoma or seroma formation, can cause marked cicatrisation. The resultant stellate distortion is characteristically planar rather than vol-

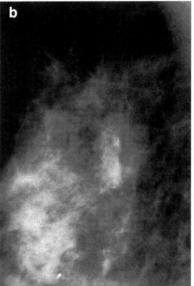

Fig. 11. **a**. A large diffuse area of slightly increased density is present in the upper half of the right breast.
b. Paddle view reveals extensive underlying distortion and histology was of a 40mm ILC.

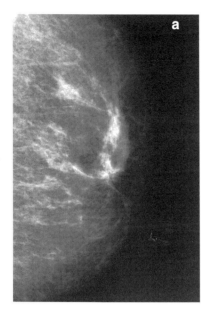
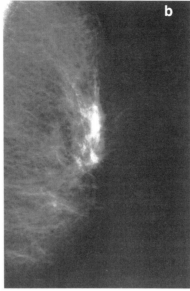
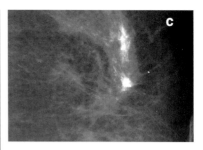

Fig. 12. **a**, **b** + **c**. Microcalcification and increasing density is noted over 5 years at the site of a previous microdochectomy (performed 10 years previously).
Histology revealed a15mm IDC.

umetric (that is, much more obvious in one view than two) (Fig. 13) and, radiographically, fat may be seen centrally within the scar.[19] Ring calcification may be evident in the walls of lipid cysts due to fat necrosis and coarse, rounded, benign-type calcifications can develop in 25% of irradiated breasts by 6 years after irradiation.[20]

These are felt to be a direct result of radiation and do not usually cause diagnostic confusion. However, suspicious microcalcifications can develop at the biopsy site after lumpectomy and radiotherapy. Many of these microcalcifications are histologically prov-

en to be benign. Unfortunately, the mammographic appearances of the calcium particles are not sufficiently specific to distinguish recurrent malignancy from benign disease.[21] It has, however, been noted that malignant microcalcifications do tend to appear sooner after the cessation of radiation than the benign ones (the mean time of appearance being 16 months compared with 32 months) and patients with new microcalcifications due to recurrent tumour tend to be younger (mean age 40 years) than those with benign microcalcifications (mean age 66 years). These benign, but morphologically suspicious, microcalci-

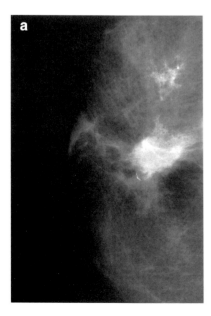
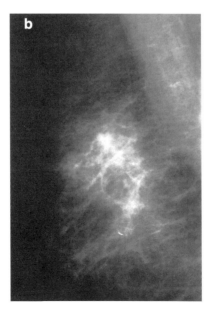

Fig. 13. This 55-year-old woman had undergone wide local excision of a carcinoma in the upper central portion of the right breast.
The spiculate mass and distortion is far more obvious on the CC view (**a**) than the oblique (**b**).

fications have been documented as developing in the breast at any time between 5 and 88 months after irradiation.

Conclusion

Distortion of architecture and asymmetry can be difficult to detect mammographically. It is important that subtle and sometimes non-specific mammographic findings are carefully correlated with clinical and ultrasound findings and that cytological or histological samples are taken to aid diagnosis.

References

1. Sloane J.P., Mayers M.M.: Carcinoma and atypical hyperplasia in radial scars and complex sclerosing lesions; importance of lesion size and patient age. Histopathology, 1993; 22: 225-231

2. Kopans D.B., Swann C.A., White G., McCarthy K.A., Hall D.A., Belmonte S.J., Gallagher W.: Asymmetric Breast Tissue. Radiology, 1989; 171: 639-643

3. Cole-Beuglet C., Soriano R.Z., Kurtz A.B., Goldberg B.B.: Ultrasound analysis of 104 primary breast carcinomas classified according to histopathologic type. Radiology, 1983; 147: 191-196

4. Paramagul C.P., Helvie M.A., Adler D.D.: Invasive lobular carcinoma: Sonographic appearance and role of sonography in improving diagnostic sensitivity. Radiology, 1995; 195: 231 - 234

5. Russell D.G., Ziewacz J.T.: Pressures in a simulated breast subjected to compression forces comparable to those of mammography. Radiology, 1995; 194: 383-387

6. Buckley J.H., Roebuck E.J.: Mammographic changes following radiotherapy. Br. J. Radiol., 1986; 59: 337 - 344

7. Dershaw D.D., Shank B., Reisinger S.: Mammographic findings after breast cancer treatment with local excision and definitive irradiation. Radiology, 1987; 164: 455-461

8. Stomper P.C., Van Voorhis B.J., Ravnikar V.A., Meyer J.E.: Mammographic changes associated with postmenopausal hormone replacement therapy: a longitudinal study. Radiology, 1990; 174: 487-490

9. Newstead G.M., Baute P.B., Toth H.K.: Invasive lobular and ductal carcinoma: mammographic findings and stage at diagnosis. Radiology, 1992; 184: 623-627

10. Hilleren D.J., Andersson I.T., Lindholm K., Linnell F.S.: Invasive lobular carcinoma: mammographic findings in a 10-year experience. Radiology, 1991; 178: 149-154

11. Ikeda D.M., Andersson I.: Ductal carcinoma in situ: Atypical mammographic appearances. Radiology 1989; 172: 661-666

12. Klein D.L., Sickles E.A.: Effects of Needle aspiration on the mammographic appearance of the breast : A guide to the proper timing of the mammography examination. Radiology, 1982; 145: 44

13. Hann L.E., Liberman L., Dershaw D.D., Cohen M.A., Abramson A.F.: Mammography immediately after stereotaxic breast biopsy: is it necessary? Am. J. Roentgenol., 1995; 165: 59-62

14. Bassett L.W., Gold R.H., Cove H.C.: Mammographic spectrum of traumatic fat necrosis. Am. J. Roentgenol., 1978; 130: 119-122

15. Wallis M.G., Devakumar R., Hosie K.B., James K.A., Bishop H.M.: Complex sclerosing lesions (radial scars) of the breast can be palpable. Clin. Radiol. 1993; 48: 319-320

16. Sickles E.A.: The subtle and atypical mammographic features of invasive lobular carcinoma. Radiology 1991; 178: 25-26

17. Cornford E.J., Wilson A.R., Athanassiou E., Galea M., Ellis I.O., Elston C.W., Blamey R.W.: Mammographic features of invasive lobular and invasive ductal carcinoma of the breast: a comparative analysis. Br. J. Radiol., 1995; 68: 450-453

18. Sadler G.P., McGee S., Dollimore N.S., Monypenny I.J., Douglas-Jones A.G., Lyons K., Horgan K.: Role of fine-needle aspiration cytology and needle-core biopsy in the diagnosis of lobular carcinoma of the breast. Br. J. Surg., 1994; 81(9): 1315-7

19. Dershaw D.D.: Mammography in patients with breast cancer treated by breast conservation (Lumpectomy with or without radiation). Am. J. Roentgenol., 1995; 164: 309-316

20. Libshitz H.L., Montague E.D., Paulus D.D.: Calcifications and the therapeutically irradiated breast. Am. J. Roentgenol., 1977; 128: 1021-1025

21. Rebner M., Pennes D.R., Adler D.D., Helvie M.A., Lichter A.S.: Breast microcalcifications after lumpectomy and radiation therapy. Radiology, 1989; 170: 691-193

Ultrasound in the diagnosis of small breast carcinomas

E. Moskovic

Introduction

Whilst mammography is the primary diagnostic tool for breast screening in the general population, high resolution breast ultrasound has become an invaluable adjunct for assessment and is now used widely in breast diagnostic units, surgical outpatient clinics, and in general radiology departments. The advantages of ultrasound are its safety, speed, cost-effectiveness and role in diagnostic biopsy/aspiration. It is used increasingly to solve problems in younger women in whom mammography is either not indicated or is not interpretable due to breast density. Most breast radiologists and indeed many surgeons are now skilled in breast ultrasound as well as mammography and this multimodality approach to the diagnosis of breast cancer can only be advantageous to the patient. The assistance of a high quality rapid cytology service is vital to the success of any breast ultrasound department; those of us who have access to such a facility appreciate it daily.

Ultrasound technology and equipment

Essentially, high frequency sound waves are emitted continuously by a hand-held transducer resting on the skin surface following application of acoustic coupling gel spread over the breast to reduce impedance created by intervening air. Sound waves emitted pass through the breast and are bounced off the various layers of soft tissue within it. Reflected sound waves are received back again by the transducer at varying frequencies according to the reflectivity or echogenicity of the tissues through which they pass. A computer assigns a visual grey scale to the frequencies obtained and constructs a "real time" picture providing a moving image on the ultrasound screen as the transducer is moved over the skin (Fig. 1). For breast work, probe frequencies of 5-8 MHz

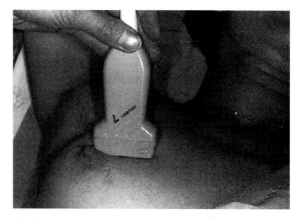

Fig. 1. High resolution ultrasound transducer placed on breast.

are used, which allows good tissue penetration of approximately 7-10 cm from the skin surface (adequate for most breast and small part work) whilst providing excellent spatial resolution in the near field.[1] Since the recent exploitation of the Doppler shift effect, velocity of blood flow in small vessels within the soft tissues can be detected using ultrasound and the vascularity of breast masses can be assessed. Neovascularity (angiogenesis) is a feature of carcinomas, and the presence of increased Doppler signals within or around a breast mass makes the diagnosis of malignancy more likely.[2,3]

Ultrasound in breast diagnosis: cystic and solid lesions

The chief role of ultrasound in the diagnosis of breast disease is the differentiation of a cystic from a solid mass. If a mass is detected on mammography, certain features may suggest a simple cyst (smooth circular contour, multiplicity) but X-ray mammography cannot be definitive since for example a low-grade carcinoma may also be well defined and circu-

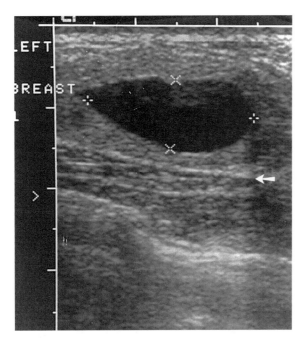

Fig. 2. Ultrasound of simple breast cyst with typical "brightup" band of sound behind it (arrow).

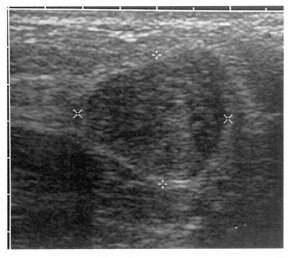

Fig. 3. Ultrasound of fibroadenoma: a solid homogeneous well circumscribed mass.

lar in shape. Because of the rapid transmission (low impedance) of sound waves through fluid, cysts are easily recognised on ultrasound as well marginated echo-free, rounded or oval lesions with a characteristic band of posterior echo enhancement. Typically, a cyst will appear as a "black hole" on the ultrasound image (Fig. 2). Sometimes a cyst contains internal debris which is seen as internal echoes within it: this can occasionally cause confusion with a solid lesion although circular contour, and through-transmission of sound, can often resolve this. A solid, non-cystic

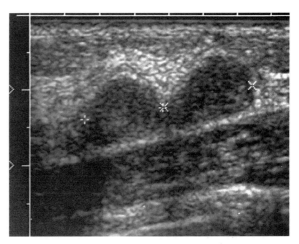

Fig. 4. Ultrasound of a lobulated/bilobed fibroadenoma.

mass attenuates sound waves and therefore will produce an image containing echoes, the appearance of which vary according to its nature. For example, a common benign solid lesion is the fibroadenoma which on ultrasound appears as a smooth, usually oval or lobulated mass which has uniform internal echoes and is of low vascularity (Figs. 3-4). Features of breast carcinoma on ultrasound include an irregular margin, strong attenuation of sound waves causing shadowing behind the lesion, disruption of surrounding tissue planes, and an increase in vascularity on Doppler. Inhomogeneity of internal echo texture in malignant masses is due to the presence of fibrosis, necrosis and calcification (Figs. 5-6).

All the features of benign and malignant breast masses described above are more obvious when the mass is large. A small breast carcinoma (less than 1 cm) may mimic a fibroadenoma especially if it is well differentiated *i.e.* low-grade and similarly a benign solid lesion can have sonographically suspicious features. The advantage of ultrasound in these circumstances is that, it lends itself easily to guided fine needle aspiration (FNA), which can be performed on the spot in most centres.

Ultrasound and breast screening

The main limitation of ultrasound in relation to early breast cancer diagnosis is that it is relatively poor at detecting fine calcification, since the density of calcium provides an interface which is "opaque" to sound waves at this frequency. Thus calcified or ductal tumours such as DCIS which have no soft tissue or invasive component are better shown by mammography and ultrasound is not used as a primary screening technique. It should be said how-

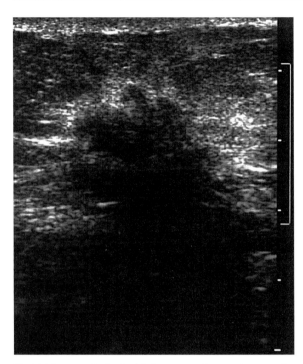

Fig. 5. Ultrasound of palpable breast carcinoma; the mass is irregular, heterogeneous and impedes sound waves posteriorly.

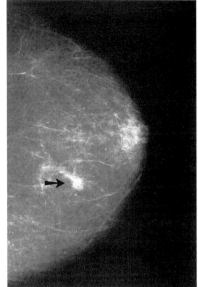

Fig. 7. Screen detected breast carcinoma; craniocaudal mammogram showing small, non-palpable mass.

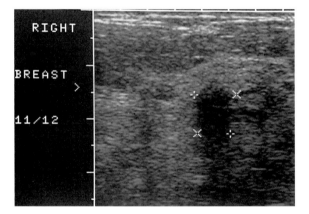

Fig. 6. Ultrasound of small, non-palpable breast carcinoma; the mass is irregular, of low-attenuation and measures less than 1 cm.

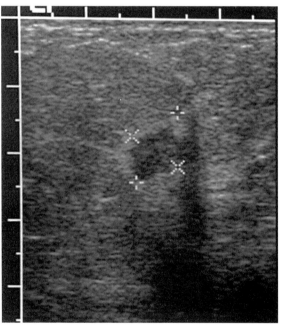

Fig. 8. Breast ultrasound of patient in Figure 7: small irregular carcinoma measuring 7 mm.

ever, that if a mammographically screen detected calcified tumour is carefully sought using ultrasound, it can normally be found, however small (Figs. 7-8).

As described, mammography is used as the primary diagnostic test in the screening population (50-65 years) and ultrasound in this cohort is used mainly to characterize masses seen on the screening mammogram and, when appropriate, to guide FNA. The benefits of obtaining accurate cytology from a non-palpable screen detected lesion without resorting to

formal biopsy are undisputed and include speed of diagnosis, lack of subsequent breast scarring and deformity, which can make future imaging difficult to interpret, and of course, low cost. In the case of a small X-ray detected breast carcinoma ultrasound can be used both to confirm the diagnosis cytologically, and if suitable, for subsequent wire localisation.[4-6] Sensitivity and specificity for ultrasound-

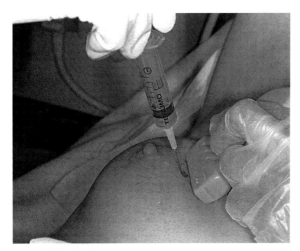

Fig. 9. Ultrasound-guided FNAC; the needle is inserted into the breast directly into the path of the beam of sound emanating from the transducer.

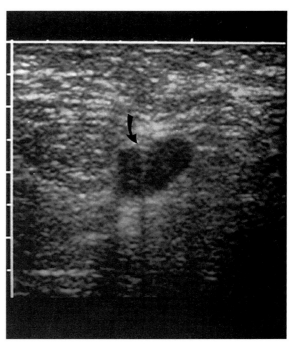

Fig. 11. Ultrasound showing indentation of the surface of the mass in Figure 10 by aspiration needle (arrowed).

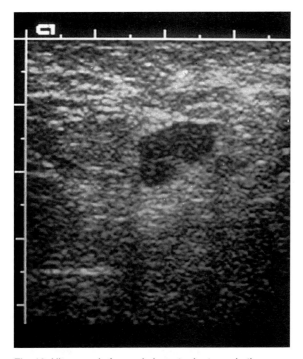

Fig. 10. Ultrasound of mass in breast prior to aspiration.

guided procedures are extremely high and in experienced hands, ultrasound-guided aspiration and localisation is at least as accurate and generally faster than mammographically-guided techniques. In particular, wire localisation using ultrasound guidance is far less traumatic for the patient since breast compression is not required and time is not spent waiting for films to be processed whilst the breast is both compressed and transfixed by a needle. If required, con-

firmation of the position of the wire tip after ultrasound-guided localisation can always be undertaken using mammography.

Technique of ultrasound-guided aspiration

Ultrasound is a highly effective method of guiding successful FNA in small breast cancers, i.e. masses well under 1 cm.[1,4,7] There is without doubt a "learning curve" for mastering this technique, requiring both training and practice but this is usually overcome particularly if there is regular communication with and feedback from the cytopathologist.

Various techniques have been described, and most operators develop their own hybrid. I shall describe the technique used at the Royal Marsden Hospital which in our experience is fast, accurate and non-traumatic. The vast majority of diagnoses in breast disease can be made with cytology alone since a result positive for malignancy is sufficient to plan surgery especially if the lesion is small and non-palpable. Our practice is to have one person assisting the procedure by scanning and locating the lesion, with the operator free to use both hands to manoeuvre the needle and apply suction to the syringe. It has not been found necessary in our practice to use commercially available needle guides attached to the ultrasound transducer. The patient has consented following explanation, and the lesion to be aspirated

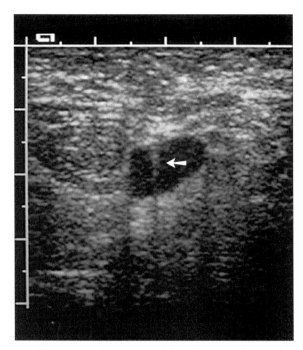

Fig. 12. The needle is passed into the mass for suction producing a shadow of the needle shaft which is easily visualised (white arrow).

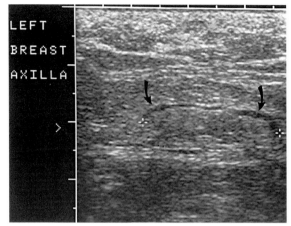

Fig. 13. Ultrasound of large, impalpable, benign, fatty axillary lymph node. The node is oval and mostly replaced by echogenic fat which is of similar reflectivity as the surrounding axillary fat. It has a thin rim of normal low-attenuation lymphoid tissue (arrowed)

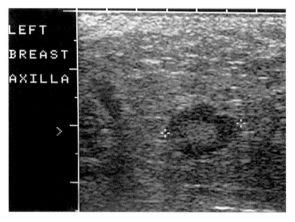

Fig. 14. Ultrasound of small (<1 cm) impalpable but abnormal axillary node. It is more irregular and circular in contour than Figure 13 and has little central fat and more peripheral lymphoid tissue. This node was aspirated using ultrasound guidance and contained metastatic carcinoma.

is located using ultrasound with the patient positioned so that the shortest distance lies between the skin surface and the mass. This often requires the patient to lie in the lateral decubitus or oblique position if the lesion lies laterally within the breast. The transducer is sterilised with an appropriate cleaning solution, and sterile acoustic coupling gel is also used. The surface marking of the underlying lesion is inked on the skin and 2 ml of 2% lignocaine is infiltrated subcutaneously into that area. It is my experience that the use of local anaesthetic is preferable, since it improves patient confidence and permits repeated needle passage if necessary without pain. It also allows the use of a wide bore 19 gauge needle for aspiration thereby improving the chances of a more cellular smear. For almost all aspirates our choice of fine needle is a simple 19 gauge hypodermic needle, universally available and inexpensive. It can be easily visualised with ultrasound due to the sharp reflecting needle bevel, air within the lumen and movement of the needle itself. For aspiration of a small solid lesion a 5 ml syringe is used; if the lesion is deep a 10 ml syringe may be required to obtain good suction; larger syringes are cumbersome and do not enhance the outcome. To facilitate expulsion of the contents of the syringe after aspiration, it helps in advance to withdraw the syringe plunger by about 1 ml prior to attaching the needle and inserting it. The assistant places the transducer slightly obliquely to

the skin surface, with the lesion to be aspirated lying in the midline of the scan so that the operator can insert the needle vertically into it under direct vision (Fig. 9). Once the needle tip is seen within the mass, the operator simultaneously applies maximum suction to the plunger whilst moving the needle to and fro and angling it in a fanlike fashion throughout the mass, observing the screen all the while so that the needle tip does not exit the region of interest (Figs. 10-12). Suction on the syringe is terminated before the needle is withdrawn from the mass, so that the contents of the needle lumen and syringe are not contaminated by normal overlying tissue or blood. The contents of the syringe and needle are discharged onto a series of dry microscopic slides and smeared so that their adequacy can be assessed. We have not found it necessary to have the cytopathologist on hand to assess the sample obtained; with practice the operator is able to judge the adequacy of a cytological sample; the usual reason for failure in our experience is that of inadequate suction on the syringe whilst moving the needle in a controlled manner. Lesions which are technically hard to aspirate successfully include fibro-adenomas, scarred or irradiated tissue and lesions near vital structures such as the chest wall or a breast prosthesis. However, with practice all of these can be sampled satisfactorily. If in doubt, it is far better to repeat the whole manoeuvre a second or even third time if required, rather than waste time bringing the patient back for a further attempt. The slides are either air dried or fixed with spray according to the preference of the cytology department. The syringe and needle are then washed with 5 ml of normal saline and the contents sent in a sterile bottle along with the slides.

Simple pressure followed by a small plaster applied to the aspiration site is all that is needed after the procedure, which is tolerated well in all circumstances. Intercurrent medication with Warfarin is not a contra-indication to FNA; a 20 or 21 gauge needle may be preferred in this circumstance, and pressure on the skin for a full 5 minutes after the procedure is advisable.

Large-core needle biopsy can also be guided with ultrasound using spring-loaded automatic biopsy devices (*e.g.*: Biopty gun, Bard Urological, Covington, GA); this is usually reserved for larger, palpable tumours in which information about the histological grade is required, or in patients in whom primary chemotherapy is the planned treatment.

Ultrasound assessment of regional nodes

No diagnostic imaging modality including ultrasound has yet been able to identify tumour metastasis in normal sized axillary nodes with accuracy but the axilla is always interrogated as part of an ultrasound scan of the breast whether for suspected benign or malignant breast disease.

Ultrasound with guided FNA of lymph nodes can be important in making management decisions in exceptional circumstances if the need for an axillary dissection is in doubt. In early breast cancer, nodes are usually normal with less than 20% of stage 1 tumours under 2 cm having axillary metastases. If the axilla is clinically normal, ultrasound will always identify small lymph nodes but their pathological significance if normal in size and shape on ultrasound criteria cannot be ascertained since the presence of microscopic metastatic disease is beyond the resolution of the scan. However, two recent studies have shown that incorporating colour Doppler scanning of axillary nodes improves detection rate of metastatic disease with sensitivies of 70-75% for involvement and specificity of 98-100%, yielding a positive predictive value of 96-100%.[8,9] As a general rule, certain sonographic features of nodes may be considered normal and abnormal. A normal axillary node is oval in shape, contains echogenic hilar fat and has a rim of more sonolucent lymphoid tissue. Benign nodes are usually small (less than 1 cm) but may attain larger sizes up to 2 cm perhaps due to chronic breast inflammation (Fig. 13).

Pathological nodes are always visible on ultrasound if palpable, and have certain characteristic features. They are often multiple, round rather than oval, are echo-poor and have little or no hilar fat, the lymphoid tissue and fat having been destroyed by tumour. They are usually vascular and are not usually tender whereas reactive nodes tend to be sensitive to pressure[1] (Fig. 14). Other areas of nodal involvement such as the infra- and supraclavicular regions can easily be examined and needled using ultrasound if appropriate; however metastases to these sites are very uncommon in early breast cancer. The other important main route of lymphatic spread, the internal mammary chain, is less accessible to ultrasound although careful scanning of the intercostal parasternal spaces may sometimes reveal an enlarged node.

References

1. Tohno E., Cosgrove D.O., Sloane J.P.: Ultrasound Diagnosis of Breast Diseases, Edinburgh, Churchill Livingston, 1994
2. Cosgrove D.O., Kedar R.P., Bamber J.C., Al-Murrani B., Davey J.B.N., Fisher C. *et al.*: Breast diseases: color Doppler US in differential diagnosis. Radiology, 1993; 189: 99-104
3. Holcombe C., Pugh N., Lyons K., Douglas-Jones A., Mansel R.E., Horgan K.: Blood flow in breast cancer and fibroadenoma estimated by colour Doppler ultrasonography. Br. J. Surg., 1995; 82 (6): 787-788
4. Fornage B.D., Coan J.D., David C.L.: Ultrasound-guided needle biopsy of the breast and other interventional procedures. Radiologic Clinic North Am., 1992; 30(1): 167-185
5. Sneige N., Fornage B.D., Saleh G.: Ultrasound-guided fine needle aspiration of non-palpable breast lesions: cytologic and histologic findings. Am. J. Clin. Pathol., 1994, 102 (1): 98-101
6. Rissanen T.J., Makarainen H.P., Mattila S.I., Karttunen A.I., Kiviniemi H.O., Kallionen M.J., Kaarela O.I.: Wire localised biopsy of breast lesions: a review of 425 cases found in screening or clinical mammography. Clin. Radiol., 1993; 47 (1): 14-22
7. Schiller V.L., Gurfinkel F., Wolke J., Kushwaha D.: Ultrasound diagnosis of mammographically occult minimal carcinoma of the breast. J. Diagn. Med. Sonog., 1995; 11: 3
8. Dixon J.M., Walsh J., Paterson D., Chetty U.: Colour Doppler studies of benign and malignant breast lesions. Br. J. Surg., 1992; 79 (3): 259-260
9. Walsh J.S., Dixon J.M., Chetty U., Patterson D.: Colour Doppler studies of axillary node metastases in breast carcinoma. Clin. Radiol., 1994; 49 (3): 189-191

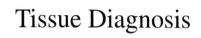
Tissue Diagnosis

Fine needle aspiration cytology

J.G. McKenzie, J. Dalrymple

Introduction

The use of fine needle aspiration cytology (FNAC) in the diagnosis of palpable breast lesions is well established and has superceded the need for diagnostic biopsy with frozen section in most cases. The relative merits of the two techniques were described by Trott and Randall in 1979 and are shown in Table I.[1] Following the Forrest report which recommended the use of FNAC in the triple approach for the assessment of screen detected lesions its use has become widespread in Assessment Centres where experienced cytopathologists are in post.[2]

In this unit, following ten years of experience of FNAC work on palpable lesions, this technique has been used in the screening programme which started in 1987. FNAC has been accepted as a valuable diagnostic aid which is cost-effective and has enabled the planning of surgical treatment in advance, with appropriate counselling of the patient.

There is continuing debate about who should undertake the aspiration, surgeon, radiologist or pathologist, but in the final analysis the quality of the aspirate is all important and obviously reflects the expertise of the aspirator. The cytopathologist can only report on the material present on the slide. It is important to remember that a positive result is of significance whereas a negative one may not be so. The reasons for this will be discussed later in the chapter.

For cytology to be of benefit in the Breast Screening Programme the inadequate rate and benign biopsy rate must be as low as possible. Inadequate aspirates usually need to be repeated, adding to the cost and causing unnecessary patient anxiety. Benign biopsies add to the surgical cost, cause anxiety and trauma to the patient and may affect the appearance of future mammograms.

In this unit the cytological opinion is considered as part of the triple approach in the assessment of screen detected lesions, and weekly multidisciplinary meetings are held where the relevant findings can be reviewed and discussed.

Preparation of material and staining

The aspirate is either directly smeared on slides or put in saline and cytospin preparations made. The latter are not used in this unit as the cytospin preparation appears to alter the 'architecture' of the aspirate which may be helpful in the interpretation of the smear. In addition they are expensive in technical time.

Table I. Merits of fine needle aspiration cytology and surgical biopsy.[1]

	Surgical biopsy	Fine needle aspiration cytology
Diagnosis	Histopathological	Cytopathological
Diagnostic facility	Narrow	Broad
Anaesthetic	Yes	No
Length of procedure	More than 5 minutes	Less than 5 minutes
Report	Long (1-2 days)	Short ($\frac{1}{2}$ hour if necessary, reduces patient anxiety)
False positives	None	Rare
False negatives	Few	Some
Cost	High	Low
Specimen obtained	In operating theatre	As outpatient anywhere
Trauma	Yes	Little, if any

This department prefers two direct smears from each case, one air dried and one fixed specimen. It is essential that fixation should be immediate and air drying be facilitated by gently waving the slide in the air, thus preserving cellular material and minimising artefact. All slides are labelled with the patient's name and number and are carefully matched with the request form. The fixed slide is stained with Haematoxylin and Eosin (H & E) and the air dried slide with May Grunwald Giemsa using automatic staining machines. Other centres use the Papanicolau stain rather than an H & E stain and it is a matter of personal preference which stains are employed. We feel that as the majority of breast carcinomas are of glandular origin an H & E stain is preferable and cytological appearances easily compared with subsequent histology. The use of the Giemsa and H & E stains is helpful and the appearances are complementary. The air drying process results in enlargement of cells but cellular detail and in particular nuclear detail is preserved, critical in the evaluation of whether an aspirate is malignant. Wet fixation results in reduction in cell size but minimizes artefact and cellular preservation is good. Some centres offer instant reporting in the assessment clinic. This unit is a busy district hospital pathology department and it has not been possible to offer this facility on a regular basis due to restricted technical and medical time, although a quick technical and medical result in approximately half an hour can be given if requested by the clinician in a specific case. Slides are double screened by two pathologists and reported without prior knowledge of the radiological appearance to avoid bias. Whilst obviously positive or negative reports are straightforward there are a significant proportion of aspirates from impalpable lesions that need careful, quiet consideration and discussion. In our opinion the additional pressure for instant results makes the reporting of these latter cases particularly difficult and will increase the number of unhelpful and possibly incorrect reports. Technical staff who undertake the staining of the aspirates are encouraged to look at cases, after reporting, and there are several in this department who are able to offer a valuable opinion. This is important in maintaining the level of interest in the service.

General diagnostic patterns

The criteria used for distinguishing between a benign and malignant aspirate are given in Table II. A wide range of histological appearances is seen in the breast and this is reflected in the cytological appearances. Some of the more difficult diagnostic categories and their cytological appearances are described in more detail later.

Reporting categories

The Marsden grading is used in this unit:

C1 Inadequate

C2 Benign

C3 Suspicious probably benign

C4 Suspicious probably malignant

C5 Malignant

The C1, C2 & C5 categories are relatively straight-forward diagnostic groups, however the C3 & C4 categories are the most difficult for the cytopathologist to interpret. These categories in particular require careful discussion at the multidisciplinary meetings where the radiological, cytological and clinical appearances are considered together and appropriate action taken. The C3 category is a particularly difficult grade and we would prefer the description "*Atypical probably benign*".

Aspirates obtained from palpable lesions are usually representative of that lesion with a relatively uniform population. Aspirates from impalpable lesions may include cells through which the needle has passed and therefore a dual population of both benign and malignant cells in a single aspirate is not uncommon. This makes reporting more difficult.

Many mammographic abnormalities show microcalcification of both benign and malignant type. The absence of microcalcification in the aspirate from such a site may be significant and indicate that the needle is not in the lesion. It is our aim to provide a useful result wherever possible giving a definitive diagnosis of malignancy or benignity with the object of keeping the benign biopsy ratio to a minimum.

C1 Inadequate

An aspirate may be inadequate for a variety of reasons:
a. Poor cellularity with less than five epithelial cell clusters.
b. Artefacts making interpretation difficult. These include heavily bloodstained smears, thick smears or unevenly spread smears, air drying artefact and artefact due to vigorous spreading. The reason for inadequacy must always be stated in the report.

C2 Benign (Figs. 1-5)

The components of a benign aspirate include:
a. Bare nuclei (bipolar cells or myo-epithelial cells);

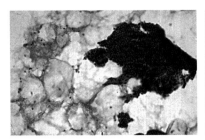

Fig. 1. H.E.×20. Monolayered sheet of cohesive, uniform benign epithelial cells including apocrine cells. Background bare nuclei.

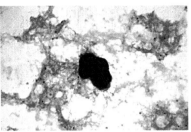

Fig. 2. H.E.×20. Cluster of benign epithelial cells with microcalcification. Background bare nuclei.

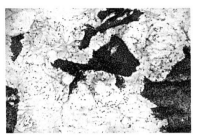

Fig. 3. H.E.×20. Fibro-adenoma – papillary monolayered fragment, abundant background bare nuclei.

b. Stromal fragments;
c. Cohesive clusters of uniform epithelial cells with benign cytological features.

If the aspirate is from an area of breast tissue showing benign fibrocystic change then the aspirate may also show:

a. some background debris with foamy macrophages;
b. apocrine cells: apocrine cells may show cytological atypia with variably sized nuclei and prominent central nucleoli with some cell dispersion. The recognition of cytoplasmic granularity and staining characteristics, slate blue on Giemsa and red on H & E should identify the cell type.

Table II. General diagnostic criteria for the recognition of benign and malignant conditions.[3]

Criterion	Benign	Malignant
Cellularity	Usually poor or moderate	Usually high
Cell to cell cohesion	Good with large defined clusters of cells	Poor with cell separation resulting in dissociated cells with cytoplasm or small groups of intact cells.
Cell arrangement	Even, usually in flat sheets (monolayers)	Irregular with overlapping and three-dimensional arrangement
Cell types	Mixtures of epithelial, myo-epithelial and other cells with fragments of stroma	Usually uniform cell population
Bipolar (elliptical) bare nuclei	Present, often in high numbers	Not conspicuous
Background	Generally clean except in inflammatory conditions	Occasionally necrotic debris and sometimes inflammatory cells including macrophages
Nuclear characteristics		
Size (in relation to RBC diameter)	Small	Variable, often large depending on type of tumour
Pleomorphism	Rare	Common
Nuclear membranes (PAP stain)	Smooth	Irregular with indentations
Nucleoli (PAP stain)	Indistinct or small and single	Variable but may be prominent, large and multiple
Chromatin (PAP stain)	Smooth or fine	Clumped and may be irregular
Additional features	Apocrine metaplasia, foamy macrophages	Mucin, intracytoplasmic lumina

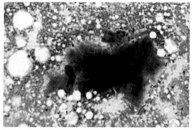

Fig. 4. Giemsa ×40. Fibroadenoma- myxo- id stroma.

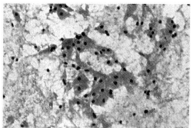

Fig. 5. H.E. ×20. Granular cell tumour- groups and single epithelial cells with eosi- nophilic granular cytoplasm and indistinct cell borders.

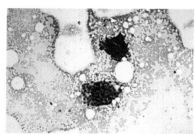

Fig. 6. Giemsa ×20. 'C3' – Upper cluster shows nuclear enlargement but normal chromatin pattern, scanty background bare nuclei.

Other features may also be seen in the aspirate if it is from a discrete entity such as a fibroadenoma; c) microcalcification.

C3 Atypical probably benign (Figs. 6-8)

This is perhaps the least helpful category for the radiologist/surgeon but it is nevertheless on occasion necessary to report smears as such and it is our aim to keep this category to a minimum. The aspirate will show benign features but, in addition may also show the following:
a. increased cellularity;
b. nuclear cytological atypia with nuclear irregular- ity, overlapping and nuclear enlargement;
c. some loss of cohesion with dispersion;
d. only scanty 'bare' bipolar nuclei;
e. changes due to treatment or hormonal effect, e.g. HRT, irradiation or even pregnancy.

It appears that aspirates from breast tissue show- ing epithelial hyperplasia often show the above fea- tures and it has to be accepted that this is a 'grey area' for the pathologist and the limitations of cytology in this area become apparent. It may be that with time and experience we may learn to recognise

particular cytological appearances for this diagnostic group.

C4 Suspicious of malignancy (Figs. 9-11)

The aspirate though suspicious is not diagnostic of malignancy. This may be for a variety of reasons.
a. A scanty specimen showing malignant features.
b. Artefactual changes due to poor preservation or preparation making a definite opinion difficult.
c. An aspirate with a predominantly benign pattern but with very occasional malignant cells.
d. Aspirates from well differentiated carcinomas, e.g. tubular and lobular where the epithelial cells are small and relatively uniform and cytological atypia is not marked.

C5 Malignant (Figs. 12-18)

The aspirate shows the cytological features of malignancy (see Table II). Malignant cells should be present in significant numbers. It is important to appreciate that in our experience it is not possible to distinguish between in situ and invasive lesions. Some pathologists have reported that malignant cells seen in stromal fragments indicate invasion. In our

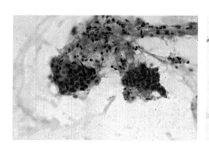

Fig. 7. H.E. ×20. 'C3' – 2 epithelial groups, one cluster showing nuclear enlargement but normal chromatin pattern.

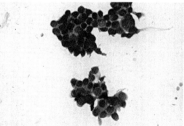

Fig. 8. Giemsa ×40. 'C3' – Clusters show variation in nuclear size and shape but normal chromatin pattern.

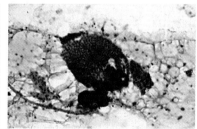

Fig. 9. H.E. ×20. 'C4' – Dual population with a predominence of benign epithelial cells. A small cluster of larger epithelial cells with suspicious nuclear characteris- tics. Dirty background with scanty bare nuclei.

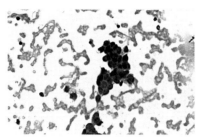

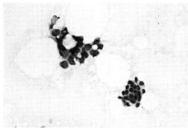

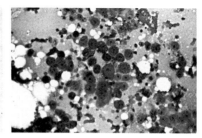

Fig. 10. Giemsa ×40.'C4' – Large epithelial cells with some dissociation. Nuclear atypia but cells not clearly malignant.

Fig. 11. Giemsa ×40. 'C4' – Larger cluster shows highly suspicious features but poor preservation.

Fig. 12. Giemsa ×40. 'C5' - large dissociated malignant cells with prominent nuclear cytological atypia, nucleoli and mitotic figures.

opinion this is not reliable. In many aspirates from malignant tumours of the breast, stroma is scanty and sometimes even absent.

In the reporting of malignant aspirates some helpful suggestions can be made with regard to the particular type of cancer.

However it is important to remember that the aspirate may not be representative of the entire lesion and mixed tumours do occur:

a. an assessment of cell size may indicate whether the tumour is of large cell or small cell type;
b. the arrangement of cells in tubular or 'Indian file' profiles suggests tubular or lobular differentiation;
c. the presence of abundant mucin is suggestive of colloid carcinoma;
d. abundant lymphocytes associated with large pleomorphic epithelial tumour cells suggests a medullary carcinoma (Figs. 19-20). Lymphocytes may also be seen in association with other tumour types.

At present this unit does not apply formal grading systems to cytological samples, however well differentiated and poorly differentiated features are commented on.

Immunocytochemical techniques are not routinely performed but are at present used as a research tool.

Diagnostic difficulties leading to a potentially false positive result

There are a number of conditions which make the reporting of aspirates difficult and must always be remembered when reporting.

'Hyperplasia'

It is our experience that one of the most difficult areas is in the interpretation of aspirates from hyperplastic lesions. The aspirates invariably are responsible for the C3 category and occasionally C4. False positive diagnosis can be avoided if the strict diagnostic criteria are adhered to.

It is particularly important to discuss these cases carefully with the surgeon and radiologist. These lesions are one of the major causes of benign diagnostic surgical biopsies.

Fibroadenoma

The interpretation of aspirates from fibroadenomas can be difficult. They are usually extremely cellular with some cell dispersion and cytological atypia but the presence of abundant bare bipolar nuclei and myxoid stroma should avoid a false positive diagnosis.

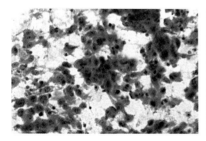

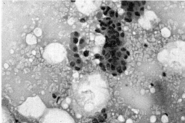

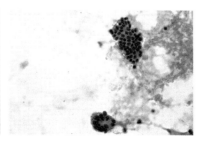

Fig. 13. H.E. ×40. 'C5' - large dissociated malignant cells with prominent nuclear cytological atypia, nucleoli and mitotic figures. Small cell carcinoma.

Fig. 14. H.E. ×40. Epithelial cells show dispersion with Indian file formation.

Fig. 15. H.E. ×20.Tubule formation.

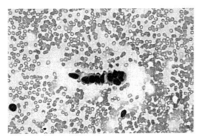

Fig. 16. Giemsa ×40. Indian file with moulding of cells.

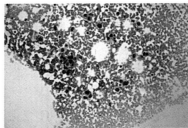

Fig. 17. Giemsa ×20. Dissociated small epithelial cells.

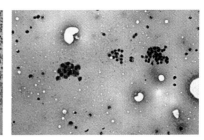

Fig. 18. Giemsa ×20. Dissociated small epithelial cells with intracytoplasmic vacuoles. Medullary carcinoma.

Papillary tumours

Aspirates from intraductal papillomas can be very cellular with papillary aggregates and can be difficult to distinguish from *in situ* and invasive papillary carcinoma. The presence of bare nuclei strongly suggests benign papilloma, while nuclear pleomorphism, necrosis, the absence of bare nuclei and apocrine cells favour a malignant diagnosis.

Apocrine cells

These can show a variable appearance particularly in hyperplastic lesions and complex sclerosing lesions/radial scars. It may not always be obvious that the cells are of apocrine origin.

Granular cell tumours

These lesions are composed of cells with indistinct cell membranes with prominent granular cytoplasm which is eosinophilic on the H & E preparation.

The nuclei can be variable in size and show some nuclear atypia. Positivity with an S100 immunohistochemical stain and PAS positivity confirm the diagnosis.

Adenomyoepithelial lesions (Fig. 21)

These lesions are uncommon and as yet incom-

pletely understood. Aspirates from these lesions can show suspicious features with high cellularity, a tendency to dispersion of rather pleomorphic cells which are actually myoepithelial. Obvious benign epithelial cell clusters and normal bare bipolar nuclei are also present.

Radiotherapy

Aspirates from breast tissue which has been irradiated are usually of low cellularity and can show prominent irradiation fibroblasts which can be mistaken for malignant cells. In addition epithelial cell changes occur, marked nuclear pleomorphism and dissociation can be present. Caution should always be taken when reporting such aspirates.

Diagnostic difficulties leading to a potentially false negative result

The commonest cause of a false negative result is when the needle is not in the lesion resulting in an aspiration miss. If the mammographic abnormality is microcalcification and this is not seen in the aspirate, it suggests that the needle may not be in the lesion and the aspirate may therefore not be representative of the abnormality. There are particular tumours which may produce a false negative result.

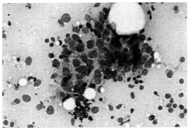

Fig. 19. H.E. ×40. Large malignant epithelial cells with associated lymphocytes.

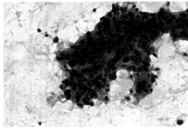

Fig. 20. Giemsa ×40. Large malignant epithelial cells with associated lymphocytes.

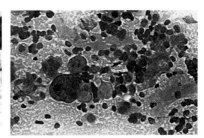

Fig. 21. Giemsa ×40. Globules of basement membrane material with dissociated myoepithelial cells and epithelial cells.

Well differentiated carcinomas (Figs. 14-18)

Tubular carcinomas, cribriform carcinomas and lobular carcinomas will by definition yield aspirates which show, on initial inspection, much in common with benign aspirates. Important features to look for include:
a. absence of bare nuclei;
b. individual cells and small groups with cytoplasm;
c. tubular profiles and 'Indian files';
d. intracytoplasmic lumina. (lobular carcinomas);
e. mild cytological atypia.

Such tumours may also result in a C3 or C4 diagnosis.

Sclerotic carcinomas

These tumours, by definition, have abundant fibrous stroma and therefore may yield either an acellular aspirate or stromal fragments only.

Table III. Cytology results in prevalence and incidence rounds.

	Prevalence Round (%)	Incidence Round (%)	Suggested Minimum Value
Absolute sensitivity	71.8	69.6	>60
Complete sensitivity	87.2	88.8	>80
Specificity (full)	74.7	78.3	>60
Positive predictive value (C5)	100.0	99.1	>95
False negative rate	6.2	3.1	<5
False positive rate	0.00	0.6	<1
Inadequate rate	12.6	8.0	<25

Table IV. Biopsy results 1987-1994.

Year	Benign (B)	Malignant (M)	Total	M/B Ratio
1987/8	24	50	74	2.0
1989	28	100	128	3.5
1990	21	106	127	5.0
1991	13	82	95	6.3
1992	13	60	73	4.6
1993	16	45	61	2.8
1994	5	42	47	8.4

Other lesions

Lymph nodes

It is always important to remember that intramammary lymph nodes are present within the breast and that they can be benign or malignant. The recognition of a lymphoid origin is important. It is also important to remember that some *in situ* and invasive carcinomas are associated with a lymphoid response, without necessarily being typical of a medullary carcinoma.

Metastatic carcinoma in lymph nodes may be the presenting feature of breast cancer when the primary tumour may be small and undetected. Lymph nodes can be almost entirely replaced by metastatic tumour and an aspirate may not show an obvious lymph node origin.

Primary lymphoma of the breast does occur as well as lymphomatous involvement. Clinical information is all important and immunocytochemistry will be helpful in such cases.

Metastatic tumours

Metastatic oat cell carcinoma (small cell carcinoma) of lung has been seen rarely in breast aspirates. Metastatic melanoma has also been reported and careful attention to the cytological appearance and pattern must be given, especially if melanin pigment is absent.

Other metastatic tumours have been reported such as ovarian and renal carcinomas.

Stromal lesions

Fibromatosis does occur in the breast and typical fibroblasts, spindle in shape with regular nuclei, are present in the aspirate. Malignant stromal tumours occur but are rare.

Metaplastic carcinomas would be more common and considered first in any aspirate showing sarcomatous features.

Phyllodes tumours

The benign variants will show cytological appearances similar to a fibroadenoma; however a clue to the diagnosis is an excess of bare bipolar nuclei, cellular stromal fragments with myxoid material.

Malignant variants will show benign epithelial cells with malignant characteristics in spindle-shaped cells.

Results

FNAC has been used in this unit since November 1987. Table III shows an analysis of the cytology results for the Prevalence Round (1987-1990) and an Incidence Round (1991-1993). The suggested minimum values shown are taken from the NHSBSP Publication.[3] It is reassuring to note that in comparing the prevalence and incidence round, the inadequate and false negative rates have improved and that sensitivity and specificity rates are well above recommended minimum values.

Table IV shows the biopsy results since 1987. The malignant to benign ratio illustrates the learning curve in the early years and emphasises the small number of benign biopsies since 1991.

Conclusion

The use of fine needle aspiration cytology has been shown to decrease the benign biopsy rate, to assist in the early diagnosis of breast cancer and to allow planned cost effective treatment in the Breast Screening Unit. In addition, for the patient, it reduces the number of operations and allows pre-treatment discussion and counselling.

References

1. Trott,P.A.: Fine needle aspiration cytology. The Lancet 2:253
2. The Forrest report 1986.
3. Guidelines for Cytology Procedures and reporting in Breast Cancer Screening. Cytology Sub-Group of the National Coordinating Committee for Breast Screening Pathology. NHSBSP Publication no.22. September 1992

Diagnostic biopsies

M.W.E. Morgan

One of the major morbidities of a screening programme is the number of diagnostic and benign biopsies carried out. Forrest[1] laid down recommendations in the NHS Breast Screening Programme that every effort should be made to reduce the number of unnecessary biopsies without compromising the cancer detection rate and increasing the number of interval cancers. Since the advent of the National Health Breast Screening Programme in the United Kingdom in 1987 an obvious increasing number of patients have been discovered with screen detected lesions that would require further investigations. These patients are acutely anxious and every effort should be made in the assessment clinic, with counselling, to allay their fears, for the psychological trauma produced by the diagnosis of breast cancer is well documented.[2] Improvement in screen detected breast cancer survival depends on early detection and definitive diagnosis.[3] Lack of specificity of mammography alone has meant an increase in the number of biopsies. Studies have shown that only about 10% of these are for malignant lesions.[4]

In non-palpable lesions mammography alone has only a 20% to 30% positive predictive value,[5,6] although studies have shown an improvement in the positive predictive value of various mammographic abnormalities following the assessment process. The assessment will include triple or quadruple assessment, i.e. clinical examination, further mammographic views, fine needle aspiration cytology or core biopsy with or without ultrasound.

In any screening programme benign biopsies are inevitable and the malignant to benign biopsy rate varies considerably.[4,5,6,7,8,9]

Tissue diagnosis of the breast can be carried out by one of four available techniques:
1. Fine needle aspiration cytology (FNAC);
2. Core breast biopsy (CBB);
3. Incisional biopsy;
4. Excisional biopsy.

Fine needle aspiration cytology

FNAC is a well tried and tested procedure that has been used for many years and was first popularized in Scandinavia,[10] although it has never achieved the same popularity in the United States. It is an effective, simple and cheap procedure to perform, relatively painless and therefore rarely requiring local anaesthesia. It is usually carried out in out-patients and has the advantage of instant definitive reporting thereby allowing planned treatment to be immediately discussed. Uncommon complications are usually haematoma and mastitis and rarely pneumothorax. FNAC is not a biopsy procedure because it does not provide a histological diagnosis but it is probably the best way to avoid unnecessary benign open biopsies.

It is however very operator dependent[11,12] with a high sensitivity rate of over 80% and a specificity of 89% to 100%.[11-13] A significant reduction in benign breast biopsies has been achieved in many breast units since the introduction of FNAC.[14] False negative rates vary between 3% and 9% and many are due to sampling errors, missing small lesions of less than 0.5 cm or specific histological types, e.g. tubular carcinomas and papillary carcinomas.[15,16] In impalpable lesions FNAC can be carried out either with stereotaxis or ultrasound, achieving the same diagnostic accuracy as that of palpable lesions.[17]

Core breast biopsy

As with FNAC, CBB may be performed with or without stereotaxis depending to a large extent on whether the lesion is palpable or not.

A variety of needles are available based on the Tru-cut principle of cutting a solid core of tissue sufficient for paraffin embedded histological examination.

Many of the needles have a spring-loaded or trigger firing system and, in some, suction is used to retrieve the specimens.[18] Diagnostic accuracy increases with the number of samples taken and three is usually sufficient. The optimum needle size 14 achieves the best results.[19,20] CBB cannot be performed without a local anaesthetic and with palpable lesions can be performed in out-patients. With impalpable lesions, however, a stereotactic method must be utilised and is usually performed with the patient sitting up but this is cumbersome and difficult both for the patient and the operator.[21]

More recently, specific prone mammogram stereotactic localisation tables have been developed (Mammotest Stereotactic System, Fischer Imaging, Denver, Colorado) in which the breast hangs free beneath the table allowing the operator easy access to carry out CBB. The cost of these tables however may preclude their general use in district general hospitals and would be best preserved for specialised breast units. Despite its advantage of obtaining histological material, some carcinomas can be missed[21,22] and if the tissue obtained by stereotactic core biopsy does not correlate with the mammographic abnormality excision biopsy is recommended. CBBs are routine for the diagnosis of microcalcification where the adequacy of sampling can be checked by immediate X-ray of the CBB and repeat sampling may be carried out if the mammogram fails to reveal areas of calcification.

Very recently the same specific prone mammogram stereotactic localisation tables developed for CBB have been upgraded to carry out stereotactic minimally invasive excision biopsies using 5, 10, 15 or 20 mm instruments and this procedure is carried out under local anaesthetic as an out patient. At present the experience with this very interesting technique is extremely limited but the very high cost of the equipment may preclude its general use.

Incisional biopsy

During this procedure a portion of the mass is excised usually under general anaesthesia although local anaesthetic may be used for smaller masses. It is usually performed when there is an index of suspicion either mammographically or cytologically that cannot be confirmed by both modalities. Common situations in which this would arise are:
1. widespread mixed calcification;
2. spiculated masses with benign cytology;
3. areas of increased density with atypical cytology;
4. where the CBB or FNAC does not correlate with the mammographic abnormality.

Excisional biopsy

This approach is frequently used for small localised lesions and again it can be carried out under local anaesthetic for superficial lesions or general anaesthetic for those lesions that are more deeply placed. It is recommended in a number of situations:
1. *Patient desire.* Despite counselling and reassurance a number of patients will not rest until a mammographic lesion has been removed.
2. *Lesion increasing in size* despite benign cytology, *e.g.* fibroadenoma.
3. *Radial scars.* Although a histological diagnosis, mammographically frequently mimic small invasive tumours.
4. *Small expanding lesions* in which the cytology may not be representative in view of their small size.
5. *Lesions radiologically and cytologically suspicious* without definite evidence of malignancy.

Operation

Prior to the operation, indeed ideally at the assessment visit, the patient will have been counselled to allay fear and explain the operative procedure and reassured that nothing more than the procedure for which she has consented will be carried out. On the day of the operation the patient must be examined by the operating surgeon and palpable lesions marked accurately. Impalpable lesions will have been localised with a guide wire either by stereotaxis or ultrasound or by measurement marking using the true lateral and cranio-caudal view and allowing the surgeon to place the needle at the point of surgical incision.

Occasionally two guide wires are used to mark the distal limits of more extensive lesions, thus allowing, after X-ray confirmation of the specimen, more adequate total excision of the abnormality. When in the operating theatre the current mammogram must be available and mounted on a viewing box in the operating theatre. This allows review of the mammogram during the operative procedure and when excision of the mammographic abnormality is carried out with X-ray confirmation of the specimen, a specimen X-ray mammogram may be compared for adequacy of excision.

When excising benign lesions within 5 cm of the areola, a peri-areolar incision not encompassing more than half the circumference of the areola will allow good access and the lesion is easily removed either with skin retraction or by tunnelling through the subcutaneous breast tissue and this usually results in an excellent scar.

When operating on any breast mass with a suspicion of malignancy one must always place the incision such that it would not compromise the incisions for a mastectomy which may be advised following the result of the diagnostic biopsy.

For lesions more than 5 cm from the areola or lesions with a suspicion of malignancy a curvi-linear incision over the mass and parallel to the areolar will allow good access and heal well. More peripheral lesions in the medial and lateral sixths are best approached via a radial incision for reasons mentioned above. Of particular difficulty are lesions inferior to the nipple close to the periphery of the breast. Better cosmetic results are sometimes obtained with these via a radial incision.

Biopsy excision technique

Excision of palpable lesion

The mass will have been marked pre-operatively. It is necessary to re-examine the breast on the unprepared patient in the operating theatre to reorientate oneself with the clinical picture. It is remarkable how difficult it can be to palpate the lump intraoperatively. With lumps that are difficult to feel it is sometimes helpful to insert a 21gauge hypodermic needle through the skin into the mass thereby fixing it and using this needle as an intra-operative guide.

The skin and subcutaneous tissue are incised and all bleeding points secured. The mass is palpated, the

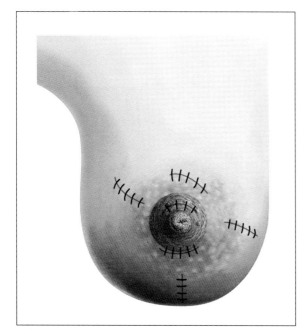

Fig 1. Acceptable incisions for breast biopsies.

extent assessed and the mass excised. Depending on the size of the residual cavity the breast tissue may be opposed with absorbable sutures and unless the cavity is very small all wounds are best drained for 24 hours.

Excision of impalpable lesion

The lesion will have been marked with a guide wire pre-operatively. An incision is made close to the guide wire, the subcutaneous tissue dissected and the guide wire delivered into the wound. A small self-retaining retractor is placed into the wound and the incision with a knife carried down into the breast tissue adjacent to the guide-wire until the lesion is reached. If there is a high degree of suspicion the lesion is excised together with a 1 cm clearance of normal breast tissue around the lesion. If the index of suspicion is low then simple excision alone is sufficient.

One should avoid using cutting diathermy as this frequently scars the margins and makes histological interpretation difficult and also if the diathermy touches the guide wire it will either melt or vaporise. Similarly scissors should be avoided as these can frequently cut through the guide-wire. The size of the residual cavity will dictate whether the breast tissue should be closed and whether the wound should be drained. The specimen removed from the patient is marked. Many methods have been described but the simplest is to place a nylon suture at the nipple end of the specimen and a silk suture at the skin surface of the specimen which is then sent for immediate X-ray to confirm that the mammographic abnormality has been removed. The specimen is then sent fresh without fixative to the pathology department.

Antibiotics

Antibiotics are rarely used in diagnostic biopsies although there may be clinical situations in which they are needed, *e.g.* diabetes, immuno-compromised patients, HIV, and concomitant use of steroids.

Day surgery

It is not good policy to admit to Day Surgery Units as this removes the patient from the team support that is so essential and it is unlikely that specimen X-rays will be available on Day Surgery Units. However, the operation may be performed as a day case within the Breast Unit environment.

Conclusions

In a Breast Screening Programme it is imperative to keep to a minimum the number of benign diagnostic open biopsies. These women would not have undergone a surgical procedure had it not been for the degree of suspicion generated by the screening process.

FNAC and CBB are acceptable diagnostic tools that over the years have proved their reliability and cost-effectiveness in avoiding unnecessary open biopsies. The very recent minimally invasive stereotactic radiological excision biopsy instruments are very much more expensive in comparison to FNAC and CBB. The solution is not to excise with minimally radiological tools all radiological lesions but to increase the sensitivity and specificity of the combination of mammography, ultrasound and cytology to reduce to virtually nil the number of benign biopsies.

References

1. Breast Cancer Screening: Report of the Health Ministers of England, Wales, Scotland & Northern Ireland by Working Group chaired by Professor Sir Patrick Forrest, DHSS, HMSO 1987
2. Ellman R., Angel N., Christians A., *et al.*: Psychiatric morbidity associated with screening for carcinoma. Br. J. Cancer, 1989; 60:781-784
3. Tabar L., Gadd A., Holmberg L.H., *et al.*: Reduction in the mortality from breast cancer after mass screening with mammogaphy: randomised trial from the breast cancer screening working group of the Swedish National Board of Health & Welfare. Lancet, 1985; 1: 829-832
4. Choucair R.J., Holcomb M.B., Matthews R., Hughes T.G.: Biopsy of non-palpable breast lesions. Am. J. Surg., 1988; 156: 453-456
5. Tinnemans J.G.M., Wobbes T., Hendricks J.H.C.L., *et al.*: Localisation and excision of non-palpable breast lesions: a surgical evaluation of three methods. Arch. Surg., 1987; 122: 802-806
6. Rissanen T.J., Makarainen H.D., Mattila S.J., *et al.*: Wire localised biopsy of breast lesions: A review of 425 cases found in screening or clinical mammography. Clin. Radiol., 1993; 47: 14-20
7. Burrell H.C., Pinder S.E., Wilson A.R.M., *et al.*: The positive predictive value of mammographic signs: A review of 425 non-palpable breast lesions. Clin. Radiol., 1996; 51: 277-281
8. Warren R.: Film reading and recall of patients. This volume, pp.61-63
9. Finlay M.E., Liston J.E., Lunt L.G., *et al.*: Assessment of the role of ultrasound in the differentiation of radial scars and stellate carcinomas of the breast. Clin. Radiol., 1994; 49: 52-55
10. Zajicek J.: Aspiration biopsy cytology, part 1: mammographs in clinical cytology. Basle: Karger, 1974
11. Dixon J.M., Anderson T.J., Lamb J., *et al.*: Fine needle aspiration cytology in relationship to clinical examination and mammography in the diagnosis of solid masses. Br. J. Surg., 1984; 71: 513-596
12. Vural G., Hagmar B., Lilleng R.: A one year audit of fine needle aspiration cytology of breast lesions. Factors affecting adequacy and a review of delayed carcinoma diagnosis. Acta. Cytol., 1995; 39: 2021-2025
13. Kline T.S.: Fine needle aspiration biopsy of the breast. Am. Fam. Physician, 1995; 52: 2021-2025
14. Green B., Dowley A., Turnbull L.S., Leinster S.J., Winstanley J.H.: Impact of fine needle aspiration cytology ultrasonography and mammography on biopsy rate in patients with benign breast disease. Br. J. Surg., 1995; 82: 1509-1511
15. Kreuzer G., Zajicek J.: Cytological diagnosis of mammary tumours from aspiration biopsy smears. Studies of 200 cases with false negative and doubtful cytological reports. Acta. Cytol., 1972; 16: 249-252
16. Wollenberg N.J., Caya J.B., Clowry L.J.: Fine needle aspiration cytology of breast. A review of 321 cases with statistical evaluation
17. Nordenstrom B., Zajicek J.: Stereotactic needle biopsy and pre-operative indications of non-palpable mammographic lesions. Acta. Cytol., 1977; 21: 350-355
18. Parker S.H.: Stereotactic large core breast biopsies. In: Parker S.H., Jabe W.E., (Eds.) *Percutaneous breast biopsy*. New York, Raven Press, 1993; 61-79
19. Brenner R.J., Fajardol L., Fisher P.R., *et al.*: Percutaneous core biopsies of the breast: Effect of operator experience and number of samples on diagnostic accuracy. Am. J. Roentgenol., 1996; 166: 341-346
20. Nath M.E., Robinson T.M., Tobon H., *et al.*: Automated large core needle biopsy of surgically removed breast lesions: comparison of samples obtained with 14, 16 & 18 gauge needles. Radiol., 1995; 197: 739-742
21. Parker S.H., Louin J.D., Jobe W.E., *et al.*: Non-palpable breast lesions: stereotactic automated large core biopsies. Radiol., 1991; 180: 403-407
22. Elvecrogel E.L., Lechner M.C., Nelson M.T.: Non-palpable breast lesions: correlation of stereotactic large core needle biopsy and surgical biopsy. Radiol., 1993; 188: 453-455

Pre-operative localization of impalpable breast abnormalities

G. Querci della Rovere, A. Patel

Introduction

The detection and excision of impalpable breast abnormalities is a common event due to the growing number of abnormalities identified with breast screening mammography. Pre-operative localization of impalpable breast lesions enables the surgeon to excise them adequately and with minimal cosmetic deformity.

Historical notes

The technique of localization of impalpable breast abnormalities was first described by Dodd *et al.* in 1966.[1] In 1976, Frank *et al.*[2] first proposed the combination of needle and hook wire for the pre-operative localization of impalpable breast abnormalities. This technique involved localization being done in the radiology department immediately prior to the operation.

The hooked wire and needle were introduced through a small skin incision in a direction perpendicular to the chest wall. The outer needle was withdrawn and the inner hookwire left *in situ*. Several techniques of pre-operative localization have been described, involving either positioning of a needle,[3,4,5,6] hook wire[2,7-10] or a dye injection[11,12] done with either stereotaxic devices,[13,14] perforated grids,[15,16] or radiological and clinical measurements.[17] Ultrasonography[18,19] and computed tomography[20] have all been used for localization of impalpable breast abnormalities if they can be visualized with these techniques. Several types of hook wires are available. We prefer the Cook breast localization needle Hook Type B DHBL - 22 - 9 William Cook Europe A/S wire because:
- It is fine and relatively pain-free.
- No need for local anaesthetic.
- No need for sterile gloves.
- Insertion takes only seconds.
- Easily replaced if necessary.
- There is a selection of introducing needles (gauge 18-23).
- It is graduated so as to recognise the distance from the tip.
- Two lengths of needles and wires are available for small or large breasts.

Needle insertion by most authors, mostly radiologists using a perforated plate, is done in a plane parallel to the chest wall. The needle and wire are inserted whilst the breast is compressed in the mammography machine, through a perforated plate for localization. Depending on the site of the lesion the wire can be introduced in a craniocaudal or in a lateral direction. However often the wire enters the skin at a site which is relatively distant from the skin projection of the mammographic lesion (the more so, the more central and close to the chest wall the lesion is) and follows a course which is parallel to the chest wall due to the compression of the breast. Localization of lesions lying centrally and close to the chest wall are associated with wire entry at the extreme periphery of the breast disc (Fig. 1).

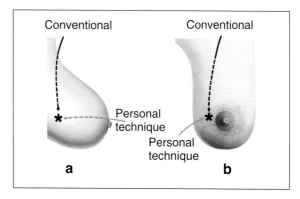

Fig. 1. **a.** True lateral view of the breast showing the direction of the wire with the conventional and with our personal technique. **b.** View of the breast and the point of entry of the wire with the two methods of insertion of the wire.

We do not favour this technique, as the surgeon when excising the abnormality has either to tunnel along the wire for a long distance leading to a poor cosmetic result, or guess where the lesion is and make a surgical incision in the proximity of the tip of the needle and then search for it. This can lead to cutting through tumour. Instead, we recommend insertion of the needle perpendicular to the chest wall. Gisvold et al.[21] and Frank et al.[2] have also recommended insertion of the needle perpendicular to the chest wall.

Technique of localization

We use a method that consists of radiological and clinical measurements. On two mammography views, true lateral and craniocaudal, we measure the distance of the lesion from the nipple line (Fig. 2).

These measurements are then transferred on to the breast itself. The resulting point then represents the skin projection of the lesion. This point is essential because it provides the surgeon with the most direct access to the breast lesion. This is the site where the surgeon would have chosen to make the surgical incision had the lump been palpable, and this is the point where the localization wire is inserted. The wire insertion is carried out without a need for a local anaesthetic and with no undue discomfort for the patient.

With the patient lying on her back and hands behind her head, the needle is inserted through the established point at an angle which follows the line of the two intersection planes with a direction perpendicular to the chest wall. Women with large breasts, which fall laterally, are asked to turn slightly to the opposite side far enough so that the breast lies almost on a flat surface. After the wire is inserted, further X-rays are taken (craniocaudal and true lateral) to check the distance of the wire from the lesion (Figs. 3-4). We believe it is acceptable if the wire is within a radial distance of about 2 cms for excision of carcinomas, and of about 1 cm for diagnostic biopsies.

Excision of these abnormalities is carried out with an incision made through or near the point of entry of the localizing wire, keeping in mind the need for radical surgery. If for cosmetic reasons the incision is in proximity to the wire, the wire can be brought into the surgical field by undermining the skin edge in the direction of the wire. The dissection is carried out with a scalpel avoiding the use of scissors which can cut the wire. The direct contact of the diathermy with the wire can cause it damage and diathermy should be used with caution.

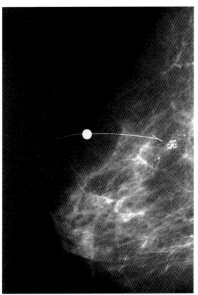

Fig. 3. Post-localization film; true lateral view.

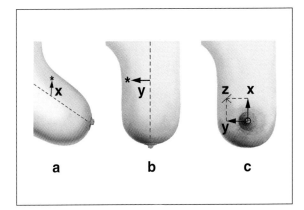

Fig. 2. Radiological clinical measurement; a. measurement of distance (x) of lesion from the nipple plane on true lateral view; b. measurement of distance (y) of lesion from nipple plane on craniocaudal view; c. the 2 measurements x and y are transferred on the patient's breast: the resulting point (z) is the skin projection of the lesion.

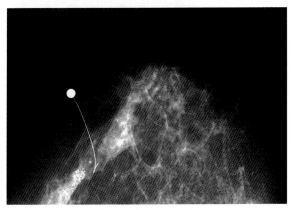

Fig. 4. Post-localization film; craniocaudal view.

The technique for excision depends on whether or not the wire goes through the lesion.

If the wire is not through the lesion, we dissect the breast tissue so as to expose all the length of the wire. In so doing, we have created one of the planes of excision. Once this is done, knowing the direction and distance of the lesion from the wire, the lesion can easily be excised (Fig. 5).

If the wire is through the lesion, the wire itself is excised with an appropriate amount of breast tissue around it (Fig. 6). In the case of diagnostic biopsies one can at first dissect along the wire and once judged to be in proximity of the lesion, extend the dissection around the wire. This will avoid removing an unnecessary amount of normal breast tissue. For diagnostic biopsies care is taken to see that the specimen does not exceed 20 gms. Once the specimen is excised, it is marked for orientation. We use a black silk suture to mark the skin surface and a nylon suture to mark the nipple margin. All specimens are sent for specimen radiography, which is then compared with the clinical mammogram to confirm adequacy of excision, while the patient is still under a general anaesthetic.

Results and complications

In the period 1 November 1987 to 31 March 1995 in the Breast Screening Programme at St. Margaret's Hospital, Epping we have screened 88,562 women (prevalence screen 46,817, incident screen 41,745) and detected 465 carcinomas. Of the carcinomas 276 (59%) cases were impalpable and of the benign biopsies 96 (80%) cases were impalpable. Furthermore we carried out 144 excisions of impalpable lesions referred from other screening districts. The senior Author has in addition carried out 149 excisions of impalpable lesions at the Royal Marsden Hospital, Sutton, UK. In total we have carried out 665 localizations and excisions for impalpable breast lesions (Table I).

Out of a total of 665 excisions of impalpable lesions, the localizing wire was introduced with radiological control in 600 cases (90%), and with ultrasound control in 65 (10%) of cases. We had to reposition the localizing wire in 26 (4%) cases. The lesion was excised with the first biopsy in 658 (99%) cases, with the second biopsy in 4 (0.7%) cases, and

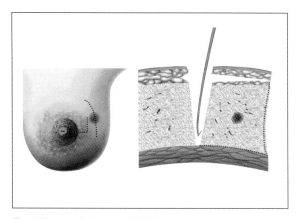

Fig. 5. Removal of impalpable lesion with wire near the lesion. Skin incision in proximity to the wire, possibly over impalpable lesion; wire found in the subcutaneous tissue and brought into the wound; dissection of breast tissue so as to expose all the length of the wire down to pectoral fascia. This creates one of the planes of excision. Once this is done, knowing the direction and the distance of the lesion from the wire, the lesion can easily be excised.

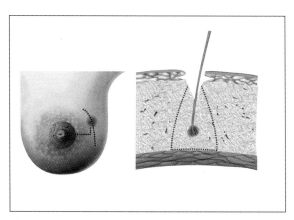

Fig. 6. Removal of impalpable lesion with wire in the lesion. Skin incision through the point of entry of the wire. The wire itself is excised with an appropiate amount of breast tissue around it.

Table I. Breast Screening Service, St. Margaret's Hospital, Epping, Essex UK, November 1st 1987-March 31st 1995.

Women screened	88,562
Prevalence screen (322 ca. - 6.8/1000)	46.817
Incident screen (143 ca. - 3.4/1000)	41.745
Carcinomas (impalpable)	465 **276**
Benign Lesions (impalpable)	120 **96**
Other screening districts impalpable lesions	144
Royal Marsden cases done by Mr. G. Querci della Rovere at the Royal Marsden Hospital, Sutton, Surrey from 1.1.94 - 31.3.96	149
Total impalpable lesions	665

Table II. Results of excision of impalpable breast lesions (665 cases).

Wire repositioned	26	4.0%
Lesions excised first biopsy	658	99.0%
Lesion excised second biopsy	4	0.7%
Lesion excised third biopsy	3	0.3%
Migration of wire	2	0.3%
Transection of wire	0	
Pneumothorax	0	

with the third biopsy in 3 (0.3%) cases, all under the same general anaesthetic. No patient left the operating theatre without the lesion removed (Table II).

Migration of the wire occurred in two cases; one wire was retrieved from the breast laterally and the second from the posterior triangle of neck. Migration has been reported into the left pleural space,[22] and into the posterior paracervical region.[23] We have not seen a pneumothorax[24] or transection of wire,[25] as reported in the literature.

Conclusion

The management of impalpable breast lesions requires careful consideration. The majority of these patients are asymptomatic women called for further assessment following a screening mammography. Some of them will have benign lesions and others very early and potentially curable breast cancers. Every effort should be made to avoid unpleasant scars and deformity of the breast after surgery.

We would like to stress the importance of close co-operation between surgeon, radiologist and pathologist to achieve what, in the end, has to be the best result for the patient.

References

1. Dodd G.D., Fry K., Delany W.: Pre-operative localization of occult carcinoma in the breast. In: Nealon T.F (Ed.) *Management of the Patient with Cancer*. Philadelphia, 1966; 88-113
2. Frank H.A., Hall F.M., Steer M.L.: Pre-operative localization of non palpable breast lesions demonstrated by mammography. New Eng. J. Med., 1976; 295: 259-260
3. Threatt B., Appelman H., Dow R., O'Rourke T.: Percutaneous needle localization of clustered mammary microcalcifications prior to biopsy. Am.J.Roent. Radium.Ther.Nucl.Med., 1974; 121: 839-842
4. Libshitz H.I., Feig S.A., Fetouh S.: Needle localization of non palpable breast lesions. Radiology, 1976; 121: 557-560
5. Schwartz G.F., Feig S.A., Rosenberg A.L., Patchefesy A.S., Shaber G.S.: Localization and significance of clinically occult breast lesions. Experience with 469 Needle Guided Biopsies. Rec. Res. in Can. Res., 1984; 90: 125-132
6. Marrujo G., Jolly P.C., Hall M.H.: Non palpable breast cancer needle localized biopsy for diagnosis and consideration for Treatment. Am. J. Surg. 1986; 151: 599-602
7. Kopans D.B., De Luca S.A.: A modified needle-hookwire technique to simplify pre-operative localization of occult breast lesions. Radiology, 1980; 134: 781
8. Kopans D.B., Meyer J.E.: Versatile spring-hookwire breast lesion localizer. Am.J. Radiol.: 1982; 138: 586-587
9. Homer M.J., Pike-Spellman E.R.: Needle localization of occult breast lesions with a curved end retractable wire. Technique and Pitfalls. Radiology, 1986; 161: 547-548
10. Homer M.J.: Localization of non palpable breast lesions with the curve-end retractable wire leaving the needle *in vitro*. Am. J. Rad., 1988; 151: 919-920
11. Egan J.F., Sayler C.B., Goodman M.J.: A technique for localizing occult breast lesions. Ca.CancerJ.Clin., 1976; 26: 32-37
12. Czarnecki D.J., Feider H.K., Speltgerber G.F.: Toluidine blue dye as a breast localization marker. AJR., 1989; 153: 261-263
13. Nordenstrom B., Azileck J.: Stereotaxic needle biopsy and pre-operative indication of non palpable mammary lesions. Acta Cy., 1977; 21: 350-351
14. Svane G.: A sterotaxic technique for pre-operative marking of non palpable breast lesions. Acta. Radiol. Dign. Stock., 1983; 24: 145-151
15. Parekh N.J., Wolfe J.N.: Localization device for occult breast lesions: Use in 75 Patients. AJR, 1987; 148: 699-701
16. Goldberg R.P., Hall F.M., Simon M.: Pre operative localization of non palpable breast lesions using a wire marker and perforated mammographic grid. Radiology, 1983; 146: 833-835
17. Querci della Rovere G., Benson J.R., Morgan M., Warren R., Patel A.: Localization of impalpable breast lesions: A Surgical Approach. Eur. J. Surg. Onco., 1996; 22: 478-482
18. Schwartz G.F., Goldberg B.B., Rifkin M.D., D'Orazio S.E.: Ultra-sonographic localization of non palpable breast masses. Ultra-sound Med. & Biol., 1988; 14: 23-25
19. Weber W.N., Sickley E.A., Callen P.W., Filly R.A.: Non palpable breast lesion localization: limited efficacy of sonography. Radiology, 1985; 155: 783-784
20. Dixon G.D.: Pre operative computed tomographic localization of breast calcifications. Radiology, 1983; 146: 836
21. Gisvold J.J., Martin J.K.: Pre biopsy localization of non palpable breast lesions. AJR, 1984; 143: 477-481
22. Bristol J., Jones P.A.: Transgression of localizing wire into the pleural cavity prior to mammography. Br. J. Radiol., 1981; 54: 139-140
23. Davis P.S., Wechsler R.J., Feig S.A., March D.E.: Migration of breast biopsy localizing wire. AJR, 1988; 150: 787-788
24. Tykka H., Castren-Person M., Sjoblom M., Roiha M.: Pneumothorax caused by hook wire localization of an impalpable breast lesion detected by mammography. The Breast, 1993; 2: 52-53
25. Homer M.J.: Transection of the Localizing Hook Wire during Breast Biopsy. Am. J. Radiol., 1983; 141: 929-930

ABBI: Advanced Breast Biopsy Instrumentation

G.A. Farello, A. Cerofolini

The progressive lowering of the threshold for identification of abnormalities in the breast as a result of the widespread use of mammography and the development of methods for breast imaging is associated with different diagnostic difficulties; the increased detection rate of breast lesions means that a sample of cells/tissue must be taken ever more commonly since this is the only way in which morphologically non-specific lesions can be identified.

Furthermore taking cell/tissue samples from the breast is controversial at present because there are so many technical options available (fine needle biopsy, core biopsy, minimally invasive breast biopsy) and the indications for each, and their reliability, are still under discussion. Fine needle biopsy and core biopsy are purely diagnostic procedures, whereas taking a sample by means of Advanced Breast Biopsy Instrumentation (ABBI) is clearly different from these two methods because its purpose is twofold, ie diagnostic and, especially, therapeutic.

Fine needle aspiration (FNA) has progressed considerably over the last ten years and, in expert hands, it has been shown to be highly sensitive and specific. Nevertheless, operators are often reluctant to take definitive decisions on the basis of cytology because FNA is associated with the possibility of false negatives due to sampling errors; furthermore, it is difficult to discriminate between hyperplasia with atypical features, DCIS and micro-invasive carcinomas. The advent of core biopsy led, gradually and progressively, towards percutaneous mini-invasive biopsy. By comparison with FNA, core biopsy allows a more precise morphological profile of a breast lesion to be drawn; it can distinguish between benign and malignant forms and between infiltrating and *in situ* lesions. Core biopsy is not however immune from false negatives, also due to sampling errors. If however hyperplasia with atypical features or a carcinoma *in situ* are found, the lesion as a whole must be examined and so surgical biopsy is required.

From the diagnostic point-of-view, the characteristic features of sampling with ABBI are high sensitivity and specificity, with a predictive value similar to that of open surgical biopsy (there are no artefacts in the sample which is readily legible even at the periphery), and much less breast tissue is removed.

Diagnosis, however, is not an end in itself but it should obviously be a basis for treatment and it is only helpful if it enables subsequent action to be planned and modified.

Lesions of the breast can be classified into three groups, those which are definitely benign, those which are definitely malignant, and borderline lesions (focal hyperplasia without atypical features, ductal and/or lobular atypical hyperplasia, and lobular carcinoma *in situ*) which suggest progression of a benign disorder to malignancy. When identified, pre-cancerous lesions probably reflect a greater risk of tumour development and may therefore suggest a particular approach to treatment. This is not an insignificant problem because the majority of borderline lesions are not palpable and they are likely to be found increasingly commonly. In non-palpable lesions, ABBI resolves the diagnostic problem accurately and definitively and governs the choice of treatment and methods for subsequent diagnosis. This is particularly obvious in non-palpable lesions in the presence of:
- hyperplasia with atypical features;
- carcinoma *in situ;*
- carcinoma of low malignant potential.

In the event of hyperplasia with atypical features, complete removal of the area concerned means that, not only can the presence of any foci of transformation be excluded, but also that the patient is protected against any progression of that lesion (although the risk of developing breast cancer is still considerably higher than in the normal population).

In the case of ductal carcinoma *in situ*, it provides

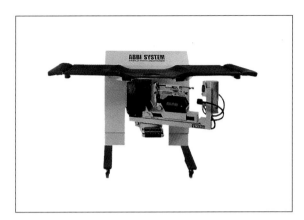

Fig. 1. The table consists of a paddle area with a circular opening, 25 cm in diameter.

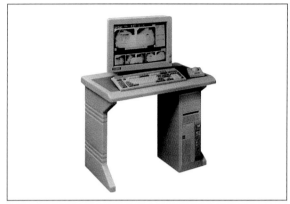

Fig. 2. The system for calculating the coordinates.

a reliable and full diagnosis and can exclude the presence of areas of micro-invasion; thereafter either simple mastectomy or a wide excision with or without radiotherapy can be carried out according to the extent and the histological grade of the DCIS.

Very small, low grade invasive carcinomas, complete excised will require no further surgical treatment to the breast.

The ABBI system consists of permanent apparatus and a disposable "trocar". The permanent apparatus consists of:
- a table;
- a control console;
- a system for calculating the coordinates.

The table (Fig. 1) consists of a flat padded area which supports the patient during the procedure; the breast is brought through a circular opening 25 cm in diameter into the operating area which is below the flat part of the table. At each end there is a support which can be pulled out so that the patient can be positioned with her head to one side or the other and so that either breast can be approached from any direction (360°).

This feature means that the breast can also be entered from below, which shortens the computed track of the needle through the gland. The prone position reduces the danger of vagal reactions and allows the doctor to work out of the patient's line-of-sight so that she is not subjected to unnecessary anxiety-inducing stimuli. In the operating area below the flat part of the table there is a C-shaped arm which supports the tube producing the X-rays, the image recorder, the apparatus for stereotactic direction-finding and the breast compressor.

The arm of the tube and of the compressor can be rotated together around the central axis of the table from 0° to 180°. The direction-finding apparatus is used to position the tip of the needle in accordance with the coordinates calculated by the computer. The digital system for image recording means that radiological images of the breast can be acquired without using radiographic film. The image is passed to the computer in 5 seconds where it can be processed. Using digital images reduces the overall duration of the operation. The controls for regulating the tube which is the source of the X-rays are placed on the control console.

The system for calculating the coordinates consists of a computer (Fig. 2) with a screen on which the operator can show the site of the lesion directly. The apparatus calculates the coordinates in three spatial planes and then transmits them to the direction-finding system. Images can also be memorized, recalled and stored.

The disposable trocar (Fig. 3) is placed on the direction-finding device and is composed of a cannula (available in various diameters: 5, 10, 15, 20 mm) containing a narrow circular blade, a snare at the distal end to which an electrical diathermy can be attached and a central coaxial needle at the tip with T-shaped arrester. The trocar allows removal of a cylinder of tissue at the centre of which is the lesion identified by the T-piece on the needle.

The operation is carried out on an outpatient basis under local anaesthesia and lasts for 25 minutes on average. Recovery is immediate and the patient can be discharged within a couple of hours.

The point of entry and the direction of the trocar are governed by the site of the lesion which has been localised previously by mammography. The breast is compressed and immobilised (Fig. 4). A sterile transparent cover is placed over the working area to retain sterility during use of the manual controls. The site of the lesion is checked by stereotactic imaging. The surgeon identifies the target area on the monitor. The

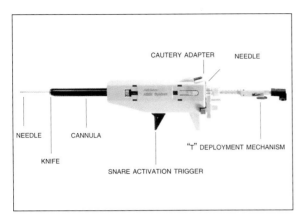

Fig. 3. The disposable trocar.

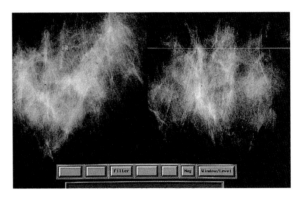

Fig. 4. The breast is compressed and immobilised.

digital system automatically calculates the X, Y and Z coordinates of the lesion with an accuracy of ±1 mm (Fig. 5).

These coordinates are passed to the guidance system on which the trocar is fixed. The guidance system operates automatically on the X, Y, and Z coordinates to line up with the area of interest on horizontal and vertical axes. Moderate local anaesthesia is inserted at the point at which the needle is to be inserted (Fig. 6).

A small incision in the skin is made with the blade and the needle is inserted to the required depth. A stereotactic image is taken to establish the position of the needle, at which point the T-shaped guide wire is advanced to stabilise the tissue. At this stage, local anaesthesia must be extended to the deeper layers. The skin incision is lengthened to permit insertion of the trocar. The cannula is advanced to the skin incision and guided by the surgeon to the required depth (Fig. 7).

The instrument isolates the piece of tissue within the cannula by slight oscillation of the surgical blade. A stereotactic image is used to check that the snare is beyond the point of insertion of the T-shaped guide wire. The diathermy on the snare is then used for cutting. The cannula and the whole sample of tissue are carefully removed. Pressure with a piece of gauze at the site of insertion prevents any blood loss. The piece of tissue is taken out of the cannula and sent for histology (Fig. 8).

The needle with the T-shaped guide wire allows correct pathological orientation (Fig. 9).

The patient is rolled over on to her back. Any bleeding can be controlled with pressure, diathermy and/or suturing by hand (Fig. 10).

The small incision in the skin is sutured with a few stitches. A pressure dressing is applied.

The method has many advantages: it removes the whole piece of tissue in one operation (locali-

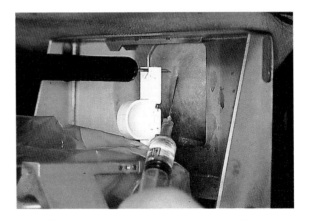

Fig. 5. The digital system automatically calculates the x,y and z coordinates of the lesion with an accurancy of ± 1 mm.

Fig. 6. Moderate local anaesthesia is inserted at the point at which the needle is to be inserted.

sation is no longer necessary); it allows correct orientation of the piece of tissue; it identifies accurately the objective to within ±1 mm so that the surgeon has to remove a smaller amount of healthy tissue; the smaller incision results in a better aes-

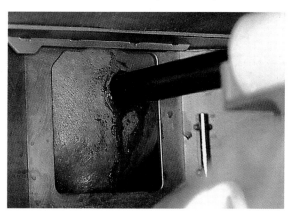

Fig. 7 The cannula is advanced to the skin incision and guided by the surgeon to the required depth.

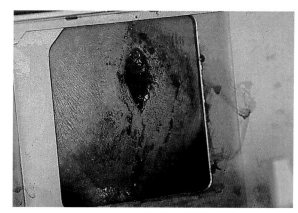

Fig. 10 Any bleeding can be controlled with pressure, diathermy and/or suturing by hand.

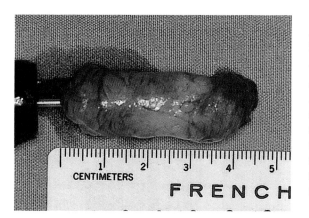

Fig. 8. The piece of tissue is taken out of the cannula and sent for histology.

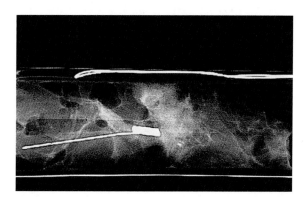

Fig. 9. The needle with the T-shaped guide wire allows correct pathological orientation.

thetic result, and scars and disfigurement are avoided; there is less anxiety and emotional and physical trauma since an operation is avoided; it reduces operating theatre costs.

On the other hand, the procedure is not always possible because digital imaging heightens the contrast and facilitates identification of microcalcifications but localising small solid nodules is made more difficult because definition is poorer. Deep-seated lesions close to the pectoral muscle or in the axillary extension and peripheral lesions (close to the nipple), especially in patients with small breasts, are difficult to aim at. Long-term results are not available, of course: the consequences of the procedure on the radiological "legibility" of the breast should be examined.

Complications are very few; occasionally a haematoma may occur especially if the lesion is deep, the breast large and the course of the trocar particularly long.

This is a new and extremely promising method which appears to be able to modify treatment of non-palpable lesions of the breast in the future. Its recent introduction, however, and the consequent shortage of cases do not yet allow it to be established in a particular place within the choice of methods for diagnosis and treatment.

Conclusions

The ABBI system could play a major role in the management of screen-detected lesions but should not be a substitute for FNA cytology which, if positive, is cheap and allows definitive treatment. The main indications for ABBI are:
1. mammographic lesions suspicious, but not positive, on cytology;
2. mammographic lesions, proven to be carcinoma on FNA which do not require axillary dissection.

The Pathology of Breast Cancer

Normal breast and benign breast lesions

K. Agarwal

Mammary glands are distinguishing features of mammals. The term "mammal" is derived from the Latin word "mamma", the breast. The mammary gland and breast are not synonymous: the latter includes the connective tissue and fat which surrounds and supports the gland. The female breast is unusual in the species in that it develops without the stimulus of copulation or pregnancy. Although present in both sexes, the breast remains rudimentary in the male.

Embryology

The breasts are highly specialised apocrine sweat glands developed from ectoderm, and as down growth from the skin they first appear at 8 mm embryo stage (5-week human foetus) when there is bilateral longitudinal thickening along the ventral body wall from the axillae to the medial aspect of the proximal part of the thigh; these are known as mammary lines-milk lines. In humans they regress and disappear except in the area of the thoracic region and, in the 20 mm embryo stage, only one persists at the definite site of the adult nipple and is the precurser of the future mammary gland.

In the fifth or sixth month of foetal life the cords of epithelium extend into the underlying mesoderm as solid epithelial columns comprising 15-20 branches which form the outline of lactiferous ducts. These are surrounded by invading mesenchyma which later develops into the fat and connective tissue. During the last eight weeks of foetal life these epithelial cords become canalised and acquire lumina. The epidermis at the point of origin of the gland forms a depression which is called "the mammary pit" into which these lactiferous ducts open.

At the time of birth this pit evaginates to form the nipple, the epithelium responds to the circulating maternal hormones with occasional secretion of milk,

i.e. witch's milk. Congenital anomalies can be explained by these developmental processes.

Anatomy

The adult human female breast has a distinctive and uniquely protuberant form; it extends from the 2nd/3rd rib to the 6th rib below. Its medial border extends to the lateral edge of the sternum and the lateral border extends up to the mid-axillary line. It is important also to note that the breasts extend superolaterally as a projection into the axillae. The breast consists of glandular tissue which is concentrated in the centre and upper outer half. The glandular tissue is composed of milk-producing lobular units, a system of branching ducts which in turn connects them to the nipple areola complex. Adipose and connective tissue surround these functional units and form the bulk of the breast. Dense connective tissue bands extend from the underlying pectoral fascia to the skin; these ligaments (Cooper's ligament) hold the breast upwards and their lengthening is responsible for ptosis of the breast with age. In the centre is the nipple which is elevated and pink in colour in nulliparous women, surrounded by the areola.

Development of the breast

The life cycle of the breast consists of three main periods, development (and early reproductive life), mature reproductive life and involution.

The female human breast undergoes two separate phases of growth and maturation. The first occurs in foetal development, resulting in the formation of a rudimentary organ which consists of simple branched ducts. The breasts are identical in boys and girls in childhood, are inactive and consist of sparse ducts lying in stroma. The second period of growth occurs at puberty in females when the ducts elongate, divide and form specialised terminal structures, *i.e.* terminal duct lobular units. The onset of puberty varies amongst different races, though in the western world it can start from the age of 9-10 onwards.

The breasts are integral parts of the reproductive system and with the onset of puberty major changes take place in the female breast, both in size and shape as well as morphologically. There is enlargement of the breast with increase in volume of connective tissue and fat. There is elongation, reduplication branching and budding of the epithelial ducts with formation of new lobules. The nipple and areola show alteration in shape and pigmentation.

All these changes are hormone-induced, particularly related to the release and production of oestrogen and progestogen; both stimulate and promote growth in the breast parenchyma and are released after the onset of ovulation along with general growth hormones. By the onset of menstruation the breasts are often well developed and a normal adolescent protruberant form takes shape.

After the breast has developed, it undergoes regular changes in relation to the menstrual cycle, and responds to repeated hormonal stimuli. In recent years several authors have commented on and described subtle underlying changes taking place.

During the luteal phase the ductules are small and surrounded by condensed intralobular stroma containing plasma cells. In the secretory phase there is an increase in the size of lobules and ductules, the stroma becomes loose, and oedematous. There is vacuolation of the basal cells in the late secretory phase. In the premenstrual phase there is a peak in the number of mitoses, lymphocytic infiltration and apoptosis following the onset of menstruation.

Fully functional differentiation is said not to occur until the breast is subject to the stimulus of pregnancy.

Pregnancy results in a series of changes in the breast that culminate in the fully differentiated state of lactation. These changes take the form of external appearance with enlargement, vascularity and pigmentation of the areola and nipple and doubling of weight at term.

In the breast parenchyma, there is marked proliferation and enlargement of the lobules in pregnancy with diminution of the intralobular as well as interlobular stroma. The secretory activity starts with supranuclear vacuolation in the early stages, to collection of colostrum in the lumen and abundance of lipid inclusions, fat globules and vesicles in the later stages. The myoepithelial cells show slight elongation.

With the onset of lactation, there is even greater distension of the glandular lumina with obliteration of the stroma (Figs. 1, 2).

Interlobular ducts and lactiferous sinuses are markedly dilated. These changes are not uniform, some acini showing minimal activity.

After pregnancy and lactation the involutionary changes take place, the rate and degree varying between individuals. After a period of three months or so the breast returns to "resting phase".

The term "involution" is used however to describe post-menopausal atrophic changes in the breast which involve lobules, ducts and stroma. In the nulliparous woman these changes begin after the age of 30. There is a gradual decrease in the amount of lobular component, with both stroma and epithelium being involved. The stroma converts into dense hyaline collagen and resembles ordinary connective tissue. The basement membrane of acini becomes thickened, the epithelium shrinks and becomes flattened and the luminal space becomes narrow, almost obliterated, with cessation of secretions (Fig. 3).

Some acini may coalesce with formation of small cysts (microcysts) which may later shrink and be replaced by fibrous tissue. The interlobular ducts are also affected, some disappear, some show shrinkage with irregular loss of elastic tissue and prominent myo-epithelial layer. These changes are not uniform and may vary from segment to segment. The stroma is replaced by fat, the breast becomes less radiodense, softer and droopy, hence more amenable to mammographic screening and examination.

It is extremely important to be familiar with and

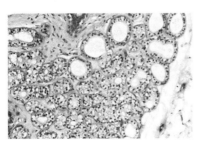

Fig. 1. Lactating breast.

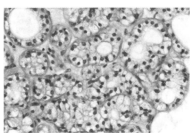

Fig. 2. Lactating breast (high power).

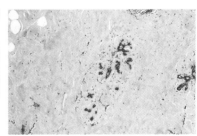

Fig. 3. Normal atrophic lobules.

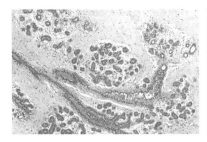 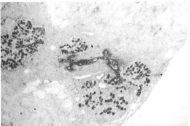 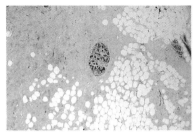

Fig. 4. Normal lobules and terminal ducto-lobular units.

Fig. 5. Normal lobules.

Fig. 6. Normal lobule.

to appreciate the various changes which affect breast parenchyma in order to understand the various breast conditions which occur during one specific period of life and are so common that they are best considered as aberrations rather than disease. This is particularly true when considering the benign fibro-cystic disease.

Histology: normal structure of breast

The functional unit of the breast is the terminal duct lobular unit (TDLU) and is composed of lobules and terminal ducts which drain via a branching duct system to the nipple (Figs. 4, 5).

Under the microscope, the lobule is seen to consist of a collection of small blind-ending epithelial structures variously termed acini, alveoli or ductules and embedded in connective tissue stroma. The number of acini varies from less than 15 to more than 100 (Fig. 6). The acini are lined by two cell layers, the inner luminal layer consisting of epithelium either cuboidal or columnar in type and the outer layer consisting of myo-epithelial cells which lie beneath the epithelium and are discontinuous; hence, some epithelial cells reach the basement membrane . The myo-epithelial cells are spindle-shaped and contain small nuclei and clear cytoplasm (Figs. 6a, b). These cells can be difficult to demonstrate in H & E preparations; however the immuno-histochemical stains

facilitate the identification of these cells. Epithelial cells can be stained by antibodies to epithelial membrane antigen (EMA) and by anticytokeratin antibodies especially to low molecular-weight cytokeratins. Myo-epithelial cells can be demonstrated by various stains in fresh tissue and in formalin-fixed paraffin embedded tissue (Figs. 7, 8). Smooth muscle actin is a useful marker. S100 protein can also be localised in these cells.

The lobular stroma is very distinct from the periductal stroma, both in type and in cellularity. It is highly specialised, richly vascular and contains fine collagen fibres and abundant reticulin. It also constitutes the major bulk of the lobule, is mucoid and more cellular. A mixture of cells, including lymphocytes, histiocytes, plasma cells and mast cells is found in addition to blood vessels and nerves.

In contrast the extralobular stroma is more compact and contains elastic tissue which becomes more abundant with ageing and lobules of fat which make up the bulk of breast tissue (Fig. 9). This stroma also contains supplying blood vessels, lymphatics and nerves of the breast.

The extra lobular terminal ducts lead to larger ducts, eventually to segmental ducts and ultimately to collecting ducts (Fig. 10). The proximal part of collecting ducts is lined by stratified squamous epithelium which is continuous with the skin, but the distal part shows abrupt transition and is lined by two cell layers like the rest of the glandular epithelium,

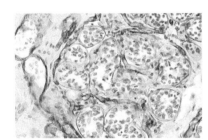 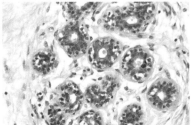 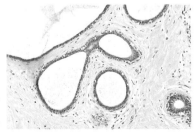

Fig. 6a. Normal lobule staining for basement membrane.

Fig. 6b. Normal lobule high power view showing double cell layer and basement membrane.

Fig. 7. Immunostaining for myoepithelial cell layer.

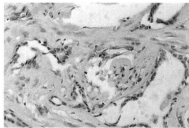
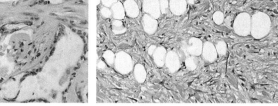
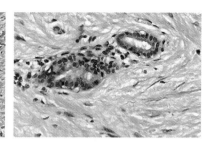

Fig. 8. Immunostaining for the myoepithelial cell.

Fig. 9. Fat, stroma and fibroblasts.

Fig. 10. Ductal system in fibrous stroma.

the only difference being that the myo-epithelial layer is continuous.

The collecting ducts are continuous with the lactiferous sinuses. It is important to note that in the resting state there is marked papillary infolding of the wall of the lactiferous sinus, and to distinguish this normal appearance from intraduct papilloma or papillomatosis.

About 15-20 collecting ducts converge under the areola on to the surface of a nipple through separate orifices. Nipple and areola have distinctive histological appearances, the nipple being covered by stratified squamous keratinised epithelium, while the subcutaneous tissue contains irregularly arranged smooth muscle fibres which have an erectile function (Fig. 11). The areola has numerous sebaceous glands, many of which are not associated with hair follicles and discharge directly on to the nipple. Apocrine sweat glands are also normally present and should not be mistaken for apocrine metaplasia resulting in breast lobules.

Non-neoplastic conditions
(Miscellaneous benign conditions)

There are several conditions which are poorly understood but are clinically of great importance as they mimic carcinoma although they are benign in nature.

Duct ectasia

The major subareolar ducts dilate and shorten during involution and a minor degree of such change is commonly seen in breast biopsies as an incidental finding.

Post-mortem findings have indicated that it is present in almost 40-50% of the women aged 60 years or more.

The term "duct ectasia" i.e. dilation of ducts, coined by Hagenson in 1951, is a poorly-understood condition which is also variously known as plasma cell mastitis, comedo mastitis, obliterating chronic mastitis. Its aetiology is unknown; some suggest that the dilatation is the primary event with the inflammation being secondary, perhaps due to a leak of the contents; others suggest that the inflammation is the primary process leading to fibrosis and duct dilatation with destruction of periductal elastic tissue.

Clinically it is a disease of mature women, who present with nipple discharge, nipple retraction, or a pale mass that may be hard or doughy. The discharge is usually cheesy, which may cause eczematous reaction, and the nipple retraction is "slit-like" classically. These features may clinically mimic carcinoma or Paget's disease. Mammographically, features like calcification of the ducts in duct ectasia may resemble the pattern of calcification seen in comedo carcinoma.

Pathologically, the subareolar zone is firm, the

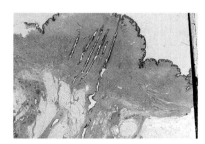
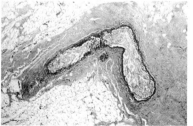
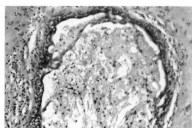

Fig. 11. Normal nipple and major ducts.

Fig.12. Dilated duct with reactive macrophages in the lumen.

Fig. 13 Dilated duct (high power).

ducts are dilated, filled with greenish brown tenaceous fluid or more commonly paste-like material.

Duct ectasia is a ductal disease, the hallmark of disease being dilated ducts filled with pasty material, periductal inflammation and fibrosis. In the early stages, the dilated ducts contain amorphous eosinophilic debris, some lipid-filled foamy cells and occasional crystalline material (Figs. 12, 13).

The epithelium may be attenuated, deformed or absent. There may be replacement by granulation tissue which also contains giant cells, foamy cells and myofibroblasts.

There is a periductal inflammatory cellular infiltrate which mainly consists of plasma cells, lymphocytes and histiocytes.

In the later stages, there is predominant periductal fibrosis, which may be irregular, resulting in distortion and obliteration of the ducts. Finally, there may be calcification.

Fat necrosis

Traumatic fat necrosis is another uncommon yet benign condition which is frequently mistaken for carcinoma. It is most commonly encountered in elderly women, with voluminous pendulous breasts. It is post-traumatic and a history of trauma can be elicited in 50% of the cases. Focal ischaemia is a possible aetiological factor or cause.

Clinically it can present as a firm ill defined, indurated mass, with pain, redness of the overlying skin and cutaneous retraction.

Macroscopically, the breast tissue shows an indurated zone with a bright yellow/opaque area of fat necrosis, which is quite different from the adjacent unaffected fat. In some patients it can form a cystic mass. In advanced cases there may be fibrosis and calcification.

Histologically, there is necrosis of adipose tissue with an inflammatory cell infiltrate which is rich in lymphocytes, plasma cells and histiocytes. There is release of fat from adipose tissue with empty spaces surrounded by macrophages, with foamy cells and multinucleated giant cells of foreign body type.

In the later stages, the granulomatous and fibroelastic reactions progress, resulting in fixation to the overlying skin. Granules of lipofuscin and haemosiderin pigment can be demonstrated by special stains. Sclerosis progresses and calcification can occur.

Aberration of normal development and involution (ANDI)

Benign, non-neoplastic conditions of the breast show a wide variety of proliferative and regressive changes in the breast parenchyma, epithelial elements and stroma; some form distinct entities but most have been grouped together and various terms have been used in the past to describe these changes collectively. These include chronic mastitis, interstitial mastitis, benign mammary dysplasia, mazoplasia, cystic mastopathy, fibroadenosis, Reclus disease, Schimmelbusch disease, and the most common term used, fibrocystic disease. Clinically, fibrocystic disease refers to a condition of painful nodularity and histologically to a picture of fibrosis, adenosis, apocrine metaplasia, epithelial hyperplasia, and cyst formation.

Cyclic pain and nodularity is extremely common in women of reproductive age and is regarded as physiological rather than pathological. Focal nodularity is seen in women of all ages and is the most common cause of a breast lump, yet when excised and examined a normal evolutionary process in the form of fibrosis or sclerosis is seen, and no pathological abnormality is found. Similarly these changes have been found in the breasts of women without any clinical disease in autopsy studies. All these observations have led to questioning the concept of 'disease' and the term fibrocystic change has been suggested which appears more appropriate. As already mentioned, fibrocystic change histologically includes cysts, apocrine metaplasia, adenosis and epithelial hyperplasia. In addition, to encompass all the clinico-pathological changes, the aberration of normal development and involution (ANDI) concept has been proposed as a framework to classify benign breast disorders, a concept which is comprehensive, based on pathogenesis and important for rational management.

The spectrum of change for each disorder varies from normal to mild abnormality and only in some cases progresses to disease.

Apocrine metaplasia

The term apocrine change/metaplasia denotes the presence of pink apocrine cells which resemble apocrine sweat glands (Fig. 14).

The cells are large, mostly columnar in shape and contain abundant granular eosinophilic pink cytoplasm and basal nuclei. The cells show apical snouts, i.e. rounded protrusions (Fig. 15).

The cytoplasmic granules stain with Sudan Black B and are PAS positive after diastase digestion. The nuclei are round, basal and show prominent nucleoli. Nuclear pleomorphism is a common feature, but is not regarded as atypical (indeed the presence of apocrine change denotes benignity). The apocrine change may present as a single layer of cells but most

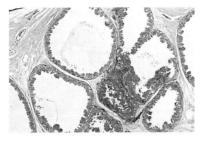 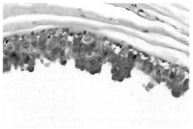 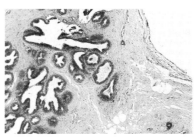

Fig.14. Apocrine metaplasia (low power).   Fig. 15. Apocrine metaplasia (high power).   Fig. 16. Blunt duct adenosis.

commonly they form papillary projections. These changes are most frequently seen in the cysts and lobules.

Adenosis

Adenosis is a term used to describe an increase in the number of acini or ductules in a lobule, thus resulting in the expansion of the lobule and alteration in its architecture. Two forms are recognised, blunt duct adenosis and microglandular adenosis.

Blunt duct adenosis

In blunt duct adenosis the acini show marked dilatation and an irregular outline. Two cell layers are present. There is hypertrophy of the epithelium as well as the myoepithelium (Figs 16-18). The inner epithelial cells show apocrine snouts. There is an increase in the specialised stroma; these changes are described as organoid lobular hypertrophy. Some acini show considerable dilatation resulting in microcysts.

Microgranular adenosis

This is a rare condition which histologically can be mistaken for a well-differentiated carcinoma, particularly tubular carcinoma. It can be an incidental finding in a biopsy or can present as a lump. Their size can vary from 0.3 cm to 1.3 cm in diameter.

Microscopically, there are foci of numerous small rounded acinar/glandular structures infiltrating and present in breast adipose tissue. The acini are lined by a single layer of uniform small cells, many containing PAS positive material. No myo-epithelial cells are present, but basement membrane is present and can be demonstrated by Reticulin stain and with type IV Collagen. The stroma consists mainly of adipose tissue.

Epithelial hyperplasia

Epithelial hyperplasia is described as benign, non-papillary intraluminal epithelial proliferation which can affect any part of the glandular system but most frequently involves the terminal duct lobular unit or the interlobular ducts (Fig.19). Larger ducts are rarely involved.

The affected structures are expanded. There is multilayering (more than four cells in thickness) but there is no cytological atypia. Two-cell type differentiation is present. The epithelial cells are uniform, cohesive and often appear syncitial. The nuclei are normochromatic and vesicular, nucleoli are inconspicuous. Mitotic activity is usually low and no abnormal forms are seen. Myoepithelial cells are present, intermingling with proliferating epithelial cells and can be demonstrated by special stains already mentioned. Epithelial hyperplasia is described as mild, moderate or florid depending on the degree of proliferation.

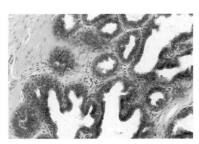 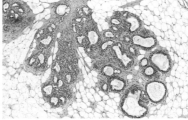 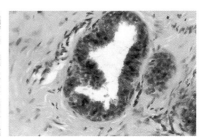

Fig. 17. Blunt duct adenosis and ductal hyperplasia.   Fig.18. Blunt duct adenosis.   Fig. 19. Ductal hyperplasia (usual type).

Fibroadenomatoid hyperplasia

The term is used to describe a fibroadenoma-like change in individual lobules; occasionally these lobules may be loosely coalescent, thus forming an ill defined irregular mass. Depending on the size, it may or may not be clinically detectable. Macroscopically as well as microscopically, there is no clear demarcation between the lobules showing fibroadenomatoid hyperplasia and the surrounding breast tissue. Very often the breast tissue nearby shows fibrocystic change.

Cysts

Cysts are round or spherical structures derived from lobules and are defined by the presence of walled space filled with fluid. Cysts are often multifocal, bilateral and are usually found in clusters. Small cysts (microcysts) seen in breast biopsies represent an involutionary process but several microcysts may expand and coalesce to form a solitary large cyst (Fig. 20).

Large cysts (macrocysts) commonly present as discreet, palpable, smooth, sometimes painful lumps, which may or may not be fluctuant. Cysts constitute up to 15% of all discreet breast lumps and are common in pre- and peri-menopausal women, the median age being 40-60 years. They are uncommon after the age of 60 years (but are important because of associated intracystic papilloma).

They vary in size and can measure up to several centimetres, but cysts less than 1 cm are not usually palpable.

They are readily diagnosed by ultrasound and mammography. The diagnosis is confirmed by aspiration of contents and cytology.

The larger cysts have rounded contours and bluish colour (blue domed cyst).

The cyst fluid can be thin, yellow in colour but more often is turbid, thick and varies in colour from dark green to brown, occasionally being blood stained.

The cysts are usually lined by epithelium which may be flattened, attenuated or even absent, particularly if the contents are under pressure. However, myo-epithelial cells can be demonstrated by special stains.

Many cysts are lined by an apocrine type of epithelium which forms small papillae.

Rupture of the cyst results in inflammatory response with collection of lymphocytes, plasma cells and histiocytes in the adjacent stroma. Foamy macrophages can be seen in the lumen as well as in the wall with dense fibrosis.

Aberration of stromal involution

Aberration of stromal involution includes the development of localised areas of excessive sclerosis. These lesions, though benign have the capacity to infiltrate locally but are not known to metastasize or have any premalignant potential. However they are of clinical importance as they cause diagnostic problems both clinically and mammographically. Excision biopsy is usually required to make a definite diagnosis. Two separate conditions belong to this group.

(a) Sclerosing adenosis

This is the most widely recognised form of organoid lobular proliferation in which the increased number of acini show elongation and distortion with spiky infiltrative margins. The lobular proliferation is multifocal and, with coalescence of lobules, can present as a painful palpable mass. The term "adenosis tumour" has been used to describe such lesions. The condition affects pre- or peri-menopausal women, is most common in the age group 30-45 years, and is thought to recede after the menopause. Incidence of sclerosing adenosis has been described between 12.5-25% of all benign biopsies.

Macroscopically, it can form a mass with well defined borders and is firm (not hard) in consistency. On slicing, it can mimic carcinoma, particularly when yellow streaks of elastosis are present.

Microscopically, characteristic changes are present on low power examination which is of great value in making the correct diagnosis. Enlarged nodular units show a whorled pattern of compressed tubules. Normal lobular architecture is retained, though there is myo-epithelial and stromal hyperplasia. The early proliferative and later fibrotic/sclerotic phase can be recognised. The proliferative process involves the epithelial and myoepithelial cells and results in compression and distortion of ductules with obstruction of the lumen (Figs. 23-25).

However, normal two-cell population (double cell layers) can be recognised in the tubules, there is no cytological atypia, cells have uniform small nuclei, and no abnormal mitotic figures are seen (Figs. 26-29). Myo-epithelium is abundant in the proliferative phase and can be demonstrated by special stains, *i.e.* PAS or by immunocytochemical methods (Fig. 8). Proliferating units extend and infiltrate not only stroma but also the nerves and vessels, but two-cell layers can be demonstrated confirming the benign nature of the condition. Incidence of vascular and perineural infiltration varies and has been described between 3.9 and 10%. In areas apocrine metaplasia is seen.

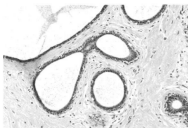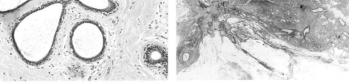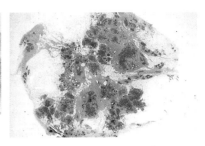

Fig. 20. Early stage of cyst formation.   Fig. 21. Radial scar.   Fig. 22. Radial scar (low power).

In later stages there is evidence of elastosis and the lumina of tubules contain calcispherules.

The main differential diagnosis is with carcinoma of the breast including tubular carcinoma from which it can easily be differentiated by lack of cytological atypia, normal organoid lobular pattern and the presence of normal two-cell layer in the acini.

(b) Radial scar/complex sclerosing lesion

Radial scar (RS) is yet another proliferative lesion with pseudo-infiltrative growth pattern. These lesions over the years have been described under several names, which include infiltrative epitheliosis, sclerosing papillary proliferation, complex compound heteromorphic lesion, benign sclerosing ductal proliferation, non-encapsulated sclerosing lesion, rosette-like lesion, indurative mastopathy, radial sclerosing lesion and proliferation.

Radial scars are usually less than 1 cm in diameter; larger lesions greater than 1 cm are termed complex sclerosing lesions. They rarely present as palpable mass. The reported incidence varies between 1.7% of benign surgical biopsies to as much as 28% but they are becoming more and more common since the implementation of mammography as a diagnostic tool for screening women for cancer.

They present as a stellate mammographic abnormality but their greatest importance is due to their ability to mimic carcinoma mammographically and even histologically.

Macroscopically, small lesions may be difficult to see but if viewed by a hand lens an irregular stellate shaped area is seen, yellow streaks and flecks of calcification may be apparent and again these features may mimic a malignant lesion.

The histological changes depend on the stage of development and maturation. The mature fully developed lesion clinically consists of a central area of fibro-elastic tissue which shows entrapped tubules with proliferating epithelial elements radiating out at periphery. This appearance has been described descriptively as "flower head", "daisy head" or floret manner (Figs. 21, 22).

The dense fibro-elastic tissue in the central core stains pink by H & E and black by Weigert stain, but also shows entrapped tubules which are angulated randomly and distributed in a non-organoid manner (Fig. 30). It is this pattern that can mimic a well differentiated tubular carcinoma. The epithelial tubules in RS still show a normal two-cell layer. The myoepithelial layer as well as the basement membrane can be demonstrated both by conventional stains (*i.e.* PAS) or by immunocytochemical stains. The epithelial element at the periphery shows variable proliferative changes. There is epithelial hyperplasia, which may be papillary, solid or cystic and may contain intraluminal calcispherules. There is no cytological atypia.

Complex sclerosing lesions (CSL) are larger than 1 cm and have all the features of radial scars though on a greater scale.

Macroscopically, they may appear as a nodular mass with a central area of fibrosis, though occasion-

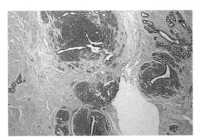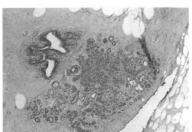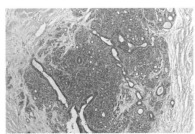

Fig. 23. Sclerosis adenosis.   Fig. 24. Sclerosis adenosis   Fig. 25. Sclerosis adenosis.

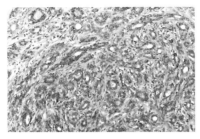

Fig. 26. Sclerosing adenosis.

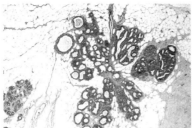

Fig. 27. Radial scar and blunt duct adenosis.

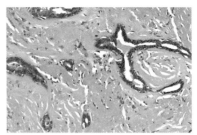

Fig. 28 Radial scar (high power).

ally they give the impression of a mass, which is due to coalescence of several small adjacent sclerosing lesions. Like RS they may mimic carcinoma on naked eye examination.

Besides being larger in size than RS these lesions show in addition more disturbance of structure and other additional changes, *i.e.* apocrine metaplasia, papilloma formation and sclerosing adenosis at the periphery resulting in nodule formation. As with RS epithelial atypia is lacking, the two-cell layer and basement membrane are present and can be demonstrated by special stains.

As with other lesions, the most important differential diagnosis is from tubular carcinoma. The epithelial tubules in carcinoma are lined by a single cell layer, the basement membrane is absent and there is infiltration of fat.

Benign tumours

Fibroadenoma

Fibroadenomas (FA) are benign circumscribed tumours of the breast, composed of varying amounts of epithelial and stromal components (Fig. 31). Although described as benign tumours these lesions are thought to be a benign malformation/aberration of normal development. They arise from a single lobule and not a single cell and like the rest of the breast are under the same hormonal control, they lactate during pregnancy and undergo involution in the perimenopausal stage and may be calcified. Their incidence is variable; overall they account for 13% of all palpable breast lumps, though the relative incidence in different age groups varies, *i.e.* accounting for 60% in the younger age group (15-25 years) to 15% in women of 30-40 years of age. They are much less frequently found in the breasts of older women. The autopsy incidence varies from 9% to 28% in different series. They are said to occur more frequently in Afro-Carribean populations. They are usually solitary but sometimes can be multiple and bilateral.

Clinically, they present as a palpable breast lumps. The majority are located in the upper outer quadrant of the breast. Classically the lump is discrete, smooth, mobile and not painful. The clinical diagnosis of FA must be confirmed by aspiration cytology.

Most fibroadenomas grow to a size varying from 1-3 cm, some stay stationary in size but many regress and even disappear; a few grow larger (giant fibroadenoma). Several follow-up studies have confirmed this behaviour and this is the reason why, after confirming the diagnosis of fibroadenoma, many hospitals and units allow the patient the choice of excision or observation. However, if there is increase in size or other unusual features they are excised and examined histologically.

Four separate clinical entities are described: common fibroadenoma, giant fibroadenoma, juvenile fibroadenoma and phyllodes tumour.

FA exhibit a wide variety of histological and

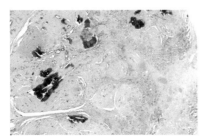

Fig. 29. Sclerosing adenosis and micro-calcifications.

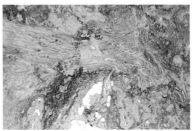

Fig. 30. Complex sclerosing lesion. Stained with EVG.

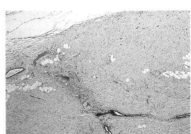

Fig. 31. Fibroadenoma.

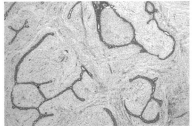

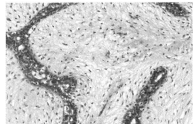

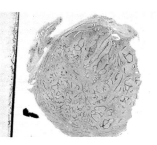

Fig. 32. Fibroadenoma (high power).   Fig.33. Fibroadenoma with ductal hyper-   Fig. 34. Fibroadenoma, intracanicular type.
plasia (usual type).

cytological changes, as already mentioned, both ep-ithelial and stromal component being present. The epithelium is usually two-cell layer but may be multilayered (Figs. 32, 33).

The stroma is rather loose, myxoid and consists of spindle cells. Rarely other mesenchymal elements, *i.e.* fat, muscle or, rarely, bone is present. Two types of growth pattern are described, *i.e.* pericanalicular and intracanalicular (Figs. 34, 35).

In the pericanalicular type the epithelial compo-nent consists of rounded duct-like structures sur-rounded by stroma which is arranged in a concentric manner. In the intracanalicular type the epithelial element shows considerable thinning, elongation and distortion with prominent intervening stroma. In any fibroadenoma usually both patterns are present.

The older lesions show atrophy of epithelium, hyalinisation and sometimes calcification of the stro-ma. They can undergo infarction.

As they arise from lobules, other histological changes, *i.e.* apocrine metaplasia, epithelial hyper-plasia and sclerosing adenosis which affect the lob-ule, can also be seen in a fibroadenoma. Rarely, *in situ* malignant changes can also be seen.

Papilloma

Papilloma is a term which refers to a distinct villous lesion with an arborescent fibrovascular stro-ma covered by a double layer of epithelium, outer myo-epithelial and inner epithelial layer. Papillomas can be microscopic or macroscopic (Fig. 36).

Solitary papillomas occur centrally and are found most frequently in large collecting ducts beneath the nipple. They are relatively uncommon, can appear at any age, may be seen in adolescents or in elderly women, but occur most commonly in middle age.

They are the commonest cause of nipple dis-charge and 80% of the patients present clinically with this symptom. The discharge can be scrosanguinous or blood stained. A mass can be felt sometimes but nipple retraction is uncommon. They can be shown by galactography.

Papillomas can be small, a few millimeters in diameter when they appear as an elongated structure extending along a major duct and are only seen on microscopic examination.

However, they can be larger, form a spheroid mass which is soft and friable, present in a major duct which results in dilatation and distension of the ducts, assuming a cyst-like appearance (hence the name intracystic papilloma) and may be filled with blood. The size even when large is rarely greater than 3 cm in diameter.

Sections show a true papilloma with a stalk which is attached to the duct wall. It shows a distinct arborescent configuration with branching fibrovas-cular stroma, usually well developed, and contains blood vessels and collagenous stroma. These are covered by epithelium. The epithelium is the normal

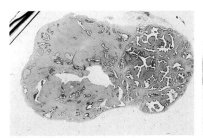

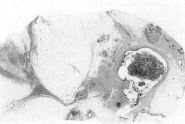

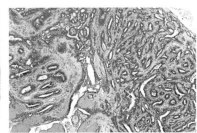

Fig. 35. Fibroadenoma with some leaf-like   Fig. 36. Intraduct papilloma (low power).   Fig. 37.   Sclerosing intraduct papilloma
structures (on the right hand side).   (high power).

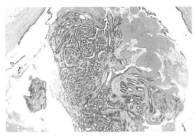 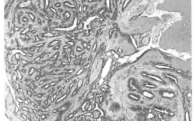 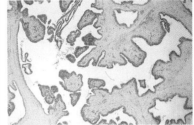

Fig. 38. Sclerosing intraduct papilloma (low power).

Fig. 39. Sclerosing intraduct papilloma (high power).

Fig. 40. Benign phyllodes tumour.

two-cell layer, an essential feature of a benign papilloma, with outer myo-epithelial and inner luminal epithelial layer.

The cells are either cuboidal or columnar, the nuclei are vesicular with inconspicuous nucleoli and normochromatic. The nuclear/cytoplasmic ratio is low, mitoses are usually infrequent, and no abnormal forms are seen (Figs. 37-39).

There may be foci of epithelial hyperplasia which is without atypia.

Other features are also seen: apocrine metaplasia is a frequent finding, squamous metaplasia is also seen sometimes, particularly near areas of infarction. Haemorrhage and sclerosis are very common. Periductal fibrosis and sclerosis may result in entrapped epithelium which may be distorted and may be mistaken for infiltration or invasion. In spite of this appearance of pseudo-infiltration, the two-cell layer is retained and myo-epithelial cells can be demonstrated by special stains, particularly by Alpha smooth muscle actin antibody.

All the features present in a lesion should be taken into account to confirm the diagnosis of a benign papilloma.

Multiple papillomas are found at the periphery, distant from the nipple, they involve the terminal duct lobular unit and form an integral part of fibrocystic change.

Phyllodes tumour (cystosarcoma

phyllodes)

Cystosarcoma phyllodes is a tumour with the basic structure of a fibroadenoma but is characterized by marked proliferation of connective tissue stroma and has potential for local recurrence and metastasis.

The name cystosarcoma phyllodes was given to the tumour by Muller in 1838, describing a large fleshy tumour with a papillary "leaf-like" appearance on the cut surface.

These tumours have been described as giant fibroadenoma, adenomyxoma, pseudosarcomatous adenoma and papillary cystofibroma. As most of the tumours are benign, the term "sarcoma" has caused considerable confusion. The WHO classification adopts the term phyllodes tumour which is widely used nowadays. The biological behaviour of these tumours is unpredictable; even the histological appearance is not a good prediction of subsequent behaviour but many Authors classify them as neither benign nor malignant.

The tumours appear in middle-aged women with maximum incidence in the fifth decade, although they have been reported in adolescent as well as in elderly women. The most common age of phyllodes tumour is 10 years later than that of fibroadenoma.

Characteristically it grows slowly at first, then rapidly attains a large size. Although they are usually larger than fibroadenoma, size is not an acceptable

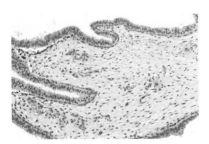

Fig. 41. Benign phyllodes tumour. Double cell layer and cellular stroma.

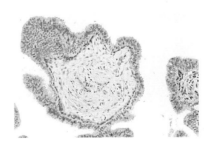

Fig. 42. Benign phyllodes tumour (high power).

criteria for diagnosis. Clinically a large spherical well-circumscribed tumour is present in the breast. It can be 10-20 cm in diameter. Cutaneous ulceration may be present but is a late manifestation. Bilateral tumours are very rare.

The tumour is well-circumscribed, grey to white in colour, firm and generally larger than 5 cm in diameter. Cut surface shows clefts and cystic spaces, and loose myxoid areas may be seen. Larger tumours are soft, fleshy and may show areas of haemorrhage or necrosis.

Sections show a tumour with basic growth pattern of an intracanalicular fibroadenoma. There are leaf-like epithelial-lined papillary projections into the cystic spaces (Fig. 40). The main changes are seen in the stroma which is abundant, prominent and shows both increased cellularity as well as variation in appearances within the same tumours.

The cells may show the appearances of uniform spindle-shaped fibroblasts, but also nuclear hyperchromasia, marked pleomorphism and mitotic activity. The stromal cells usually aggregate around the epithelium and sometimes around blood ves-

sels. The cellularity of the stroma may vary from a cellular fibroma to a fibrosarcoma (Fig. 41). Hyalinisation and myxoid change are common. Adipose tissue, smooth muscle cartilage and bone may be seen.

Epithelium is composed of two-cell layers but may show hyperplasia (Figs. 41, 42). Other changes, *i.e.* apocrine metaplasia and sclerosing adenosis are not commonly seen in phyllodes tumour. Phyllodes tumours must be differentiated from FA because of the different clinical behaviour.

Further reading

1. Rosen P.P., Oberman H.A.: Atlas of tumor pathology: tumors of the mammary gland. IFIP, Washington DC. 1992
2. Rosen P.P.: Rosen's Breast Pathology. Philadelphia, Lippincott-Raven, 1997
3. Bland K.I., Coleland E.M.: The Breast. Philadelphia,Saunders, 1991
4. Hughes L.E., Mansel R.E., Webster D.J.T.: Benign disorders and diseases of the breast. London, Bailliere Tindall, 1989
5. Harris J.A., Lippman M.E., Morrow M., Hellman S.: Diseases of the breast. Philadelphia, Lippincott-Raven, 1996

Risk factors, prognostic indicators and staging

S.E. Pinder, I.O. Ellis

Risk factors

Risk factors may be defined as those characteristics which impart a greater chance of developing a disease over the risk of the general population. The biological risk factors for the development of breast cancer are complex, multifactorial and remain poorly understood. Several factors for breast cancer are, however, well recognised including family history of breast cancer, reproductive hormone and radiation exposure, diet/nutrition and morphological factors within the breast itself. It is not appropriate in this chapter to cover all of these and only those of particular relevance to early breast cancer or which are presently under debate will be addressed here.

At the present time there is much interest in the effects of hormone replacement therapy and the contraceptive pill on a woman's risk of developing breast cancer. It has been suggested that prolonged exposure to normal levels of oestrogens and progesterones may be significant at an early stage in the development of breast cancer by stimulating epithelial proliferation. Thus an association with the known risk of early menarche, late menopause and nulliparity may be explained. The role of exogenous hormones in the development of breast cancer is, however, less clear. Whilst hormone replacement therapy (HRT) may have an influence on the interpretation of mammograms affecting both the background diffuse density and the size of focal lesions such as fibroadenomas,[1] much of the epidemiological data has been derived from studies in which oestrogen-only hormone supplements were used. Some of these series have suggested an increased risk of breast cancer with oestrogen-only HRT of at least 15% after 10 years use.[2] The risks associated with combined oestrogen and progesterone HRT are less clear; Bergkvist *et al.*[3] in a series including 23,244 women found a relative risk of 4.4% of developing breast cancer for patients on combined HRT but this was derived from only 10 women. Other studies have found no association between the oral contraceptive pill or HRT of combined type and breast cancer.[4] Overall the reported increased risk of breast cancer in association with exogenous hormones is small and appears to be related to length of exposure to steroid hormones both in the form of oral contraceptives[5] and hormone replacement therapy.[6] The large Nurse's Health Study found a small increased risk for women on either oestrogen or combined HRT of 1.32% and 1.41% respectively but the increased risk associated with 5 or more years postmenopausal use was greater for older patients. Further studies including stringent risk benefit analysis are required to evaluate the apparent small increased risk of developing breast cancer in balance with the protection from heart disease and osteoporosis gained from long term use of HRT. The issue has also been complicated by the suggestion that xeno-oestrogenic compounds present in the general environment, possibly derived from herbicides, pharmaceuticals and other chemicals, can experimentally induce mammary carcinomas and may have a role in the induction of breast cancers in humans[7] but this requires further investigation.

Radiation exposure causing DNA damage either secondary to atomic bombs or radiation therapy is known to be associated with an increase in breast cancer which may be particularly significant if the exposure is during infancy. The risks associated with radiation are important with respect to the possible risk of induction of breast carcinomas by mammography itself. Although it is widely agreed that the risk of induction of breast cancer with a 3-year interval between screens, as is used in the UK, is exceeded by the benefit of detection of carcinomas in the 50-64 year age-group,[8] other authors have suggested that the increase in the incidence of breast cancer in the USA could be linked to the widespread use of mammography.[9] It has been noted that an increased number of breast cancers has been described in women treated with ionising radiation for other breast conditions but the dose to the breast epithelium due to mammography is probably much less than has previously been suggested.[10] Bryant et al.[10] have argued that the assumption, for estimation of radiation dose, that the female human breast is composed of 50% adipose tissue and 50% "glandular" tissue by weight is incorrect. These 2 components have both been ascribed equal radiation sensitivity despite the obvious derivation of the majority of breast malignancies from the epithelial component. The average proportion of luminal epithelium by morphometric analysis in Bryant's series was 0.24% and epithelium and stroma together comprised only 16.12%; thus it seems likely that a much lower proportion of the breast tissue is at risk due to radiation than has previously been predicted and estimates of radiation risk secondary to mammography may need to be re-investigated.

It is not possible to review the genetics of breast cancer in this chapter and the reader is referred to a recent paper by van Rensberg and Ponder for a review of the genetics of familial breast carcinoma, and to the chapter by Dr. Evans in this book.[11] Only a small proportion of breast cancers are due to the inheritance of mutated autosomal dominant genes. The familial breast cancer gene BRCA1 on 17q[12] is now characterized and BRCA2 is now also localised.[13] These genes confer a very high risk of breast cancer; for individuals carrying the BRCA1 gene the risk is about 85% by age 70. The rare Li-Fraumeni syndrome with aberrant p53 tumour suppressor gene is important in few familial breast cancers but may be associated with soft tissue and bone sarcomas as well as brain tumours and other neoplasms.[14] Other genes conferring a lower risk including the ataxia telangectasia gene probably also affect a small number of patients. In the 85% of cancers which occur in women with no family history, the genetic abnormalities are also complex and no single gene appears to be of particular import; a cascade of genetic lesions, as described in colo-rectal cancers, does not appear to be of causal significance in breast disease.

It is well recognised that epithelial proliferative diseases including usual and atypical ductal epithelial hyperplasias and lobular neoplasia confer an increased risk of developing breast cancer and these lesions may be discovered coincidentally in breast screening practise. Much of the work on the risk associated with histopathological appearances has been performed by Page and Dupont and their criteria for atypical proliferative diseases in particular must be adhered to if risk estimates are to be extrapolated from their series. Fibrocystic changes are now no longer believed to be a disease but there is an increased risk of cancer in patients with usual epithelial hyperplasia amounting to 1.5 to 2.0 times that of

a reference population during the subsequent 10 to 15 years after diagnosis. A 4.6 times increased risk is found for patients with atypical ductal hyperplasia (ADH) although it is important to note that this risk falls after 10 to 15 years towards that of a control population.[15] Conversely an associated family history (at least one first degree relative) doubles the risk associated with ADH.[16] Atypical lobular hyperplasia confers a 4 to 5 times increased relative risk and lobular carcinoma in situ an 8-10 times increased risk.[16] Sclerosing adenosis is associated with a minor increased relative risk of breast carcinoma amounting to 1.7 times that of the general population[17] and fibro-adenomas confer a 2.17 times increased risk overall but this increases to 3.10 times in "complex" fibro-adenomas with foci of sclerosing adenosis or papillary apocrine change.[18]

These lesions may be excised coincidentally as a result of the Breast Screening Programme and may, if sufficiently high a risk is conferred, warrant follow up. The risk incurred by the patient with these lesions and the lifetime risk for an "average" woman (which is now reported as 1 in 8 for women in the USA[19]) must be interpreted by clinicians. The relative risk indicates the number of patients who develop breast cancer compared with that of the general population over a given period of time but the absolute risk of developing breast cancer reflects the probability of developing breast cancer for that patient and is related to the woman's age, the age specific incidence of carcinoma and deaths from other causes as well as the relative risk of that patient and is thus a more useful concept for the individual patient. Thus the relative risk of a 40-year-old woman with atypical ductal hyperplasia (ADH) of 4.5 times is reflected in an absolute risk of about 8-10% of developing invasive breast carcinoma in the following 10-20 years and for a 60-year-old with ADH a 25% chance within 20 years. In terms of absolute risk it may be easier for a patient to understand her true individual risk of developing breast carcinoma. It is also important that the relative risks described associated with epithelial proliferative diseases may not be long lasting; the increased risk associated with ADH lasts only 10-15 years and follow up ad infinitum at a high risk clinic for patients with some of these lesions and no family history may not be justified.

Prognostic indicators

There has been a great increase in interest in the prediction of behaviour of breast carcinoma by the use of prognostic indicators in recent years largely due to the recognition that breast cancer is not a single disease entity. It is also clear that screen detected lesions may be substantially different from symptomatic tumours. The range of treatment choices for patients with breast cancer has significantly widened and includes breast conserving surgery or mastectomy as well as differing adjuvant systemic therapies. Prognostic factors have been described as having 3 major functions;[20] the first being to identify patients whose prognosis is so good that they require no further adjuvant treatment. The second purpose is to identify patients whose prognosis is so poor that an aggressive approach to treatment may be required. The third reason is to identify patients who may respond or be resistant to specific therapies. Thus treatment strategies for individual patients may be significantly different and can be based on the prediction of behaviour of each individual breast tumour. Although previously the major role of the pathologist lay solely in determining the diagnosis, it is now well recognised that much prognostic information can be obtained from careful examination of well fixed resected tumour and regional lymph nodes.

Tumour size

The clinical measurement of breast tumours is inaccurate; a correlation between surgical and pathological assessment of tumour size was found in only 54% of cases by the Yorkshire Breast Cancer Group.[21] Ultrasound measurement may be more useful if an estimate of the clinical tumour size is required for planning treatment. Tumour size is assessed most accurately in the fresh state and this is then confirmed in the fixed specimen when the margins of the tumour may be better defined. If there is doubt as to the size of a carcinoma, for example with small or *in situ* lesions which form a major part of the breast screening work, tumour size should be confirmed on the tissue sections using the Vernier scale on the microscope stage.

Many studies have confirmed the prognostic significance of breast cancer size;[22] patients with small tumours have a better long term survival. Rosen and Groshen[23] found 20-year relapse free survival rates of 88% for patients with tumours less than 10 mm in diameter, 73% survival over the same time period for women with cancers measuring 11-13 mm falling to 65% and 59% for lesions 14-16 mm and 17-22 mm respectively. It is well recognised that Breast Screening Programmes identify smaller tumours than can be found in symptomatic practise and 35% percent of screen detected invasive carcinomas are less than 1 cm in maximum extent in Nottingham.

The terms "minimal breast cancer" and "minimal invasive breast carcinoma" have been used by different groups to represent lesions of varying sizes but there is little doubt that lesions which, for example, measure 10 mm or less are at an earlier stage than larger tumours; lymph node positivity was seen in approximately 15-20% compared to 40% in lesions greater than 15 mm in diameter by Rosen and Groshen.[23] Because of the recognition of the prognostic importance of tumour size the measurement of breast carcinomas has become an important quality assurance measure for radiologists in the UK NHS BSP, with a recommendation that a target of 15 minimal invasive carcinomas per 10,000 women screened should be detected.

Histological grade and type

The degree of differentiation of a breast carcinoma may be determined by the measurement of histological grade and tumour type. Both factors can be assessed by microscopical examination of routine tissue stains with the proviso that samples should be well fixed, and well defined criteria adhered to.[24] Specimens are ideally sent to the laboratory in the fresh state and immediately incised and placed in fixative to obtain optimum preservation of morphological details and mitotic figures.

Histological grade is now well recognised as a prognostic indicator and several studies have refuted earlier suggestions of lack of reproducibility if strict criteria are maintained.[25,26] Two main methods for histological grading have evolved. One is based on nuclear features alone and the other on both architectural and tumour cell features. The latter has been modified to give greater objectivity[27] and has been adopted for use in the UK NHS BSP. This method of histological grading assesses the three features of tubule formation, nuclear size/pleomorphism and mitotic count; each of these elements is scored 1-3 and the sum of the scores used to categorise the tumour. If less than 10% of the carcinoma is forming tubules a score of 3 is given, those with 10 to 75% score 2 and if more than 75% of the cancer is forming lumina a score of 1 is given. Mild, moderate and marked pleomorphism/small, medium and large nuclear size score 1, 2 and 3 respectively. For mitotic count a score is given according to the field area of the high power lens used. Apoptotic and hyperchromatic nuclei should be discounted and only nuclei with definite features of metaphase, anaphase or telophase are included. An overall sum of the three component scores of 3, 4 or 5 indicates a grade 1 cancer, a score of 6 or 7 a grade 2 tumour and 8 or 9 a carcinoma of histological grade 3.

Histological grade is a strong indicator of patient survival (Fig. 1). Patients with grade 1 carcinomas

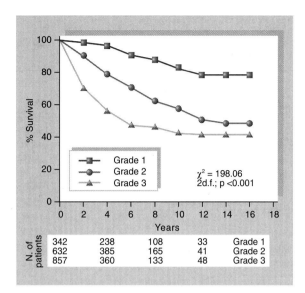

N. of patients				
342	238	108	33	Grade 1
632	385	165	41	Grade 2
857	360	133	48	Grade 3

Fig. 1. Long term survival in the Nottingham Tenovus Primary Breast Carcinoma Series (NTPBS) by histological grade.

Table II. Comparison of the proportion of histological type and stage in symptomatic and screen detected practise in Nottingham.

Types	Screen detected carcinomas	Symptomatic carcinomas
Tubular mixed	29%	14%
Ductal / NST	28%	47%
Tubular	20%	2%
Lobular	13%	15%
Medullary and Atypical Medullary	2%	5%
Mucinous	1%	1%
Others	7%	16%
Lymph node negative (Stage 1)	80%	63%

have an 85% 10-year survival compared with less than 45% for patients with grade 3 tumours. Importantly a greater proportion of well differentiated carcinomas are seen in screening compared to symptomatic practice (Table I).

Breast carcinomas show a great variety in morphological appearance and it is well recognised that some forms of primary breast cancer, the so-called "special types" carry a significantly better prognosis than the more common "no special type" (NST)/ ductal tumours. Other tumour types with varying prognoses can be determined however and 15 categories of invasive tumour type are used in Nottingham, not including the *in situ* and micro-invasive classes.[28] It is for this reason that approximately 50% of breast carcinomas are classified as of no special type (NST)/ductal in our unit; tumours which include areas of NST with for example a "special type" morphology elsewhere within the mass are placed in a separate group. These groups of tumours behave differently with a 64% 10-year survival in NST with special type tumours compared to the 47% 10-year survival of NST breast carcinomas.[28] An increased proportion of the good prognosis "special types" is

seen in screening compared to symptomatic practise (Table II).

It is not possible to describe fully the methods of classification for each tumour type group in this chapter but for prognostication purposes several of the tumour types can be amalgamated into 4 prognostic type groups according to 10-year survival.[29] Those tumour types with an excellent prognosis (>80% 10-year survival) include tubular, invasive cribriform, mucinous and tubulo-lobular carcinomas. Tumours with a good prognosis (60-80% 10-year survival) include tubular mixed, alveolar lobular, mixed ductal/NST with special type and atypical medullary carcinomas. A 50-60% 10-year survival is seen with medullary, invasive papillary and classical lobular carcinomas and a poor prognosis (<50% 10-year survival) with lesions of mixed lobular, NST, solid lobular and mixed ductal with lobular types.

Tumour type group alone provides important biological information but with the evaluation of histological grade individual tumours can be more accurately classified. This is not only true for tumours of NST/ductal morphology in which the importance of histological grade is well recognised and in our laboratory we routinely grade all breast cancers. Although, for example, the majority of lobular carcinomas are of grade 2 pattern, rarer sub-groups of both grade 1 and grade 3 lesions may be identified with better and worse survivals respectively (Fig. 2). We also recognise a category of "tubular mixed" carcinoma; this is different from the classification of "tubular variant" which other groups define as showing 75-90% tubule formation. Lesions formed of a stellate fibrous centre incorporating tubular structures (no matter what the extent) but with an infiltrating edge of carcinoma of NST are grouped as tubular mixed carcinomas.

Although it has previously been suggested that histological grade is not a reproducible technique for

Table I. Comparison of the proportion of histological grade in symptomatic and screen detected practise in Nottingham, UK.

Grade	Screen detected carcinomas	Symptomatic carcinomas
Histological grade 1	45%	19%
Histological grade 2	40%	34%
Histological grade 3	15%	47%

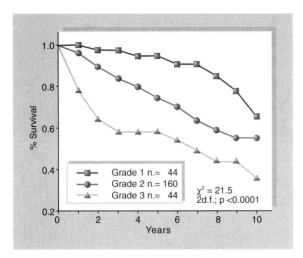

Fig. 2. Long term survival in the Nottingham Tenovus Primary Breast Carcinoma Series (NTPBS) for lobular carcinoma (all sub-types) by histological grade.

providing prognostic information it is of interest that medullary carcinomas do not have the good survival in the Nottingham Tenovus Primary Breast Carcinoma series (NTPBS)[29] which is seen in other studies. Whilst the criteria for grading breast carcinomas are now well defined, the same is less true for the determination of tumour type. The variation in survival of patients with medullary carcinoma may be a reflection of the difficulties in establishing robust diagnostic criteria for breast carcinoma type.

Nevertheless both histological type and grade provide important complementary prognostic information. Whilst in multivariate analysis (Table III), grade is of much greater importance in predicting survival than type, tumour typing provides additional information on behaviour. For example lobular carcinomas, particularly those of alveolar lobular type, are often oestrogen receptor positive[30] and may show a different pattern of metastatic disease to tumour of no special type.[31]

Staging

Staging of breast cancer is essential in the assessment of the patients, prognosis and determination of treatment options. Staging may be purely clinical, or pathological by examination of the tumour and axilla and, when appropriate, other sites such as internal mammary nodes. The TNM staging method incorporates an assessment of the primary tumour (T) including size, the regional lymph nodes (N) and distant metastases (M) and although initially proposed in 1954 several modifications have since been made.[32] However this system is complex and notoriously

Table III. Stepwise multivariate analysis in primary operable breast carcinoma for survival. Z values >1.96 significant at p=0.05 level. Z value reflects significance and B value the importance of each factor.

	B	Z
Size	0.19	4.86
Grade	0.64	6.69
Tumour type	0.29	3.47
LN Stage	0.76	11.18
Vascular invasion	0.18	3.18

inaccurate; lymph nodes may be enlarged due to reactive changes whilst nodes with metastatic tumour may be impalpable. It is however imperative that reliable staging is performed and a careful histological examination of lymph nodes should be carried out, although there has been debate over whether lymph nodes should be sampled or whether the axilla should be cleared. Arguments have been presented for both axillary clearance[33] and axillary sampling.[34] Steele et al.[34] found no difference in the incidence of lymph node positivity in patients with sampling or clearance and argued that, provided at least 4 nodes were examined, sufficient prognostic information could be provided by sampling. The greater number of nodes obtained by clearance is associated with increased post-operative morbidity including lymphoedema and reduced shoulder mobility.

Whatever the technique, all the excised nodes should be examined histologically. We take blocks by serial slicing each node along the long axis thus providing a large area of lymph node and peripheral sinus in one section. Each node is examined separately and one slice of node is examined microscopically for approximately each 5 mm of the maximum dimension. Numerous studies have shown that patients with involved lymph nodes have a poorer prognosis than those with no metastases in the loco-regional nodes. Prognosis is also related to the number of involved lymph nodes; the greater the number of nodes with metastatic tumour the poorer the progno-

Table IV. Staging of lymph node disease in primary breast carcinoma.

		Score for NPI
Stage A	Tumour absent from all nodes sampled at all three sites	1
Stage B	Tumour in a low axillary node only or in an internal mammary node only or in 3 or less nodes in axillary sample	2
Stage C	Tumour in apical node or in low axillary plus internal mammary nodes or in 4 or more nodes in axillary sample	3

sis.[35] We follow the National Surgical Adjuvant Breast Project (NSABP) in the USA and classify cancers with no loco-regional lymph node disease as stage 1, carcinomas with 3 or less nodes as stage 2 whilst tumours with 4 or more involved lymph nodes (or both axillary and internal mammary lymph nodes) are categorized as stage 3 (Table IV). The level of nodal involvement also has prognostic significance; metastatic disease in the apex carries a significantly worse prognosis[36] but may require an additional incision unless mastectomy is being performed. Screen detected breast carcinomas are more frequently stage 1 compared to symptomatic tumours (Table III).

There has been debate over the prognostic significance of micro-metastases; a definition of the maximum size of these lesions has not been agreed and different methods of examination have been used to identify these tumour deposits. Some groups have suggested that micro-metastases identified by serial sectioning of lymph nodes are prognostically significant.[37] Other authors have found that micro-metastases identified by immunohistochemical techniques are not prognostically significant in lobular carcinomas but are associated with recurrence in ductal/NST tumours.[38] It is undoubtedly true that an additional small number of cases with micro-metastases can be identified by immunohistochemical examination with anti cytokeratin antibodies which have not been found with routine stains but we have found no prognostic significance in this.[39] Given the significant increase in workload and cost to examine every case either immunohistochemically or by serial sectioning we compromise by careful examination as described above.

A few cases where features suspicious of metastatic disease are seen may be assessed immunohistochemically with anti cytokeratin antibodies. Lymph nodes containing any foci of metastatic carcinoma are classified as positive.

Vascular invasion

Apart from tumour size, histological grade and type and lymph node stage the other variable which in multivariate analysis is found to be of independent prognostic significance in predicting for survival in the NTPBS is the presence or absence of vascular (blood vessel or lymphatic space) invasion, despite the strong association with lymph node involvement.[40] Although some studies have suggested that the assessment of vascular invasion can be used, and provides information as powerful as lymph node examination,[41] this is not widely accepted. This feature is perhaps more important, however, in the

prediction of local recurrence in patients who have had wide local excision[40] and flap recurrence in patients having had mastectomy.[42] Other groups have not however found a similar correlation and a wide variation in the incidence of this feature has been reported.

This may be related to the difficulties in adhering to strictly defined criteria and obtaining good fixation of specimens which must be optimal to avoid the difficulties of retraction artefacts mimicking tumour emboli.

Whilst special techniques have been used to assess vascular invasion in breast carcinoma these have a role predominantly in distinguishing artefactual shrinkage from true vascular spaces. Elastic stains are of little help in distinguishing ducts from muscular vessels and neither lymphatics nor small capillaries have elastic lamina. At the present time we report vascular invasion in 3 categories - absent, definite or probable. Probable vascular invasion is reported when an unequivocal endothelial lining cannot be seen but when possible tumour emboli are seen in the tissue adjacent to the invasive tumour; for therapeutic purposes this category is grouped with tumours showing no vascular invasion.

Multivariate analyses showed that in the NTPBS the features which predicted for local recurrence in patients who had had wide local excision (without any selection criteria for surgery) included tumour size, the presence of vascular invasion and young age.[43]

As a result of this analysis it is now our practise to advise patients with tumour greater than 3 cm clinically or radiologically against conservation surgery, especially if they are under 40 years of age. Postoperatively conversion to mastectomy is advised if the tumour is greater than 2 cm in size, histological grade 3, node positive and shows definite vascular invasion. Thus the importance of the presence of vascular invasion in patient management lies in the prediction of local recurrence and should be routinely reported in excision specimens.

Use of prognostic indicators

Several factors provide prognostic information in patients with primary breast cancer and no single indicator is universally recognised to be of overall importance. Lymph node stage has been most consistently used as a guide for stratification in most centres for patient treatment and entry into clinical trials. This factor is believed to be time dependent but is of relatively poor discriminatory value; neither a group of patients with close to 100% mortality nor a group of very high survival can be identified by the presence or absence of lymph node metastases. The intrinsic biological "aggressiveness" of the tumour itself is also of prognostic importance, as described above. For each individual patient benefit may be gained in producing a combination of the time dependent and biological features of the tumour in order to predict prognosis. It has long been recognised that a combination of lymph node stage and differentiation is more useful than either alone in the prediction of the behaviour of many epithelial malignancies.

From multivariate analyses the variables which are of independent prognostic significance can be determined and those can be combined into a prognostic index to obtain the best prediction of survival for each individual patient. In Nottingham the factors of greatest prognostic importance in primary operable breast carcinoma have been found to be histological grade, lymph node stage and tumour size (Table III).

These have been combined, with appropriate weighting from the B value of multivariate analyses to form the Nottingham Prognostic Index (NPI): (0.2 X tumour size (in cm)) + histological grade (scored 1 to 3) and lymph node stage (scored 1 to 3). This index was initially derived from a series of 387 patients by entry of 9 separate variables in multivariate analysis and has been confirmed prospectively.[44] Further confirmation of the value of the NPI has come from other multicentre series.[45]

The NPI is used to determine patient's probable prognosis and thus to select the appropriate treatments for patients with primary operable breast cancer in Nottingham. Patients with an NPI of less than 3.4 have a comparable survival to age matched controls and thus receive no systemic adjuvant treatment. Conversely patients with a higher score receive systemic treatment based on additional data such as oestrogen receptor (ER) status. Although in multivariate analyses this is not of independent significance in survival, ER status is routinely assessed by immunohistochemical means on paraffin fixed tissue sections[46] of the resected tumour in this unit. Hormone treatment can thus be given to patients who are most likely to respond to it whilst those who have a poor chance of responding to tamoxifen can be given other treatment without delay.

The quantitative assessment of ER immunoreactivity may be performed in several ways. In its simplest form the percentage of tumour cells which show positive immunostaining is determined whilst other techniques include in addition an assessment of the degree of positivity. The modified Histochemical score (H score) is one such method and incorporates both the percentage and a semi-quantitative assessment of the degree of tumour cell immunoreactivity

scored from negative (0) to strong (scored as 3) into a formula: 0 X % negative cell + 1 X % weakly positive cells + 2 X % moderately stained tumour cells + 3 X % strongly positive tumour cell nuclei. Thus the H score ranges from 0 to 300. Tumours with an H score of greater than 50 are considered positive for therapeutic purposes and this cut-off provides a good prediction of response to hormone therapy (Table V). Many screen detected breast carcinomas, however, show good prognostic features and have an NPI score of less than 3.4 and thus, despite often showing ER positivity, receive no further systemic treatment. Many groups have suggested that in addition to ER status, progesterone receptor status or other oestrogen inducible molecules should be examined in patients with breast carcinoma to assess the functioning of the oestrogen receptor. We do not routinely perform these assays and rely on ER examination to predict response to hormone treatment.

Although subsequent analyses have demonstrated that tumour type and the presence of vascular invasion are of independent prognostic significance in predicting for survival in primary operable breast cancer, the effects of these are small in comparison to the weight of histological grade, lymph node stage and tumour size. The NPI is simple to calculate and is derived from data which is relatively easy to obtain from routine careful histological examination of sections of tumour and lymph nodes. Thus additional components have not been included which might make the index more difficult to determine or calculate. The NPI may also be used to compare groups of patients and the prognosis of symptomatic and screen

Table V. Response to tamoxifen in advanced breast cancer according to ER status assessed with the 1D5 antibody (Dako) on paraffin sections. $\chi^2 = 35.7$, 3 df, p <0.0001.

	ER negative (H score <50)	ER positive (H score >50)	Totals
Response (UICC 1+2)	2	18	20
Static disease (UICC 3)	1	17	18
Progression (UICC 4)	37	15	52
Totals	40	50	90

Table VI. Proportion of breast carcinomas in Nottingham prognostic index groups.

NPI	<3	<3.4	3.4-5.4	>5.4
Screen detected	44%	76%	20%	4%
Symptomatic	12%	29%	54%	17%

detected breast carcinomas can be compared with this technique (Table VI). Seventy-six percent of screen detected carcinomas in this unit fall within the excellent and good prognostic groups compared to only 29% of symptomatic breast cancers. Conversely only 4% of screening cancers are in the poor prognostic group compared with 17% of symptomatic tumours.

Other morphological and molecular markers of prognosis

A number of other morphological factors have been suggested as useful prognostic indicators including angiogenesis, peritumoural lymphoid infiltrate, tumour necrosis, stromal fibrosis, stromal elastosis and stromal giant cells. The former feature is of particular interest but although the hypothesis that breast cancer growth and metastasis are angiogenesis-dependent is attractive and is supported by some studies, others have failed to confirm an association with prognosis. The neovascularisation of the tumour periphery provides an increased surface area for adherence and entrance of tumour cell emboli to the circulation but the development of new vessels may occur around foci of DCIS. The growth of new vessels at the periphery of a neoplasm may thus be an early event in tumour development rather than a rate-limiting step. The assessment of angiogenesis in breast carcinomas requires the identification of so called "hot spots" and immunohistochemical staining of these areas with subsequent counting of new vessel formation. The lack of association with prognosis in several series, including a study performed in Nottingham, may be a failure to identify these areas of highest neovascularisation.[47] The role of angiogenesis in breast carcinoma is at present under investigation and it may prove to be more important and interesting as a therapeutic target rather than prognostically.

The significance of other morphological features is unclear; tumour necrosis has been reported to be seen predominantly in breast carcinomas of no special type. The criteria and techniques for the assessment of tumour necrosis have varied in studies making comparison of results difficult but the overall impression is that this is a poor prognostic feature; both early treatment failure and reduced overall survival are reported. This feature requires further investigation with strict reproducible criteria and evaluation of extent.

Many tumours show no or minimal associated ductal carcinoma *in situ* (DCIS) whilst a small proportion (approximately 10% of cases) are composed of abundant DCIS. The extent of DCIS (EIC) has been reported to be of prognostic significance. In a recent study Matsukuma *et al.*[48] reported that tumours with a less than 20% invasive component had significantly fewer lymph node metastases and a better overall 10-year survival than tumours with greater than 20% invasive elements. Other series have noted an association between a prominent *in situ* component and lower histological grade[49] and it may be that histological grade rather than the EIC is the significant feature. Multivariate analyses are required to determine if the presence of abundant DCIS is of independent significance.

The greater importance of the extent of DCIS in invasive carcinomas, we believe, is in determining management after conservation treatment. The main risk for relapse after breast conserving surgery is thought to be residual tumour burden. This may be predominantly *in situ* disease.[50]

EIC has been defined by Schnitt *et al.*[51] as the presence of DCIS amounting to 25% or more of the overall tumour mass of an invasive carcinoma and extending beyond the confines of the infiltrating component. This latter group have found that tumours with EIC have a higher local relapse rate than those without. This is not the case in the work of Locker et al in Nottingham where other features in multivariate analyses are more powerful predictors of local recurrence.[43]

Many molecular predictors of prognosis have been described including the proliferation fraction marker Ki67 (and its paraffin equivalent MIB1) as well as the more technically complex assessment of thymidine labelling, S-phase fraction and bromodeoxyuridine labelling of tumours. Whilst again these appear to be of significance in univariate analyses, in stepwise multivariate analysis, histological grade which includes a proliferation component (mitotic count) appears to be more important. Other molecular markers including growth factors and their receptors such as epidermal growth factor receptor, cerbB-2 and cerbB-3, proteases such as cathepsin D, cell adhesion markers such as E-cadherin, tumour suppressor genes such as p53 and a multitude of other factors do not show independent prognostic significance in primary breast carcinoma when morphological markers such as histological grade and type, tumour size and lymph node stage are included. Although these latter factors appear to be old fashioned and simple to assess, histological grade and tumour type are measurements of tumour morphology reflecting a variety of complex biological molecular changes within the tumour including cell adhesion and structure, DNA content and proliferation index.

Thus it is perhaps not surprising that individual biological markers cannot replace these well recognised morphological prognostic factors. The place of molecular markers may in the future be to determine treatment choices with specific molecules reflecting a probable response or resistance to a particular therapy. It is also possible that some biological features such as tumour angiogenesis may prove to be directly useful in anti cancer treatment. It is certain that the examination of the expression of many molecular pathways will aid in our better understanding of the biology of breast cancer and thus should not be ignored.

References

1. Cyrlak D., Wong CH.: Mammographic changes in postmenopausal women undergoing hormonal replacement therapy. Ajr. Am. J. Roentgenol. 1993; 161: 1177-1183

2. Steinberg K.K., Smith S.J., Thacker S.B., Stroup D.F.: Breast cancer risk and duration of estrogen use: the role of study design in meta-analysis. Epidemiology 1994; 5: 415-421

3. Bergkvist L., Adami H.O., Persson I., Hoover R;, Schairer C.: The risk of breast cancer after estrogen and estrogen-progestin replacement. N. Engl. J. Med. 1989; 321: 293-7

4. Stanford J.L., Weiss N.S., Voigt L.F., Daling J.R., Habel L.A., Rossing M.A.: Combined estrogen and progestin hormone replacement therapy in relation to risk of breast cancer in middle-aged women. JAMA 1995; 274:137-142

5. Chilvers C.E, Smith S.J.: The effect of patterns of oral contraceptive use on breast cancer risk in young women. The U.K. National Case-Control Study Group. Br. J. Cancer 1994; 69: 922-923

6. Colditz G.A., Hankinson S.E., Hunter D.J., et al.: The use of estrogens and progestins and the risk of breast cancer in postmenopausal women. N.Engl. J. Med. 1995; 332:1589-1593

7. Davis D.L., Bradlow H.L., Wolff M., Woodruff T., Hoel D.G., Anton-Culver H.: Medical hypothesis: xenoestrogens as preventable causes of breast cancer. Environ Health Perspect 1993; 101: 372-377

8. Law J.: Variations in individual radiation dose in a Breast Screening Programme and consequences for the balance between associated risk and benefit. Br. J. Radiol 1993; 66: 691-698

9. Wun L.M., Feuer E.J., Miller B.A.: Are increases in mammographic screening still a valid explanation for trends in breast cancer incidence in the United States? Cancer Causes Control 1995; 6:135-144

10. Bryant R.J., Robinson A., Stephenson T.J., Underwood A.C., Underwood J.C.E.: Determination of breast tissue composition for improved accuracy in radiation dose assessments in mammographic screening. J Path. 1995; 176: 40A

11. Van Rensberg E.J., Ponder B.A.: Molecular genetics of familial breast-ovarian cancer. J. Clin. Pathol. 1995; 48: 789-795

12. Miki Y., Swensen J., Shattuck-Eidens D., et al.: A strong candidate for the breast and ovarian cancer susceptibility gene BRCA1. Science 1994; 266: 66-71

13. Wooster R., Neuhausen S.L., Mangion J., et al.: Localization of a breast cancer susceptibility gene, BRCA2, to chromosome 13q12-13. Science 1994; 265: 2088-2090

14. Li F.P., Fraumeni J.F., Mulvihill J.J., et al.: A cancer family syndrome in twenty-four kindreds. Cancer Res. 1988; 48: 5358-5362

15. Page D.L., Jensen R.A.: Evaluation and management of high risk and premalignant lesions of the breast. World J. Surg. 1994;18: 32-38

16. Page D.L., Kidd T. Jr., Dupont W.D., Simpson J.F., Rogers L.W.: Lobular neoplasia of the breast: higher risk for subsequent invasive cancer predicted by more extensive disease. Hum. Pathol. 1991; 22: 1232-1239

17. Jensen R.A., Page D.L., Dupont W.D., Rogers L.W.: Invasive breast cancer risk in women with sclerosing adenosis. Cancer 1989; 64: 1977-1983

18. Dupont W.D., Page D.L., Parl F.F., et al.: Long-term risk of breast cancer in women with fibroadenoma. N. Engl. J. Med. 1994; 331: 10-15

19. Feuer E.J., Wun L.M., Boring C.C., Flanders W.D., Timmel M.J., Tong T.: The lifetime risk of developing breast cancer. J. Natl. Cancer Inst. 1993; 85: 892-897

20. Clark G.M.: Do we really need prognostic factors for breast cancer? Breast Cancer Res. Treat. 1994; 30: 117-126

21. Yorkshire Breast Cancer Group. Critical assessment of the clinical TNM system in breast cancer. BMJ. 1980; 281: 134-136

22. Galea M.H., Blamey R.W., Elston C.W., Ellis I.O.: The Nottingham Prognostic Index in primary breast cancer. Breast Cancer Res Treat 1992; 22: 207-219

23. Rosen P.P., Groshen S.: Factors influencing survival and prognosis in early breast carcinoma (T1N0M0-T1N1M0). Assessment of 644 patients with median follow-up of 18 years. Surg. Clin. North. Am.1990; 70: 937-962

24. National co-ordinating group for breast cancer screening: Pathology Reporting in Breast Cancer Screening. Sheffield: NHSBSP Publications, 1995

25. Robbins P., Pinder S., de Klerk N., et al.: Histological grading of breast carcinomas II. A study of interobserver agreement. Human Path. 1995; 26: 873-879

26. Frierson H. Jr., Wolber R.A., Berean K.W., et al.: Interobserver reproducibility of the Nottingham modification of the Bloom and Richardson histologic grading scheme for infiltrating ductal carcinoma. Am. J. Clin. Pathol. 1995; 103: 195-198

27. Elston C.W., Ellis I.O.: Pathological prognostic factors in breast cancer. I. The value of histological grade in breast cancer: experience from a large study with long-term follow up. Histopathology 1991; 19: 403-410

28. Ellis I.O., Galea M., Broughton N., Locker A., Blamey R.W., Elston C.W.: Pathological prognostic factors in breast cancer. II. Histological type. Relationship with survival in a large study with long-term follow-up. Histopathology 1992; 20: 479-89

29. Pereira H., Pinder S.E., et al.: Pathological prognostic factors in breast cancer. IV: Should you be a typer or a grader? A comparative study of two histological prognostic features in operable breast carcinoma. Histopathology 1995; 27: 219-226

30. Domagala W., Markiewski M., Kubiak R., Bartkowiak J., Osborn M.: Immunohistochemical profile of invasive lobular carcinoma of the breast: predominantly vimentin and p53 protein negative, cathepsin D and oestrogen receptor positive. Virchows Arch. A. Pathol. Anat. Histopathol. 1993; 423: 497-502

31. Lamovec J., Bracko M.: Metastatic pattern of infiltrating lobular carcinoma of the breast: an autopsy study. J. Surg. Oncol. 1991; 48: 28-33

32. Spiessl B., Beahrs O.H., Hermanek P.: TNM atlas. Illustrated guide to the TNP/pTNM - classification of malignant tumours. UICC international union against cancer. 3rd ed. New York, Springer-Verlag, 1989, 173-183

33. Cabanes P.A., Salmon R.J., Vilcoq J.R., et al.: Value of axillary dissection in addition to lumpectomy and radiotherapy in early breast cancer. The Breast Carcinoma Collaborative Group of the Institut Curie. Lancet 1992; 339:1245-1248

34. Steele R.J.G., Forrest A.P.M. et al.: The efficacy of lower axillary sampling in obtaining lymph node status in breast cancer: a controlled randomized trial. Br. J. Surg. 1985; 72: 368-369

35. Fisher E.R., Sass R., Fisher B.: Pathologic findings from the National Surgical Adjuvant Project for Breast Cancers (protocol no. 4). X. Discriminants for tenth year treatment failure. Cancer 1984; 53: 712-23

36. Veronesi U., Galimberti V., Zurrida S., Merson M., Greco M., Luini A.: Prognostic significance of number and level of axillary node metastases in breast cancer. The Breast 1993; 3: 224-228

37. Prognostic importance of occult axillary lymph node micrometastases from breast cancers. International (Ludwig) Breast Cancer Study Group. Lancet 1990; 335: 1565-8

38. de Mascarel I., Bonichon F., Coindre J.M., Trojani M.: Prognostic significance of breast cancer axillary lymph node micrometastases assessed by two special techniques: reevaluation with longer follow-up. Br. J. Cancer 1992; 66: 523-7

39. Galea M.H., Athanassiou E., Bell J., et al.: Occult regional lymph node metastases from breast carcinoma: immunohistological detection with antibodies CAM 5.2 and NCRC-11. J. Pathol., 1991; 165: 221-7

40. Pinder S.E., Ellis I.O., Galea M., et al.: Pathological prognostic factors in breast cancer. III. Vascular invasion: relationship with recurrence and survival in a large study with long-term follow-up. Histopathology, 1994; 24: 41-47

41. Bettelheim R., Penman H.G., Thornton-Jones H., Neville A.M.: Prognostic significance of peritumoral vascular invasion in breast cancer. Br. J. Cancer, 1984; 50: 771-777

42. O'Rourke S., Galea MH., Morgan D., et al.: Local recurrence after simple mastectomy. Br. J. Surg., 1994; 81: 386-9

43. Locker A.P., Ellis I.O., Morgan D.A., Elston C.W., Mitchell A., Blamey R.W.: Factors influencing local recurrence after excision and radiotherapy for primary breast cancer. Br. J. Surg., 1989; 76: 890-4

44. Todd J.H., Dowle C., Williams M.R., et al.: Confirmation of a prognostic index in primary breast cancer. Br. J. Cancer 1987; 56: 489-92

45. Brown J.M., Benson E.A., Jones M.: Conformation of a long-term prognostic index in breast cancer. The Breast 1993; 2: 144-147

46. Goulding H., Pinder S., Cannon P., et al.: A new immunohistochemical antibody for the assessment of estrogen receptor status on routine formalin-fixed tissue samples. Hum. Pathol., 1995; 26: 291-4

47. Goulding H., Nik Abdul Rashid N.F., Robertson J.F., et al.: Assessment of angiogenesis in breast carcinoma: an important factor in prognosis? Hum. Pathol., 1995; 26; 1196-1200

48. Matsukuma A., Enjoji M., Toyoshima S.: Ductal carcinoma of the breast. An analysis of proportions of intraductal and invasive components. Pathol. Res. Pract., 1991; 187: 62-7

49. Silverberg S.G., Chitale A.R.: Assessment of the significance of proportion of intraductal and infiltrating tumor growth in ductal carcinoma of the breast. Cancer, 1973; 32: 830-837

50. Van Dongen J.A., Fentiman I.S., Harris J.R., et al.: In-situ breast cancer: the EORTC consensus meeting. Lancet, 1989; 2: 25-7

51. Schnitt S.J., Connelly J.L., Harris J.Rea.: Pathologic predictors of early recurrence in stage I and stage II breast cancer treated by primary radiation therapy. Cancer, 1984; 53: 1049-1057

Premalignant, borderline lesions, ductal and lobular carcinoma *in situ*

C.N. Chinyama, C.A. Wells

Background

A premalignant condition is one which has the potential to develop into malignancy, and can subsequently pose a threat to life.[1] Premalignant lesions of the breast were investigated by Foote and Stewart as early as 1945 in a comparative study which attempted to assess the risk of developing invasive carcinoma when certain types of epithelial proliferations were present in both cancerous and non-cancerous biopsies.[2]

Epithelial proliferation, sometimes associated with cytological atypia, was five times more common in breasts containing cancer than in non-cancerous breasts.

This was not followed up until 30 years later when, by meticulous subgross analysis of sections, Wellings *et al.*[3] demonstrated that most epithelial abnormalities and carcinomas arise from the terminal duct-lobular unit (TDLU) rather than from the major ducts.

When assessing premalignant epithelial proliferations or non-invasive carcinoma of the breast, it is clinically useful to attempt assessing the probability of progression to invasive carcinoma. Page[1] provided useful criteria in assessing non-invasive breast proliferations by calculating the relative risk of developing invasive carcinoma.

The notion of risk factors based on histological interpretation of biopsies enables the clinician to take into account the histologically assessed risk of subsequent malignancy, in addition to the patient's age, family history of breast cancer and reproductive history, to plan suitable patient management.[4]

Screening mammography is effective in detecting non-palpable architectural abnormalities or calcifications. The biopsies of these lesions yield very small invasive carcinomas, carcinoma *in situ,* atypical or benign epithelial proliferations. Carcinoma *in situ* and various epithelial proliferations are more frequently encountered nowadays than in the pre-mammographic era. Consequently the need to assess the risk factors for developing invasive carcinoma has never been greater in order to give the patient and clinicians more information so that the most suitable treatment can be instituted.

Pathological assessment of biopsies

There is no place for frozen section examination in the management of mammographically detected impalpable lesions because of the risk of false positive diagnosis in the assessment of benign lesions such as sclerosing adenosis or radial scars. It is also important to properly assess these lesions as a whole because they are usually small and sampling for frozen section may interfere with the final diagnosis. The biopsy should be submitted to laboratory fresh and fixed for 24 hours for optimum processing. A specimen radiograph is essential prior to processing of the specimen. This enables the radiologist and surgeon to assess for adequacy of excision of the area of microcalcification or architectural distortion noted *in vivo.*

The radiograph also helps the pathologist to select the appropriate area for histological examination. The biopsy is painted with India ink or any other suitable substance to aid histological assessment of margins. The specimen is sliced in its long axis and the slices re-X-rayed if no macroscopic lesion is identified.

After description of any abnormality, tissue blocks are taken. The whole lesion is sampled if small, or a minimum of four blocks including margins. Microcalcification present in the specimen mammograph must be confirmed on histology. At all stages, cooperation between radiologist, surgeon and pathologist is vital.[5]

Lesions of doubtful malignant potential

Fibrocystic change and apocrine metaplasia

Apocrine epithelium is found lining the sweat glands of the vulva and axilla. Its presence in the breast is either thought to be of similar embryological origin to the sweat glands or arises due to metaplasia.[6] The latter view is widely held. Apocrine metaplasia is an integral part of fibrocystic change or gross cystic disease (Fig. 1). The cells are large with eosinophilic granular cytoplasm and basally located nuclei with or without apical 'snouts'. Fibrocystic change presents with an ill defined palpable mass generally between the ages of 35 and 50. There is conflicting evidence as to whether apocrine epithelium is premalignant or not.

In 1932 Dawson[6] identified apocrine epithelium in both cancerous and non-cancerous breasts but she was unable to demonstrate carcinoma arising directly in the apocrine epithelium, and hence it was felt not to be a premalignant condition. These findings were

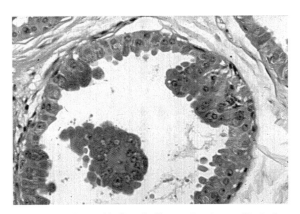

Fig. 1. Apocrine epithelium in fibrocystic change illustrating granular cytoplasm and apical snouts (H.E., 20x).

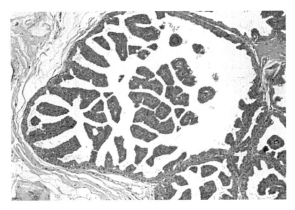

Fig. 2. Florid apocrine papillary hyperplasia (H.E., 20x).

disputed by Haagensen[7] who followed up patients whose biopsies had revealed apocrine metaplasia in gross cystic disease. His patients had a five-fold risk of developing carcinoma. The significant apocrine metaplasia in Haagensen's series had mainly a papillary configuration. Although some of these apocrine proliferations can be florid, cytological atypia is unusual (Fig. 2).

By using subgross analysis Wellings *et al.* demonstrated that apocrine metaplastic change occurred in the terminal duct-lobular unit (TDLU), the site of premalignant proliferation, and that it was a marker for increased risk for breast cancer.[8] This conclusion was based on the fact that apocrine metaplasia was more prevalent in cancerous breasts than in non-cancerous breasts; hence apocrine metaplasia was a manifestation of an unstable epithelium. In an earlier study, Page *et al.* suggested that patients over the age of 45 with papillary apocrine metaplasia had twice the relative risk of developing invasive carcinoma.[9] Seven years later, in a separate study, Dupont and Page concluded that cysts and apocrine epithelium *per se* did not increase the risk of carcinoma. However, the presence of cysts in a patient with a family history of breast cancer elevated the risk slightly to 2.7 times higher than that of women without this risk factor.[10]

Following complaints from women who were paying high insurance premiums after a diagnosis of 'fibrocystic disease', a consensus meeting was held in New York (1985) by the Cancer Committee of the College of American Pathologists.[11] They agreed to change the term to fibrocystic change and concluded that cysts and apocrine metaplasia alone were not premalignant. If the general term 'fibrocystic change' is to be used, the associated epithelial components must be specifically defined to allow an accurate assessment of the risk of subsequent cancer.

Lesions with a premalignant potential

Sclerosing adenosis (SA)

Jensen and colleagues defined sclerosing adenosis (SA) as a benign lobulo–centric lesion with a disordered increase in acinar, myoepithelial and connective tissue elements.[12] The enlargement of the lobular units due to increase in the number of acini with concomitant fibrosis often distorts the lobular architecture (Fig. 3). The significance of sclerosing adenosis lies in its ability to mimic invasive cancer clinically, mammographically, macroscopically and microscopically especially when perineural invasion is present. Sclerosing adenosis is most prevalent in perimenopausal women and its tendency to calcify makes mammographic detection easy.

Jensen *et al.*[12] followed up patients with sclerosing adenosis and they calculated the relative risk for developing invasive breast cancer to be 2.1 regardless of the presence of atypical hyperplasia. The risk decreased to 1.7 when patients with atypical hyperplasia were excluded and elevated to 6.7 when patients with atypical hyperplasia and SA only were analysed. Consequently, SA qualifies to be included in the category of proliferative breast disease without atypia with an overall cancer risk of 1.5 to 2 times that of the general population. A positive family history of breast cancer in the absence of atypical hyperplasia did not significantly elevate the risk for invasive cancer. In the same study, there was a positive association of SA and atypical lobular hyperplasia which elevated the relative risk for developing invasive cancer to 7.6. Oberman[13] and Fechner[14] independently reported an association of lobular carcinoma *in situ* and sclerosing adenosis although they did not consider SA a risk factor for lobular neoplasia. This association of lobular proliferations with SA should alert the pathologist to search for lobular neoplasia in the presence of sclerosing adenosis. Apocrine adenosis, defined as the presence of apocrine cytology in a recognizable lobular unit which may or may not be deformed, is sometimes detected on screening mammography due to the presence of microcalcification or in association with a sclerosing lesion. Because the cells are large and pleomorphic there is a risk of misdiagnosis of cancer both on cytological and histological examination.[15,16] The associated risk for developing invasive cancer with apocrine adenosis, if any, is unknown.

Multiple papillomas

Papillomas are an intraductal proliferation of villous–like or arborescent structures with a central fibrovascular core covered by a basal myoepithelial and luminal epithelial cell layer (Figs. 4, 5).

Multiple papillomas may be indistinguishable from fibrocystic change clinically. Ohuchi *et al.* demonstrated by three-dimensional reconstruction that multiple papillomas arise peripherally from the terminal duct-lobular units.[17] In 24% of cases, carcinoma *in situ* mainly of ductal type was discovered incidentally during the reconstruction. Three dimensional reconstructions also revealed that carcinomas with multifocal origin in the TDLUs were connected with peripheral papillomas. In contrast, none of the patients with solitary papillomas which arise centrally from the nipple major ducts had concomitant carcinoma. Central papillomas invariably present with a nipple discharge.

The premalignant nature of multiple papillomas was first illustrated by Muir in 1941[18] in his article on

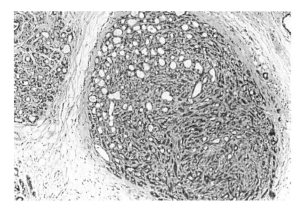

Fig. 3. Sclerosing adenosis characterised by increased lobular units and fibrosis (H.E., 10x).

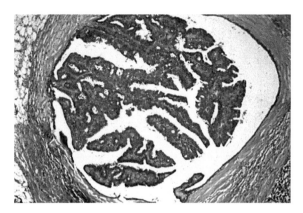

Fig. 4. Intraduct papilloma consisting of a fibrovascular core covered by two layers of cells (H.E., 10x).

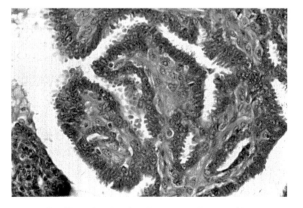

Fig. 5. Papillary fronds showing a basal myoepithelial and luminal epithelial layer (H.E., 40x).

evolution of carcinoma of the breast in which relatively young women of 50 years and below had developed carcinoma in association with multiple papillomas. The carcinoma was mainly invasive or *in situ* of cribriform type. Multiple papillomas are an infrequent condition with only 53 cases retrieved from Haagensen's files over a period of 39 years.[7] The majority of the patients were 40 years old or younger and six out of 53 developed breast cancer after a follow up of 19 years. Again, in this study, Haagensen emphasised the difference between central, solitary papillomas from multiple peripheral papillomas. Central papillomas tend to have a lower premalignant potential. Because of the frequent association of multiple papillomas with ductal hyperplasia of the usual type it is difficult accurately to ascertain the risk for developing invasive cancer in patients with multiple papillomas. Although the premalignant nature of multiple papillomas was disputed in the past, it was agreed at the consensus meeting in New York that the relative risk for developing carcinoma is comparable to that of epithelial hyperplasia of usual type which is 1.5 to two times that of the general population.[11]

Epithelial hyperplasia

The normal breast duct-lobular units are lined by two cell types consisting of an outer myoepithelial and an inner epithelial layer. Epithelial hyperplasia denotes an increase in the number of cells to more than two above the basement membrane.[19] Like most forms of epithelial proliferation, hyperplasia originates from the terminal duct-lobular units and this varies from mild through florid to atypical proliferation which may be virtually indistinguishable from carcinoma *in situ*. The relative risk for developing invasive carcinoma escalates numerically according to the degree of atypia. This was demonstrated in a large study by Page *et al.*[10] when they followed up over 10,000 women who had undergone biopsy for clinically benign breast disease. The histological slides were reviewed and the features present in biopsies of women who subsequently developed

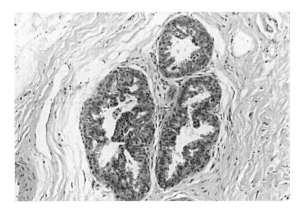

Fig. 6. Mild ductal hyperplasia with an irregular epithelial proliferation (H.E., 10x).

cancer were compared with those who did not. It was this work of Page and colleagues which led to the classification of ductal epithelial proliferations into mild, moderate or florid proliferative disease without atypia [PDWA] and atypical ductal hyperplasia (ADH). These proliferations may be identified incidentally in biopsies removed for palpable abnormalities or screen detected architectural distortion with or without calcification. ADH may also be detected as developing microcalcification in the incident round of breast cancer screening.

Although all epithelial proliferations arise from the terminal duct-lobular units the commonest pattern is known as 'ductal' or usual type to distinguish it from lobular hyperplasia.

Mild ductal hyperplasia

Mild hyperplasia is present within a duct when three or four layers of epithelium are seen above the basement membrane.[19] The proliferation may be diffuse or focal (Fig. 6). The latter gives rise to a corrugated luminal appearance. It is important not to label tangentially cut ducts as hyperplasia. Mild hyperplasia is classified as a non-proliferative disease and carries the same risk of subsequent breast cancer as the general population. Its presence or absence in biopsies is not critical to patient management.[4] A family history of breast cancer does not increase the risk of cancer in patients with mild hyperplasia.

Moderate and florid hyperplasia without atypia

Proliferative disease without atypia (PDWA) is a descriptive term indicating moderate or florid hyperplasia without associated cytological atypia. Moderate hyperplasia is characterised by the presence of five or more cell layers above the basement membrane within a duct or acinus unit.

The cells of moderate hyperplasia may be confined to the periphery of the duct and may form papillae with bridges across the ductal lumen (Fig. 7). The papillae do not have the 'rigid' appearance of micropapillary or cribriform ductal carcinoma *in situ* (DCIS) and the cells lack the monotony of *in situ* carcinoma. Florid hyperplasia is due to the expansion of the ducts by epithelial proliferation which almost completely fills the lumen with residual serpiginous slit-like lumina at the periphery (Fig. 8).

The cytomorphology of moderate or florid hyperplasia is variable and it is important not to make a diagnosis of atypical hyperplasia or DCIS. The nuclei are bland with a delicate nuclear chromatin pattern, and may be mildly hyperchromatic with

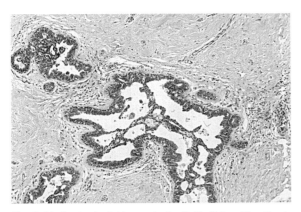

Fig. 7. Moderate ductal hyperplasia: Epithelial proliferation is present at the periphery of the duct with formation of bridges (H.E., 10x).

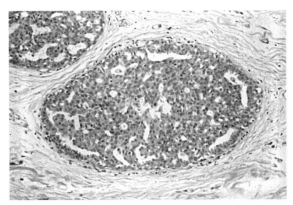

Fig. 8. Florid hyperplasia without atypia: duct completely filled by epithelial cells with serpiginous slits at the periphery (H.E., 20x).

small or inconspicuous nucleoli (Fig. 9). Mitoses may be present but are infrequent. The cytoplasm may be pale or eosinophilic and the cells may merge into an apocrine pattern with luminal 'snouts'. Only if the proliferation is completely apocrine in nature should it be designated as such. The cells can be arranged parallel to each other, a phenomenon Azzopardi termed 'streaming' or 'swirling'. Malignancy should not be diagnosed in the presence of this architectural pattern. Peripheral slit-like spaces are also a positive sign of benignity.[20] Occasionally central necrosis occurs in florid hyperplasia and this should not be interpreted as comedo carcinoma.

Moderate and florid hyperplasia is present in 20% of biopsies and its clinical significance lies in the fact that there is slight increase in the risk for invasive carcinoma of 1.5 to 2 times compared to that of the general population.[10]

Borderline lesions

Atypical ductal hyperplasia (ADH)

Atypical ductal hyperplasia (ADH) is the most controversial topic in breast pathology and scores of papers have been dedicated to the subject. This is due to the lack of definite histopathologic criteria as illustrated in the following definition of 'having both architectural and cytotogical atypia which approximates, but falls short of that seen carcinoma *in situ* (CIS).[4] This rather ambiguous definition was felt to be unacceptable by Azzopardi who stated "...the clinician should be told as unequivocally as possible whether the pathologist considers that the lesion is benign or malignant. Terms like... 'atypical hyperplasia' should be avoided as far as possible ...as such terms frighten surgeons into performing unnecessary mastectomies".[20] Over the years however, patholo-

gists have come to recognise a borderline epithelial proliferation which lies midway between PDWA and carcinoma *in situ*.

In their impressive follow up study of 10,542 women, 3.6% of which had atypical epithelial proliferations, Page *et al.*[21] illustrated that the term 'atypical hyperplasia' was appropriate for those lesions where the pattern or the cytological criteria of carcinoma *in situ* are partially met but not fully expressed. In the 1985 study Page set out criteria for identifying ADH, which he later improved in 1992.[22] In making a diagnosis of ADH, the criteria must be based on cytological features, histological pattern and anatomic extent. ADH exhibits partial involvement of basement membrane bound spaces by cell population similar to non-comedo type DCIS (cribriform). These atypical cells are evenly spaced, uniform with oval to round nuclei. The cytoplasm is pale with distinct intercellular borders. The non-atypical cells are columnar and are arranged radially at the periphery of the duct, just above the basement membrane. The histological pattern is variable. This includes

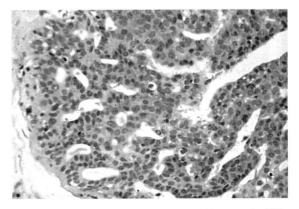

Fig. 9. Two cell types in florid hyperplasia without atypia (H.E., 20x).

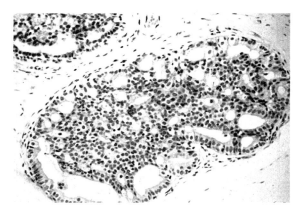

Fig. 10. Atypical ductal hyperplasia with a cribriform pattern showing partial involvement of the duct atypical cells (H.E., 10x).

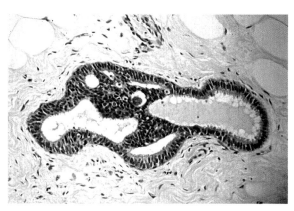

Fig. 11. Atypical ductal hyperplasia with atypical cells centrally and normal epithelium at the periphery (H.E., 20x).

secondary spaces with smooth rounded "punched-out" borders of cribriform architecture with or without rigid non-tapering bars (Figs. 10, 11). Micropapillary structures may also be present. The uniform cells must not completely involve two membrane bound spaces to qualify for ADH; if they do, DCIS is the appropriate diagnosis. ADH is usually 2-3mm in diameter.[54] The diagram in figure 12 illustrates the different features of DCIS, FHWA and ADH.

In spite of these criteria there is still a lot of inter–observer variation in the reporting of ADH as Rosai[23] found out when he distributed cases to five prominent breast pathologists in the USA. There was no consensus in the diagnosis of ADH versus CIS. The root of all this disagreement lies in the fact that it may be virtually impossible to distinguish ADH from small cell (low grade) DCIS of cribriform type. However, ADH is now a recognised entity whose relative risk

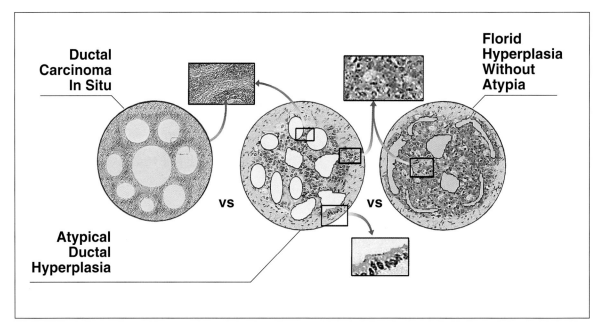

Fig. 12. Ductal Carcinoma *in situ* (DCIS) *versus* Atypical Ductal Hyperplasia (ADH) *versus* Florid Hyperplasia Without Atypia (FHWA): Cytology and Histology. DCIS features smooth, punched-out luminal borders within involved basement membrane–bound spaces. The cytologic features are regular and present throughout the entire population of at least two membrane-bound spaces. FHWA is the most densely cellular and extensive of the proliferative diseases without atypia lesions also called "papillomatosis". There are ragged, often slit-like luminal borders. The nuclei throughout the involved area show the variability and tendency to a swirling pattern, as illustrated. ADH has features predominantly of non-comedo, cribriform DCIS, but also some features of proliferative disease without atypia or normally polarised cells within the same basement membrane-bound space.

From Page and Rogers, Human Pathology, 1992, with permission of W.B. Saunders, Orlando, Florida.

of subsequent invasive cancer lies between that of PDWA and DCIS. Its presence in a biopsy should alert the pathologist to search for cancer in other sections since atypical proliferations are found more frequently in breasts harbouring cancer than non-cancerous breasts.[2] In a 15-year follow up study of women with ADH, Page and associates demonstrated a four times relative risk of developing invasive carcinoma of the breast compared to the general population. Translating this to absolute risk, approximately 10% of women with ADH will develop invasive cancer within 10-15 years of biopsy in the ipsilateral or contralateral breast. The relative risk doubles to 8-10 times if there is a family history (FH) of breast cancer (mother, sister or daughter) and hence the absolute risk is elevated to 20% at 15 years.[24] ADH is a rare lesion which often co–exists with fibrocystic change, sclerosing adenosis or multiple papillomas and is identified in 2% of non-screening biopsies.[54] The figure is much higher in screen detected lesions up to 12% in some series.[55]

Atypical lobular hyperplasia (ALH)

The histological criteria for atypical lobular hyperplasia (ALH) are met when there is partial distension of the acini in a lobular unit by a population of cells identical to those seen in lobular carcinoma *in situ* (LCIS) with residual intercellular spaces.[21] The resemblance to LCIS is striking but the acini are not uniformly distended in more than 50% of the lobular units (Fig. 13).

ALH represents incompletely developed LCIS and consequently the term lobular neoplasia is sometimes used for either LCIS or ALH.[25] ALH cells are bland and uniform with small or inconspicuous nucleoli. Pagetoid spread of atypical cells along ducts is sometimes seen in ALH as in LCIS. The latter diagnosis should not be made purely on this criterion without taking other features into consideration. Small clear spaces sometimes containing mucin may be present within the cells and these intracytoplasmic lumina or "private acini" are not true glandular lumina but represent dilated Golgi apparatus.

Like LCIS, ALH is impalpable and is usually present in biopsies removed for clinically benign conditions like fibrocystic change. The lesion is commoner in perimenopausal women with an average age of 46.[21,26] The relative risk for developing invasive carcinoma with ALH is four times that of the general population and this risk doubles when associated with a family history of breast cancer. The absolute risk for developing invasive cancer is 10% at 15 years.[25] The cancers associated with ALH are mainly lobular although ductal carcinoma can also develop and either breast is equally at risk.

Ductal carcinoma *in situ* (DCIS)

As early as 1932, Broders recognized carcinoma *in situ* (CIS) of the breast as a neoplastic epithelial proliferation confined to the ducts and acini without migration beyond the basement membrane.[27] Using subgross analysis, Wellings[3] demonstrated that carcinomas as well as other preneoplastic proliferations arise from the terminal duct-lobular units and that the histological appearance of ductal carcinoma *in situ* is due to 'unfolding' of the lobules. According to this theory, during epithelial proliferation the ductules of a lobule enlarge and the interlobular part ceases to exist. The ductules continue to dilate and incorporate themselves in a single lumen with resultant loss of the lobular architecture which is termed 'unfolding'.

Traditionally these structures have been called ducts and the term ductal carcinoma *in situ* is used to differentiate it from lobular carcinoma *in situ*. In the premammographic era ductal carcinoma *in situ* (DCIS) made up only 1 to 5% of symptomatic carcinoma.[28] In contrast to lobular carcinoma *in situ* which mainly affects premenopausal women, 70% of patients with DCIS are postmenopausal.[29] DCIS presents symptomatically as an ill defined mass, nipple discharge, Paget's disease or as an incidental finding in a clinically benign lump. In the last decade, DCIS has been more frequently seen as a non-palpable mammographically detected lesion with figures ranging from 10% to 20% depending on the breast screening unit.[30] Traditionally DCIS has been classified according to the architectural pattern into comedo and non-comedo with disregard of the cytomorphology.[19] The non-comedo type was further subclassified into cribriform, micropapillary, solid and papillary. Although, this is a useful pathological classification in terms of pattern recognition for diagnosis, it has little therapeutic or prognostic implication. Patchefsky (1989) noted the heterogeneous nature of DCIS

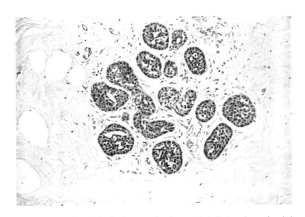

Fig. 13. Atypical lobular hyperplasia: partial distension of acini in a lobular unit by small uniform cells.

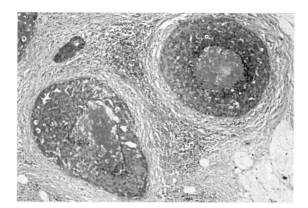

Fig. 14. High grade DCIS with central necrosis (H.E., x10).

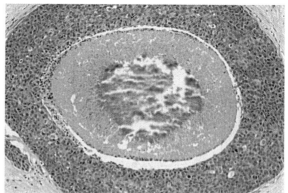

Fig. 15. Amorphous calcification of comedo high grade DCIS (H.E., 20x).

both pathologically and in biological behaviour and classified DCIS according to nuclear grade.[31]

Investigations using biological markers, three-dimensional studies, mammographic analysis and follow up of patients, demonstrated that the simple classification of DCIS according to architecture did not always correspond with the biological behaviour. Recently Holland *et al.* (1994) proposed a new classification of DCIS based on the nuclear morphology rather than on architecture and presence or absence of necrosis.[32] Using this criteria DCIS is divided into well, moderately and poorly differentiated. The only problem of using this terminology is that it may be misinterpreted by clinicians as invasive carcinoma. Similarly the United Kingdom Coordinating Group for Breast Screening Pathology classified DCIS according to nuclear grade into: high, intermediate and low grade.[54] Cytonuclear grade gives less inter-observer variation than architectural differentiation. However, there is often cytological and architectural overlap of lesions in the same breast and the *in situ* carcinomas must be graded according to the worst area. Both the new and old pathological classifications of DCIS will be discussed in relation to radiographic appearances, expression of biological markers and their behaviour.

High grade (comedo) DCIS

Comedo carcinoma is the commonest type of DCIS making up to 85% of high grade lesions.[31] It presents clinically with an ill defined mass or Paget's disease of the nipple. Radiologically it often has a linear, branching or granular pattern of microcalcification. On cut surface, breast tissue containing comedo carcinoma *in situ* reveals large ducts filled by yellow necrotic semisolid debris which is easily expressed like a 'comedone'. Histologically, high grade DCIS has a variable architectural differentiation or cellular polarization. The commonest pat-

tern is solid sheets of neoplastic cells which line the ducts with comedo central necrosis (Fig. 14). Necrosis is present in most cases but not exclusively. Pure solid DCIS is rare and is usually confined to nipple ducts in cases associated with Paget's disease. The mammographic calcification has an amorphous histological pattern (Fig. 15). Sometimes the neoplastic ducts accumulate foamy macrophages which simulates necrosis (Fig. 16). The cells may lack the solid pattern to attain a pseudocribriform or micropapillary configuration (Fig. 17). Periductal fibrosis and lymphocytic infiltration are often associated with this type of DCIS. The cells show marked variation in nuclear size and shape (pleomorphism) with a high nuclear-cytoplasmic ratio and condensation of chromatin. They are usually large with pale or eosinophilic cytoplasm (Fig. 18). The luminal layer of the epithelium is often retracted away from the necrotic debris. This distinguishes comedo necrosis from that occasionally seen in benign lesions like juvenile papillomatosis, nipple adenoma and hyperplasia of usual type.[4] Mitoses are often evident. High grade DCIS frequently demonstrates individual cell necrosis and autophagocytosis within the sheets of malignant cells.[32] When the pleomorphic cells involve recognisable lobular units, the term 'cancerization' of lobules is used (Fig. 19).

Low grade (non-comedo) DCIS

Low nuclear grade DCIS rarely presents with a palpable mass and is usually identified incidentally in a biopsy for a clinically benign lesion. Mammographic calcification is mostly granular and this is reflected histologically with a laminated crystalline pattern resembling psammoma bodies (Fig. 20). In contrast to comedo carcinoma *in situ*, low grade DCIS tends to have architectural differentiation or cellular polarization resulting in cribriform or micro-

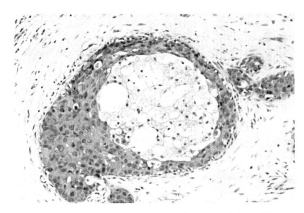

Fig. 16. High grade DCIS with central accumulation of foamy macrophages which simulates necrosis (H.E., 20x).

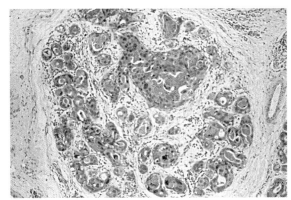

Fig. 19. Cancerization of lobules in high grade DCIS (H.E., 20x).

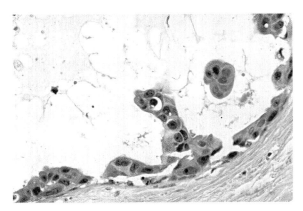

Fig. 17. High grade micropapillary DCIS (H.E., 20x).

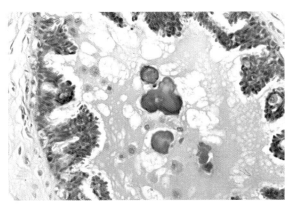

Fig. 20. Laminated calcification usually associated with low grade DCIS (H.E., 20x).

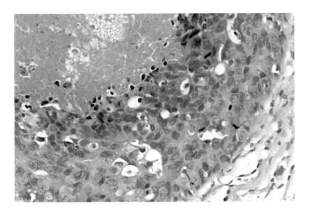

Fig. 18. Cytological features of high grade DCIS: pleomorphic large nuclei within eosinophilic abundant cytoplasm. Abnormal mitoses are common (H.E., 40x).

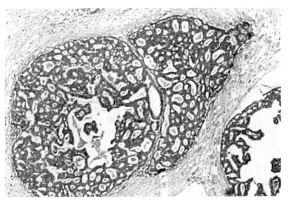

Fig. 21. Low grade DCIS with the characteristic cribriform pattern (H.E., 10x).

papillary carcinoma. The cribriform pattern consists of an intraduct proliferation of neoplastic cells separated by round or oval lumina (Fig. 21). This must be distinguished from collagenous spherulosis and adenoid cystic carcinoma. The papillae of micropapil-

lary DCIS are devoid of fibrovascular cores and are held rigidly and perpendicular to the basement membrane. Sometimes anastomosing arcades give rise to 'Roman bridges' (Fig. 22). Occasionally a single layer of neoplastic cells lines the duct lumen without

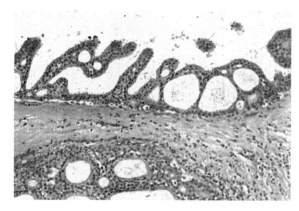

Fig .22. Low grade DCIS showing 'Roman bridges' (H.E., 20x).

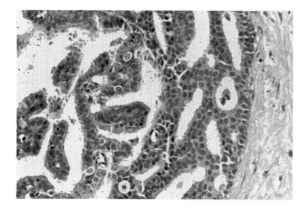

Fig. 23. The cells of low grade DCIS are uniform with small nucleoli (H.E., 40x).

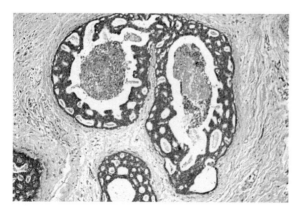

Fig. 24. Low grade DCIS with central necrosis (H.E., 20x).

projections, a pattern Azzopardi termed 'clinging carcinoma'. In cases where this is the only pattern , this would now be classified as ADH. The cells of low grade DCIS are small, monomorphic with round or oval nuclei. The nuclear membrane is smooth and the nucleolus is small or inconspicuous (Fig. 23). Mitoses are infrequent and individual cell necrosis is

not a feature.[32] Luminal necrosis is uncommon but can occur. Figure 24 illustrates clearly necrosis in low grade cribriform DCIS which would probably be termed comedo carcinoma in the old classification. Rarely, low grade DCIS exhibits solid proliferation to mimic lobular carcinoma *in situ.*

Intermediate grade DCIS

This group of DCIS cannot easily be assigned into either the high or low grade category. The architecture is variable and there is cellular polarization with micropapillae but not as marked as in low grade DCIS (Fig. 25). Solid areas with intercellular spaces may also be present. The cytomorphology of intermediate grade lies midway between that of high and low grade DCIS. The cells show moderate variation in nuclear size and shape. The chromatin pattern is coarse and the nucleoli are small. Calcification may be of mixed pattern showing both amorphous and psammomatous features in different ducts. Necrosis may or may not be present.[32] Biological markers have justified the inclusion of this third category of DCIS.[48] Clear cell and apocrine DCIS are usually of intermediate nuclear grade.

Intracystic papillary carcinoma

Intracystic papillary carcinoma is a form of ductal carcinoma *in situ* that involves a grossly dilated duct varying in size from 1 to 3 cm.[19] Irrespective of the size the important factor is that these lesions are non-invasive. Grossly the tumour may appear solid or a dilated duct filled with haemorrhagic debris may be evident. Histologically, the tumours may show a thick fibrous wall from which papillary excrescences arise (Fig. 26). The papillae consist of a fibrovascular core covered by a layer of epithelium without intervening myoepithelial cells. The cells are small, monomorphic and reminiscent of those seen in low grade DCIS (Fig. 27). The cells are so well differentiated that when Betsill (1978) reported patients with papillary intraduct carcinoma he used the term low grade and well differentiated carcinoma which would fit into the current classification of DCIS.[33] Cribriform type DCIS is sometimes present outside the 'cystic' wall where foci of micro-invasion occasionally lurk. Carter *et al.*[34] followed 29 women who had mastectomy for intracystic carcinoma and none developed metastatic carcinoma after five years of follow up. Because the cytology of intracystic carcinoma is well differentiated, these tumours should be put in the same category as low grade DCIS.

Prognostic implication of ductal carcinoma *in situ*

Because of the heterogeneous nature of DCIS, classification using cytomorphology and biological markers attempts to predict the behaviour of the different lesions. There are no long term prospective studies on the behaviour of mammographically detected DCIS and the information available is on retrospective studies on radiologically detected, symptomatic or incidental *in situ* carcinomas. Page followed up 28 patients with non-comedo DCIS identified incidentally in clinically benign lumps and treated by biopsy alone. This study predicted that 28% of women treated with biopsy alone for incidental DCIS would develop invasive carcinoma in approximately 15 years.[35] Clinically significant invasive carcinoma tends to occur proximal to the site of the original biopsy.

The calculated risk factor for developing invasive cancer following a diagnosis of DCIS is 10-11 times that of the general population.[35] The overall absolute risk of developing invasive carcinoma for both comedo and non-comedo DCIS is 30-50% at 10-18 years with 99% of the carcinoma occurring in the ipsilateral breast.[29] Invasive carcinoma occurring after mastectomy for DCIS is rare.[36] Lagios[30] followed up 79 women with mammographically detected DCIS treated by local excision alone (tylectomy). He classified the *in situ* carcinomas into four types; type I representing large cell comedo carcinoma and type IV the other end of the spectrum of small cell cribriform/micropapillary DCIS with two intermediate grades. The overall recurrence rate was 10% at 4 years. DCIS with high nuclear grade was more likely to recur than the cases with low nuclear grade and seven out of the eight recurrent cases were of high grade comedo DCIS. None of the small cell DCIS recurred and a single case of intermediate grade DCIS recurred. Price[37] recorded a higher recurrence figure of 55% at 7 years in patients with DCIS treated by local excision alone. Both invasive and *in situ* carcinoma were counted as recurrence.

Multicentricity and incompleteness of excision are usually incriminated as the underlying cause of recurrence of non-invasive carcinoma from residual carcinoma. While an occult focus of invasive carcinoma may be responsible for the development of subsequent invasive carcinoma, the majority of cases evolve from residual DCIS.[35] Rosen *et al.* demonstrated residual carcinoma in 56% of mastectomy specimens performed immediately after biopsy and 33% of these were present in quadrants other than the biopsy site.[38] In Patchefsky's study micropapillary ductal carcinoma *in situ* had a high propensity for multicentricity with more ducts involved than in any other type.[31]

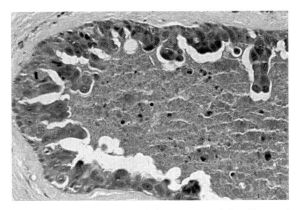

Fig .25. Intermediate grade DCIS showing partial architectural differentiation (H.E., 20x).

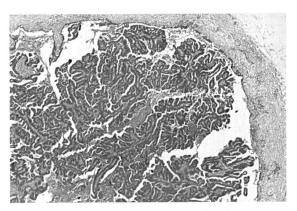

Fig. 26. Intracystic papillary carcinoma (H.E., 4x).

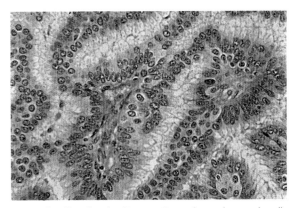

Fig. 27. Papillary fronds of intracystic carcinoma low grade cells devoid of myo-epithelial layer (H.E., 40x).

Multicentric DCIS is defined as tumour foci separated by uninvolved glandular tissue of 4 cm or more.[39] In the past multicentricity of DCIS was used as a justification for mastectomy.[37] Contrary to the widely held belief, DCIS is not always multicentric. Faverly *et al.* studied 60 mastectomy specimens using three dimensional imaging and only 8% of the cases of DCIS were multicentric. Using radiological–pathological mapping, Faverly and associates demonstrated that DCIS generally does not have a multicentric but a unicentric (segmental) distribution. DCIS tends to grow continuously by extending through the glandular tree but may also have a discontinuous or multifocal growth pattern. The latter is defined as at least two foci of tumour separated by an uninvolved portion of duct of any length less than 4 cm.[39] In this study 90% of high grade DCIS had a continuous growth pattern compared to low grade cases which had a multifocal distribution in 70% of cases.

In spite of the rare occurrence of multicentricity, DCIS tends to be extensive, hence completeness of excision is not always attainable and this is demonstrated by the frequency of recurrence following local excision.[30,37] Theoretically the assessment of margins should be more reliable in high grade DCIS which tends to have a continuous growth pattern as opposed to the multifocal nature of low nuclear grade in situ carcinoma. At the time of excision, at least 1 cm rim of normal breast tissue should be included. This approach surgically removes nearly 90% of unifocal in situ carcinoma irrespective of the histological type.[39] The use of both clinical and specimen radiographs is invaluable in assessing adequacy of excision.

DCIS and micro-invasion

Micro-invasion is defined as the presence of an invasive carcinoma not more than 1 mm in diameter (2 high power fields) outside the confines of a membrane bound lobular unit where the dominant lesion is carcinoma in situ.[5] Micro-invasion indicates the presence of a clone of cells with propensity to metastasise putting the patient at risk of a life threatening disease. The difficulty in assessing risk for metastasis is due to the different criteria used to define what constitutes micro-invasion or minimally invasive carcinoma. Hartmann defined the latter as infiltrating carcinoma equal to or less than 1 cm in greatest diameter in association with in situ carcinoma.[40] Definite micro-invasion consists of irregularly shaped and variably sized nests of cells surrounded by a 'fresh' fibroblastic proliferation that is not well orientated around individual epithelial nests.[4] However lesions which fulfill this criteria are rare and if in doubt a diagnosis of DCIS should be made. Disruption of the stromal-epithelial interface per se does not indicate micro-invasion. A prominent lymphocytic infiltrate should lead to the search for micro-invasion.[4] Basement membrane stains using immunocy-

tochemistry can aid in assessing for micro-invasion. Twenty-nine percent of patients with DCIS in Pachefsky's study had micro-invasive carcinoma and the majority were associated with comedo type DCIS (high grade). None of the solid or cribriform variants had micro-invasion.[31] Multiple sections may reveal a focus of micro-invasion. Overall, patients with high grade DCIS are at risk of harbouring micro-invasion with subsequent metastases.

DCIS in invasive carcinoma

DCIS is commonly associated with invasive carcinoma of no special type and is not a component of medullary carcinoma. The presence of in situ lesions in invasive carcinoma confirms their premalignant nature. Lampejo et al.[41] demonstrated a positive correlation between the different grades of invasive and in situ carcinomas which was prognostically significant. Low grade DCIS was usually associated with grade 1 invasive carcinoma; intermediate grade DCIS with grade 2 invasive carcinomas and high grade DCIS with either grade 2 or grade 3 cancers.

The type of the DCIS component was predictive of the outcome. None of the patients with tumours containing low grade DCIS developed recurrence after a median follow up of 13 years. Cancers containing high grade DCIS had the worst prognosis. In addition to assessing the type of DCIS present in the invasive carcinoma, it is also of clinical significance to determine the extent of DCIS outside the invasive component. The Boston group defined extensive DCIS as that consisting of more than 25% of the main invasive tumour mass and extending beyond it into the surrounding breast tissue or a tumour which shows foci of invasion within a predominantly in situ carcinoma.[42] It was agreed at the European Organisation for Research on Treatment of Cancer (EORTC) consensus meeting that the principal risk factor for local relapse following conservative surgery is a large residual burden of DCIS found adjacent to 10-15% of invasive carcinoma.[43] DCIS is commonly present beyond mammographically detected microcalcification and it is important to sample the apparently normal breast tissue to detect any extensive in situ component.

Lobular carcinoma in situ

Lobular carcinoma in situ (LCIS) was first recognised as an entity by Foote and Stewart as early as 1941.[44] This is distinguished from atypical lobular hyperplasia (ALH) by the complete distension of more than 50% of the acini in a lobular unit by uniform population of cells (Fig. 28). The cells are arranged in a regular pattern with no intercellular spaces but intracellular lumina (private acini) may be present, displacing the rather hyperchromatic nuclei eccentrically (Fig. 29). Pagetoid spread along ducts is commoner in LCIS than ALH (Fig. 30). Unlike DCIS, LCIS has no specific mammographic or clinical features and is usually an incidental finding in biopsies. Seventy percent of women with LCIS are premenopausal and the condition is present in 1% of screen detected lesions.[29]

Because of the different criteria used in different series to make the diagnosis of ALH and LCIS, the term lobular neoplasia is sometimes used for either lesion. Haagensen used the term lobular neoplasia solely for lobular carcinoma *in situ*.[7] LCIS tends to be multifocal, bilateral and predisposes to invasive cancer even after a long interval. In a 15-year follow up study of 39 patients with LCIS, Page *et al.*[25] calculated the relative risk for developing invasive cancer to be 10-11 times that of the general population. The absolute risk of developing invasive cancer in patients with LCIS is 25-30 % at 15-20 years. The risk of cancer is 50-60 % in the same breast and 40-50 % in the contralateral breast.[29] Seventy percent of the cancers are of lobular type and the remainder mixed or ductal of no special type.

In contrast to atypical hyperplastic lesions, a family history of breast cancer does not appear to have any further predictive value in identifying women who develop invasive carcinoma.[25] The effect of exogenous oestrogen in postmenopausal women is not known.

DCIS and expression of biological markers

Histological grade, lymph node status and the application of biological markers have been used in combination to evaluate prognosis in invasive carcinomas. The commonly studied biological markers are c–erbB2 and p53 proteins and oestrogen and progesterone receptors. These markers have also been applied to non-invasive carcinomas in an attempt to predict their behaviour.

The c–erbB2 gene encodes a transmembrane glycoprotein with a tyrosine kinase activity which is homologous to but is distinct from the epidermal growth factor receptor.[45] The gene is located on chromosome 17q and amplification is associated with over-expression of the protein product which can be detected by immunohistochemistry as cell membrane staining.

Over-expression of c–erbB2 in 20% of invasive carcinoma is associated with poor prognosis and most of the carcinomas are poorly differentiated

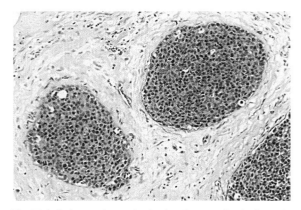

Fig. 28. Lobular carcinoma *in situ* showing completely distended acini with neoplastic cells (H.E., 10x).

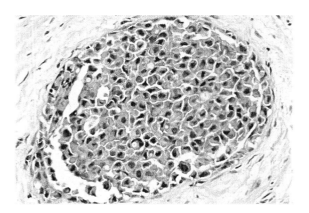

Fig. 29. Cells of lobular carcinoma *in situ* some showing eccentrically displaced nuclei and occasional intracytoplasmic vacuoles (H.E., 40x).

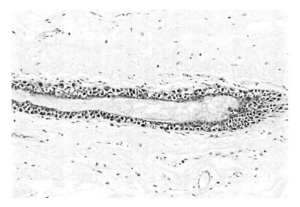

Fig. 30. Pagetoid spread within a duct by lobular neoplastic cells.

grade 3 carcinomas.[46] Approximately 60 to 80 % of high grade DCIS strongly express the c–erbB2 protein[47] (Fig. 31). None of the low grade DCIS express the c–erbB2 oncoprotein and approximately 23% of intermediate grade DCIS do.[48]

p53 is a nuclear phosphoprotein which functions

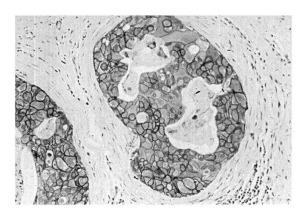

Fig. 31. High grade DCIS showing membrane staining with c–erbB2 oncoprotein antibody (20x).

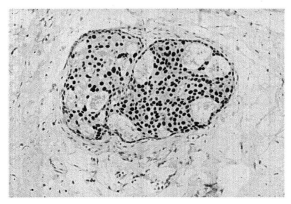

Fig. 32. Low grade DCIS positive for oestrogen receptors (wax embedded 20x).

as tumour suppressor gene and is the commonest deleted gene in human cancers.[49] The gene has been mapped on the short arm of chromosome 17 (17p13).[50] The mutant form has a longer half life than the wild type and it can be detected by immunocytochemistry[51] giving rise to positive nuclear staining. Sixty percent of high grade DCIS show positive nuclear staining for p53 protein compared to 4% of intermediate grade and none of the low grade cases.[48]

Poller et al.[52] demonstrated an inverse relationship between the expression of c–erbB2 in DCIS and hormone receptor status. A similar pattern is seen in invasive carcinoma. Majority of high grade DCIS and poorly differentiated invasive ductal carcinomas over-express c–erbB2 oncoprotein and lack oestrogen receptors. In Poller's study mostly small cell (low grade) DCIS expressed the oestrogen and progesterone receptor molecules. The latter is directly modulated by oestrogen and therefore its level of expression mirrors that of oestrogen receptor. In a separate study by Zafrani on mammographically detected DCIS, it was noted that a higher percentage of high grade cases expressed oestrogen receptors as well as c–erbB2 protein.[53] This discrepancy in the two studies may be due to the microwave antigen-retrieval method used by Zafrani. The presence of both oestrogen and progesterone receptors can now be demonstrated using immunocytochemistry on wax embedded tissue. Similar to p53, expression of these receptors is demonstrated by nuclear staining (Fig. 32).

Acknowledgements

We are most grateful to Dr. D.L. Page, Dr. L.W. Rogers and W.B. Saunders Publishers for the permission to use the diagram in Figure 12. We would also like to thank Mr. G. McPhail for assistance with photography.

References

1. Page D.L.: Cancer risk assessment in benign breast biopsies. Hum. Pathol., 1986; 17: 871-874
2. Foote F.W., Stewart F.W.: Comparative studies of cancerous versus noncancerous breasts. Ann. Surg., 1945; 121: 6-53, 197-222
3. Wellings S.R., Jensen H.M., Marcum R.G.: An atlas of the subgross pathology of human breast with special reference to possible precancerous lesions. J. Nat. Cancer Inst., 1975; 55: 231-273
4. Fechner R.E., Mills S.E.: Philosophy of risk assessment. Ductal carcinoma in situ. In: Breast Pathology, Benign Proliferations, Atypias & In Situ Carcinomas. ASCP Press, Chicago 1990; 1-3; 107-118
5. Sloane J.P.: Pathology reporting in breast cancer screening. J. Clin. Pathol., 1991; 44: 710-725
6. Dawson E.K.: Sweat gland carcinoma of the breast. A morpho-histological study. Edinburgh Med. J., 1932; 39: 409-438
7. Haagensen C.D.: Apocrine epithelium; Solitary intraductal papilloma; Multiple intraductal papilloma; Lobular neoplasia (Lobular carcinoma in situ). In: Diseases of the breast. Philadelphia, W.B Saunders Company, 1986; 82-101; 136-175; 176-191; 192-241
8. Wellings S.R., Alpers C.E.: Apocrine cystic metaplasia: subgross pathology and prevalence in cancer associated versus random autopsy breasts. Hum. Pathol., 1987; 18: 381-386
9. Page D.L., Zwaag R.V., Rogers L.W., Williams L.T., Walker W.E., Hartman W.H.: Relation between component parts of fibrocystic disease complex and breast cancer. J. Natl. Cancer Inst., 1978; 61: 1055-1063
10. Dupont W.D., Page D.L.: Risk factors for breast cancer in women with proliferative breast disease. N. Engl. J. Med., 1985; 312: 146-151
11. Hutter R.V. et al.: Consensus meeting: Is 'fibrocystic disease' of the breast precancerous? Arch. Pathol. Lab. Med., 1986; 110: 171-173
12. Jensen R.A., Page D.L., Dupont W.D., Rogers L.W.: Invasive breast cancer risk in women with sclerosing adenosis. Cancer, 1989; 64: 1977-1983
13. Oberman H.A., Markey B.A.: Noninvasive carcinoma of the breast presenting in adenosis. Mod. Pathol., 1991; 4: 31-35

14. Fechner R.E.: Lobular carcinoma in situ in sclerosing adenosis. A potential confusion with invasive carcinoma. Am. J. Surg. Pathol., 1981; 5: 233-239

15. Makunura C.N., Curling O.M., Yeomans P., Perry N., Wells C.A.: Apocrine adenosis within a radial scar: a case of false positive breast cytodiagnosis. Cytopathol.,1994; 5: 123-128

16. Simpson J.F., Page D.L., Dupont W.D.: Apocrine adenosis -a mimic of mammary carcinoma. Surg. Pathol., 1990; 3: 289-299

17. Ohuchi N., Abe R., Kasai M.: Possible cancerous change of intraductal papillomas of the breast. A 3–D reconstruction study of 25 cases. Cancer, 1984; 54: 605-611

18. Muir R.: The evolution of carcinoma of the mamma. Journ. Path., 1941; L11(2): 155-172

19. Page D.L., Rogers L.W.: Epithelial hyperplasia;Carcinoma in situ (CIS). In: Page D.L. & Anderson T.J. (Eds.) *Diagnostic histopathology of the breast*. Edinburgh, London, Melbourne, New York, Churchill Livingstone, 1987; 120-56; 157-192

20. Azzopardi J.G.: Overdiagnosis of malignancy. In: *Problems in Breast Pathology*. Philadelphia, W.B. Saunders Company 1979; 167-191

21. Page D.L., Dupont W.D., Rogers L.W., Rados M.S.: Atypical hyperplastic lesions of the female breast: A long term follow-up study. Cancer, 1985; 55: 2698-2708

22. Page D.L., Rogers L.W.: Combined histologic and cytologic criteria for the diagnosis of mammary atypical ductal hyperplasia. Hum. Pathol., 1992; 23: 1095-1097

23. Rosai J.: Borderline epithelial lesions of the breast. Am. J. Surg. Pathol., 1991; 15: 209-221

24. Page D.L., Dupont W.D.: Indicators of increased breast cancer risk in humans. J. Cell Bioch. (Supp.) 1992; 16G:175-182

25. Page D.L., Kidd T.E., Dupont W.D., Simpson J.F., Rogers L.W.: Lobular neoplasia of the breast: higher risk for subsequent invasive cancer predicted by more extensive disease. Hum. Pathol. 1991; 22: 1232-1239

26. Haagensen C.D., Lane N., Lattes R., Bodian C.: Lobular neoplasia (so-called lobular carcinoma in situ) of the breast. Cancer, 1978; 42: 737–769

27. Broders A.C.: Carcinoma in situ contrasted with benign penetrating epithelium. J.A.M.A., 1932; 99: 1670-1674

28. Rosner D., Bedwani R.N., Vana.J., Baker H.W., Harris J.R.: Non-nvasive breast carcinoma: Results of a national survey of the American College of Surgeons. Ann. Surg., 1980; 192: 139-147

29. Page D.L., Steel C.M., Dixon J.M.: Carcinoma in situ and patients at high risk of breast cancer. Brit. Med. Journ., 1995; 310: 39-42

30. Lagios M.D., Margolin F.R., Westdahl P.R., Rose M.R.: Mammographically detected duct carcinoma in situ. Frequency of local recurrence following tylectomy and prognostic effect of nuclear grade on local recurrence. Cancer, 1989; 63: 618-624

31. Patchefsky A.S., Schwartz G.F., Finkelstein S.D., et al.: Heterogeneity of intraductal carcinoma of the breast. Cancer, 1989; 63: 731-741

32. Holland R., Pertese J.L., Millis R.R., Eusebi V., et al.: Ductal Carcinoma in situ: A proposal for a new classification. Sem. Diag. Path., 1994; 11: 167-180

33. Betsill W.L., Jr., Rosen P.P., Lieberman P.H., Robbins G.F.: Intraduct carcinoma. Long term follow-up after treatment by biopsy alone. J.A.M.A., 1978; 239: 1863-1867

34. Carter D., Orr S.L., Merino M.J.: Intracystic papillary carcinoma of the breast: After mastectomy, radiotherapy or excisional biopsy alone. Cancer, 1983; 52: 14–19

35. Page D.L., Dupont W.D., Rogers L.W., Landenberger M.: Intraduct carcinoma of the breast: follow-up after biopsy only. Cancer, 1982; 49: 751-758

36. Millis R.R., Thynne G.S.J.: In situ intraduct carcinoma of the breast: A long term follow up study. Br. J. Surg., 1975; 62: 957-962

37. Price P., Sinnet H.D., Gusterton B., Walsh G., A'Hern R.P., McKinna J.A.: Duct carcinoma in situ: predictors of local recurrence and progression in patients treated by surgery alone. Br. J. Cancer, 1990; 61: 869-872

38. Rosen P.P., Senie R., Schottenfeld D., Ashikari R.: Noninvasive breast Carcinoma. Frequency of unsuspected invasion and implications for treatment. Ann. Surg., 1979; 189: 377-382

39. Faverly R.G., Burgers L., Bult P., Holland R.: Three dimensional imaging of mammary ductal carcinoma in situ: clinical implications. Sem. Diag. Path., 1994; 11: 193-198

40. Hartmann W.H.: Minimal breast cancer. An update. Cancer, 1984; 53: 681-684

41. Lampejo O.T., Barnes D.N., Smith P., Millis R.R.: Evaluation of infiltrating ductal carcinomas with a DCIS component: correlation of histologic type of the in situ component with grade of the infiltrating component. Sem. Diag. Path., 1994; 11: 215-222

42. Schnitt S.J., Connolly J.L., Harris J.R., Hellman S., Richard B.: Pathologic predictors of early local recurrence in stage I and II breast cancer treated by primary radiation therapy. Cancer, 1984; 53: 1049-1057

43. van Dongen J.A., Harris J.R., Peterse J.L., et al.: In situ breast cancer: the EORTC consensus meeting. Lancet, 1989; ii: 25-27

44. Foote F.W. Jr., Stewart F.W.: Lobular carcinoma *in situ*. A rare form of mammary cancer. Am. J. Pathol., 1941; 27: 491-495

45. Imamate T., Ikawa S., Akiyama T., et al.: Similarity of protein encoded by the human c–erbB2 gene to epidermal growth factor receptor. Nature, 1986; 319: 230-234

46. Dykins R., Corbett I.P., Henry J.A., Wright C., et al.: Long term survival in breast cancer related to overexpression of c-erbB2 oncoprotein: an immunohistochemical study using monoclonal antibody NCL-CB11. Journ. Pathol. 1991; 163: 105-110

47. Ramachandra S., Machin L., Ashley S., Monaghan P., Gusterton B.A.: Immunohistochemical distribution of c-erbB2 In: *In situ* breast carcinoma-a detailed morphological analysis. Journ. Pathol., 1990; 161: 7-14

48. Bobrow L.G., Happerfield L.C., Gregory W.M., Sprignall R.D., Millis R.R.: The classification of ductal carcinoma in situ and its association with biological markers. Sem. Diag. Path., 1994; 11: 199-207

49. Harris A.L.: Mutant p53: the commonest genetic abnormality in human cancer ? J. Pathol., 1990; 162: 5-6

50. Isobe M., Emmanuel B.S., Giro D., Oren M., Croce C.M.: Localization of gene for human p53 tumour antigen to band 17p13. Nature, 1986; 320: 84-96

51. Walker R.A., Daring S.J., Lane D.T., Valley J.M.: Expression of p53 in infiltrating and in situ breast carcinomas. Journ. Pathol., 1991; 165: 203-211

52. Poller D.N., Sneak D.R.J., Roberts E.C., et al.: Oestrogen receptor expression in ductal carcinoma *in situ* of the breast: relationship to flow cytometric analysis of DNA and expression of the c–erbB2 oncoprotein. Br. J. Cancer, 1993; 68: 156-161

53. Zafrani B., Leroyer A., Fourquet A., et al.: Mammographically-detected ductal in situ carcinoma of the breast analysed with a new classification. A study of 127 cases: correlation with oestrogen and progesterone receptors, p53 and c–erbB2 proteins and proliferation activity. Sem. Diag. Path., 1994; 11:208–214

54. Pathology reporting in breast cancer screening: National coordinating group for breast screening pathology. NHSBP Publication No. 3; 2nd ed., 1995

55. Owings D.V., Hann L., Schnitt S.: How thoroughly should needle localization breast biopsies be sampled for microscopic examination? Am. J. Surg. Pathol., 1990; 14: 578-585

Invasive carcinoma of breast

M. Letcher

Pathologists attached to Breast Screening Units and Centres find that the traditional practices used for the diagnosis of breast cancer have to be extensively modified if they are to provide a satisfactory service. The incidence of the various histological types of cancers of the breast found in patients referred from Breast Screening Programmes (screen detected cancer) differs from those of cancers found by the patient ("symptomatic cancer") although the overall pathological diagnoses are all familiar. The tumours are frequently difficult to find in operative specimens. The Breast Screening Programme demands far more exactly quantified information than has often been offered in the past.

Pathologists participating in a Breast Screening Programme must be prepared to widen traditional attitudes. They should be involved as part of the Breast Screening team and learn to appreciate at least some of their radiological and clinical colleagues techniques and approach to diagnostic problems. An approach based solely on slide diagnosis of cell type considerably limits the potential clinical value of the histopathological examination. Correlation of histological diagnosis and the behaviour of the tumour, as observed in the macroscopic and slide examinations, with the clinical diagnosis, screening mammography abnormality and cytological diagnosis improves the diagnostic quality of the whole programme.

FNA Cytology. Many Breast Screening Centres use Fine Needle Aspiration Cytology (FNAC). Histopathologists should work in close contact with their cytology colleagues and must take the time to learn at least enough of cytology to know the strengths and limitations of the technique.

Diagnostic standards

In most Centres the histopathologist's tissue di-agnosis is recognised as the "Gold Standard" by which the quality of the programme is judged. It appears self-evident that diagnostic criteria should be standardised and that local and national protocols be established.

The National Health Service Breast Screening Programme's (NHSBSP) National Coordinating Group for Breast Screening Pathology has produced a suggested standard protocol, "Pathology Reporting in Breast Cancer Screening."[1] This includes a macroscopic examination protocol and standardised histopathological diagnoses based on the WHO Classification. The group has also produced a standardised report form for data collection from the screening programme. Filling in the data, which is subsequently entered into the NHSBSP's central computer, demands a systematic approach to the observation and collection of macroscopic and microscopic histopathology data.

I find the detailed accounts of Histopathology of the Breast found in Rosen & Oberman's " *Tumors of the Mammary Gland*", Page & Anderson's "*Diagnostic Histopathology of the Breast*", and Sloane's "*Biopsy Pathology of the Breast*" generally useful.[3-5] These in combination with the descriptions in the NHSBSP Pathology protocol usually include sufficient information and references to resolve diagnostic difficulties.

Clinical pathology protocol

Surgeons associated with Breast Screening Centres will treat many of their patients by conservation surgery rather than by mastectomy. Examination of these segmental excision specimens gives particular problems to pathologists which neither the pathologist new to the technique nor the surgeon may appreciate.

Our local team aims at a one-step operation involving axillary node sampling and segmental excision at the same operation in patients with an FNA cytology or core biopsy diagnosis of malignancy established in the Breast or Assessment Clinic.

Macroscopic examination

There are few tasks in histopathology as easy as the demonstration of a tumour in a breast biopsy taken after the patient has presented with the symptom of a palpable lump. Conversely there are few tasks as difficult as finding an impalpable screen detected focus of carcinoma *in-situ* in a mastectomy specimen without access to specimen X-ray facilities.

Primary aim of the macroscopic examination

The primary aim of the macroscopic examination is to find the abnormality found by mammographic screening.

Tumours found in the screening programme are frequently small and often invisible at routine cut-up. Despite localisation techniques the surgeon may find the abnormality difficult to find at operation and, on occasion, the pathologist and thus the clinical team must be absolutely confident that an abnormality is not present in the specimen referred.

Specimen X-ray

Any histopathology laboratory attached to a major Breast Screening Centre must have easy access to specimen X- ray facilities. All specimens treated by conservative surgery referred from breast screening must have a specimen X-ray available to the pathologist in the specimen cut-up room for direct comparison with the specimen (Fig. 1).

Many samples are received with specimen X-rays taken at operation but will also need subsequent tissue slice or paraffin block X-rays. General clinical breast mammographic apparatus is frequently inaccessible to pathology laboratories and the facility is best provided by apparatus located in the pathology laboratory.

I disagree with the view of the coordinating group that this procedure[1] is only necessary for impalpable lesions. The specimen X-ray not infrequently reveals additional information even in obvious lumps (i.e. calcifications elsewhere in specimen).The pathologist is frequently not told the screening history and / or clinical status of the specimen when the specimen is referred.

If no abnormality is found during the initial cut-up then slice X-rays should be prepared and tissue blocks taken oriented to any abnormality found (Figs. 2, 3).

Specimen types

Biopsies. The diagnosis in the majority of patients is best obtained by FNAC or core biopsy. Open biopsy of the breast to get a tissue diagnosis is now unusual. *Frozen Sections* are rarely requested by surgeons specializing in breast disease since the biopsy / FNAC diagnosis would normally be made pre-operatively. The Epping breast team aim to carry out definitive surgery, including lymph node sampling, at the time of the patient's first and only admission to hospital. Many other Centres have similar treatment regimens.

Localisation biopsy

Biopsies or segmental excision samples from impalpable mammographically located lesions are often received with a guide wire *in situ*. These are inserted pre-operatively under mammographic control and placed to guide the surgeon to the area where the tumour is located and do not locate the lesion for the pathologist. From the pathologist's view it is far

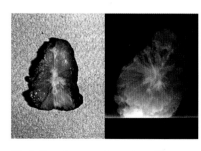 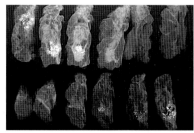 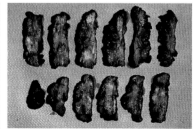

Fig 1. Specimen and specimen X-ray.   Fig. 2. Slice X-ray.   Fig. 3. Specimen slices of Fig. 2.

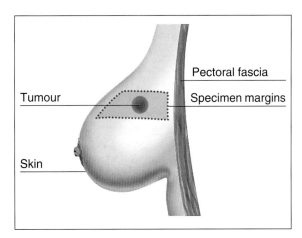

Diagram I. Schematic lateral view of breast to show surgical excision margins in a segmental excision specimen. Note that these will include all breast tissue between subcutaneous fat and pectoral fascia.

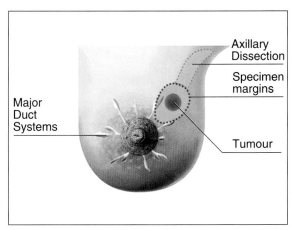

Diagram II. Schematic AP view of breast to show excision margins in segmental excision of upper quadrant.

better if the guide wire is not implanted in the lesion since cutting out the firmly implanted wire often causes artefactual damage to tumour pathology particularly to small lesions.

Segmental excision

Pathologists should appreciate fully that adequate surgical primary treatment by segmental or wide local excision is a cancer clearance operation which aims at cure and involves a complete dissection from subcutaneous fat to pectoralis fascia.

This is the preferred technique for conservative surgical treatment of suitable breast cancers and needs a completely different pathological approach to traditional methods of examining open breast biopsies or mastectomies.

Note that the specimen will include enough of one quadrant of breast to (hopefully) give a margin of at least 1cm around tumour margins and to clear the draining lactiferous ducts of the area. The specimen may include an axillary node dissection in continuity or separately.

It is extremely unlikely that early tumours clinically assessed as suitable for local excision will transgress the normal boundaries of specialized breast tissue. It is thus highly unlikely that tumour will involve subcutaneous fat or pectoral fascia. Tumour at, or very close to, margins adjoining breast tissue proper, is likely to mean that excision is incomplete and is the probable cause of the local recurrences that are a feature of conservation surgery. Early invasive carcinoma is also often associated with carcinoma *in situ* with likely spread towards the nipple.

It is essential to demonstrate the presence or

absence of tumour at the excision margins that adjoin normal breast and in particular at the nipple margin. The pathologist must be able to define these margins at the start of the macroscopic examination of the specimen.

Given the nature of breast tissue this places an obligation on surgeons to mark the margins at operation by a method previously agreed with their pathologists (Fig. 4).

The Surgeon must not incise the specimen. Formalin fixation distorts incised specimens and makes it impossible to determine the outer margins.

Demonstration of excision margins (Diag. 1, 2)

Ink or coloured solution marking is currently the method recommended by the NHSBSP Pathology fascicle.(Appendix 2)[1] We used Indian ink marking of margins from 1988 to 1993. The technique, particularly when supplemented by fast drying of the Indian ink by immersion of the specimen in Bouin's fluid, is undoubtedly effective (Fig. 5).

However we found significant disadvantages to Indian ink marking:
1. The very nature of breast tissue is to have fissures between lobules of rather loosely attached fat. These act as fjords allowing Indian ink or other fluid markers to mark areas well within the specimen and nowhere near the original surgical margin. Both pathologist and surgeon can easily be deceived by the didactic nature of the line of ink that excision is incomplete.
2. A specimen once ink marked turns into an anonymous black lump like overcooked Black Pud-

ding (Fig. 6). It becomes very difficult to orientate. Sutures used to orientate specimens by some surgeons are camouflaged and identification of the margins contiguous with remaining breast becomes extremely difficult.

3. Tissue blocks taken to demonstrate ink marked margins are taken perpendicular to the margin and thus can only sample the thickness of the slide, *i.e.* about a 4-6 micron thickness.

4. The technique is very messy and inclined to mark the fingers of the pathologist as indelibly as the specimen, enabling any latter day Sherlock Holmes to instantly identify one's profession.

In view of these considerations we have adopted a method of thin slice shave sampling parallel to the margins of the intact orientated sample into blocks orientated to the specimen before incising the sample (leaving guide wires *in situ* at this stage). Blocking a 2 mm shaving of the edge of the specimen seems likely to demonstrate tumour or multifocal disease within 1 mm of the margin over a much wider area than our previous method (Fig. 7). The method is the pathological equivalent of tumour bed biopsy advocated by some surgical teams,[6,7] and has the advantage of precise localization which can be lost when tumour bed biopsies are received separately from the main specimen.

After the essential preliminaries the whole sample is sequentially sliced at about 4-5 mm intervals and the slices laid out as for a formal brain examination. Even with thin macroscopic slices it is possible to miss a 4-5 mm tumour although tumours of 10mm diameter are easily found.

Needle or core biopsy track haemorrhage may be helpful in locating very small tumours particularly in mastectomy specimens. In *in situ* disease there may well be no macroscopic abnormality necessitating tissue slice X-ray. We usually mark the film with the block number. Particularly when looking for DCIS we have found it an advantage to take at least one large block as described by the Guildford team. Only if all these methods fail do we start to take multiple blind samples.

Axillary nodes. These are usually received marked for the highest node. I personally find it easier to detect small nodes in a well fixed sample despite the advice of the NHSBSP.[1] We do not try to detect micrometastases but do not hesitate to take more than one block from enlarged nodes. In nodes from patients with lobular carcinoma of breast it is occasionally necessary to resort to immunocytochemical demonstration of epithelial antigens to distinguish metastases from sinus histiocytosis (Fig. 8).

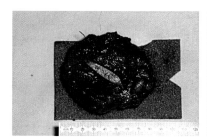

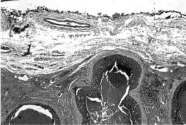

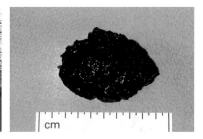

Fig. 4. Segmental excision oriented to card.

Fig. 5. Ink marked excision margin clear of DCIS.

Fig. 6. Indian ink marked localisation / segmental excision specimen.

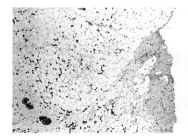

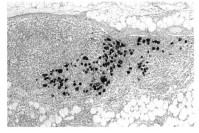

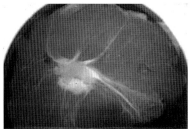

Fig. 7. Slice margin excision. Cells of infiltrating lobular carcinoma. Immunocytochemical reaction for Cam 5.2 MP.

Fig. 8. Atrophic axillary lymph node. Occult metastasis of lobular carcinoma. Immunocytochemical reaction for Epithelial Membrane Antigen. MP.

Fig 9. Specimen X- ray of 15 mm ductal carcinoma with stellate or crab-like outline.

Notes. All photomicrographs stained by Haematoxylin except where stated.
LP = x 16 - x 63 original magnification; MP = x 100 - x200 original magnification;HP = x 250 - x400 original magnification.

This would be a prohibitively expensive routine procedure in a district general hospital (DGH) histopathology laboratory.

If no nodes can be demonstrated it is necessary to clear the whole specimen in xylene (preceded by alcohol) This has helped find lymphoid foci but not yet led to the demonstration of metastases.

The pathology report should include a note on the total number of nodes sampled and on the number and site(s) of nodes showing metastasis.

Mastectomy. Treatment by mastectomy remains necessary for a substantial number of tumours and for those patients who prefer not to have breast conservation surgery.

I agree entirely with the recommendations in the NHSBSP Pathology protocol. I find it an advantage to take samples into block from small suspicious areas or small tumours during the initial examination of the fresh specimen since these are easy to palpate in the fresh sample but can be difficult to distinguish from fibrous breast when well fixed.

Mastectomy is increasingly performed for multifocal ductal carcinoma *in situ* (DCIS) which may very well be macroscopically undetectable. In this situation there is usually a previous biopsy cavity to guide the selection of blocks but the facility to X- ray whole slices through the specimen is virtually mandatory if a DGH department is to remain within budget and detect widespread DCIS. (And allow pathologists and laboratory staff to retain their sanity!)

Histology

Classification of invasive carcinoma of breast*

- **Invasive ductal carcinoma (Ductal carcinoma NOS or NST)**
- **Invasive ductal carcinoma with predominant intraductal component**
- **Invasive lobular carcinoma**
- **Medullary Carcinoma**
- **Mucinous (Colloid) carcinoma**
- Invasive papillary carcinoma
- **Tubular carcinoma**
- Adenoid cystic carcinoma
- Secretory (juvenile carcinoma)
- Apocrine carcinoma
- Carcinoma with metaplasia (Metaplastic carcinoma)
- Carcinoma with endocrine differentiation
- *Invasive cribriform carcinoma*
- *" Mixed" Carcinoma.*
- *Micro-invasive carcinoma*
- *Interval carcinoma*

The brief descriptions of these tumours given here do not pretend to be a substitute for the much more comprehensive and authoritative descriptions given in standard texts (*see* refs. 1,3,4,5) and concentrates on the tumours commonly found in a breast screening population in a DGH setting.

Introduction

Breast Carcinoma tends to have a heterogeneous histology. For example it is not unusual to find tumours showing some areas with apparently pure lobular differentiation and other areas showing mucoid change.

The diagnoses in the classification refer to the slide histological appearances of the majority of the area of the tumours. For example mucoid or tubular carcinomas should have at least 75% of the tumour showing mucoid or tubular differentiation (Figs. 20, 23).

However the terms **"Ductal"** and **"Lobular"** carcinoma can be misleading. In practice the lobular carcinoma group is defined by tight slide criteria. Invasive ductal carcinoma is diagnosed by exclusion. It is believed that both these major types of invasive breast carcinoma arise from the same area of the breast in the terminal ductulo-lobular units.[8] Conventionally any tumour not fitting the fairly rigid criteria for the defined varieties is diagnosed as a "ductal carcinoma of no specific type" (NST). Given the tendency to a heterogeneous histology the **"Ductal carcinoma NST"** group of tumours forms the majority of invasive carcinomas in all published series. The major differences from symptomatic carcinomas in this series, as in others, is the 15-20% incidence of *in situ* carcinoma and the high incidence of tubular and "other" carcinomas in the invasive carcinomas. Most of the "other" carcinomas in this series are variants of small cell carcinoma and carcinomas of mixed histology.

Invasive ductal carcinoma
Ductal carcinoma NST

In a non-screened populatio n the incidence is quoted as 65-80% of all breast cancers.

Our figures over the years 1987 - 95 show 230 of 427 (55%) invasive carcinomas were classified as Ductal NST (Tables I, II). This is by far the largest individual group of the invasive cancers in the screened population as in the symptomatic cancers.

Macroscopic examination

The classic type of breast carcinoma with a stellate or crab-like outline (Figs. 9, 10).

(* The categories in normal type correspond to the WHO Classification. Those in bold are described in this chapter. Those in bold italics are described and are recognised and normally used by pathologists in Breast Screening Centres).

Table I. Overall incidence of carcinomas in the Epping series 1987-95.

Carcinoma	All	*In situ*	Invasive	% *In situ*
Total	515	89	427	17%

Table II. Overall incidence of invasive carcinoma 1987-95.

Tumour Type	Ductal NOS	Tubular	Lobular	Other Ca	Total
Patient (n)	230	41	67	83	427
% incidence	55	10	15	19	

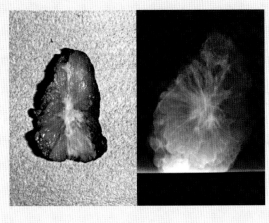

Table III. Prognostic differences between tubular, lobular and ductal invasive carcinomas.

Prognostic Features	Tumour Diam	+ve Nodes %	Vasc. Inv.	MF %
Tumour Type				
Tubular	11.6mm	8%	0%	1%
Ductal	17mm	27%	21%	30%
Lobular	18.4mm	21%	18%	32%

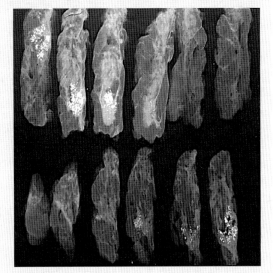

(MF = Multifocal involvement, Vasc. Inv = Lymphatic or vascular space invasion)

The cut surface of the tumour tends to be firm and flecked with a definite if spiculate edge and a gritty feel when the examining knife is dragged across its surface. A minority are softer, rounded and quite sharply outlined. Small tumours found in the screened population are usually quite easy to find in the specimen. A significant proportion of these tumours show calcifications both on specimen X-ray and histology (Fig. 2).

Microscopy

Despite the heterogeneous low power appearance implicit in the definition, the tumours show more similarities than differences. Invasive tumour cells tend to be set in a fibrous stroma and often aggregate in small and large groups. The majority of tumours showing definite gland or tubule formation are of ductal type as are most of the high grade (grade III) tumours. Screen detected invasive ductal carcinomas are frequently associated with the presence of DCIS. Calcifications are frequently present either in the invasive tumour or in the associated DCIS. The fibrous scarring tends to distort the normal architecture of the breast often producing an effect like a

contracture. The combination of this stellate scarring and calcification aids the mammographic detection of this type even when small.

Association with DCIS (41% in this series) in the screening population produces an increase in the incidence of multifocal disease.

High power. The different types of ductal carcinoma tend to show cells with prominent nucleoli, definite and often irregular nuclear membrane, variation in nuclear diameter and, usually, larger nuclei than in lobular carcinoma. The cell cytoplasm is usually more obvious than in lobular carcinoma. The cells may show mucin secretion. The stroma may also show dense elastosis. Areas of necrosis and calcifications are common features (Figs. 11-15).

Prognosis. Behaviour of ductal vs the other common types of invasive carcinoma in screen detected cancers in the Epping series is summarized in Table III.

Invasive carcinoma with extensive intraduct component. Screen detected carcinomas are frequently associated with ductal carcinoma *in situ*. 41% of the invasive ductal carcinoma in this series show some

182   M. Letcher

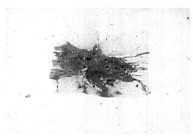

Fig. 10. Whole mount of same ductal carcinoma as in Fig 9.

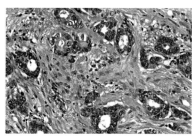

Fig. 11. Ductal carcinoma. Tubule formation in Grade I tumour HP.

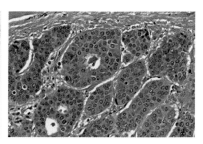

Fig. 12. Ductal carcinoma. Regular nuclei in aggregates. Grade I HP.

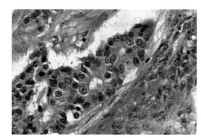

Fig. 13. Ductal carcinoma. Grade II HP.

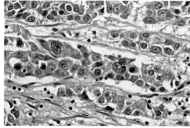

Fig. 14. Ductal carcinoma. Frequent mitoses and pleomorphic nuclei grade III HP.

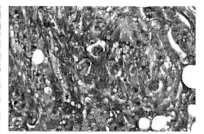

Fig. 15. Mucin secretion in ductal carcinoma. PAS/ Alcian blue MP.

Table IV. A comparison of histological type in interval and screen detected carcinoma.

Diagnosis	Ductal	Tubular	Lobular	Other	Medullary	Total
Interval Ca.% Hist. Type	66%	6%	20%	9%		
Breast Screening Service Ca.% Hist. Type	55%	10%	16%	19%		
Interval Ca. (n)	82	7	25	11	0	125
Breast Screening Service Ca. (n)	236	41	67	80	3	427

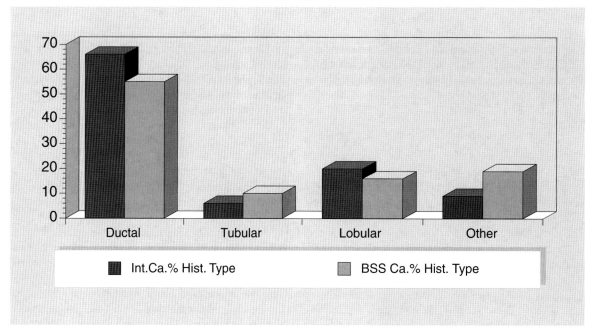

Interval Ca. *vs* BSS Ca.

(unquantified) DCIS. Extensive DCIS is associated with a high risk of local recurrence in patients treated by conservation surgery,[10] and pathologists should ensure that their reports clearly state the extent of any associated DCIS.

Infiltrating lobular carcinoma

Sixty-seven of 427 (15%) consecutive screen detected tumours were diagnosed as infiltrating lobular carcinoma 1987-95. This figure is higher than that quoted in the earlier publications but in line with those in other publications.[11,22]

Macroscopic appearance

Lobular carcinoma is also associated with productive stromal fibrosis but in early and some advanced lesions this is often not so pronounced as that found in ductal carcinoma. In a significant number the tumour exhibits diffuse infiltration amongst normal structures of the breast and can be very difficult to detect even by the pathologist examining 5 mm slices at macroscopic cut-up. The surgeon can also find it very difficult to define a tumour edge at operation even in palpable lesions. The microscopic, insidious, infiltrative nature of this tumour often causes macroscopic measurement of tumour diameter to differ significantly from slide diameter measurement.

Microscopy

The infiltrating tumour may resemble grains of dust blown by the wind to stream around pre-existing ducts and acini of the breast producing the "targetoid" appearance, without the associated destruction of these structures seen in other varieties of cancer (Fig. 16). A "Line of file" arrangement is a usual feature in many areas and is also found in variant patterns. The tumour edge is very indefinite with scatterings of cells around the main mass (Fig.17).

Separate foci of tumour are common in fat apparently quite well separated from the main tumour and are not infrequently found at excision margins (Fig 7). "Pagetoid" spread within duct epithelium at some distance from the main tumour is common and may be a feature wich helps to detect the presence of invasive tumour (Fig. 18).

Individual tumour cells are small to medium sized with relatively little variation. Rounded nuclei, slightly clouded clear nucleoplasm, a delicate nuclear membrane and inconspicuous nucleoli are all characteristic (Fig. 19). Intracytoplasmic mucin vacuoles are common although I do not rely on their presence or absence for confirmation of the diagnosis. Careful observation of these cytological nuclear features is essential to confirm the diagnosis of lobular carcinoma in a tumour with the characteristic infiltrative pattern. Calcifications are seldom present. Given the nuclear features and overall arrangement these tumours are usually histologically graded as grade I or II.

Multifocal involvement by invasive carcinoma is common (32% in our series).

Lobular carcinoma variants [1,3]

Solid. Arranged in large masses with little stroma. May resemble lymphoma.
Alveolar. Arranged in small rounded groups.
Pleomorphic. With typical growth pattern but much more marked nuclear pleomorphism.
Tubulo lobular.[12] Although composed of the characteristic cells and showing a diffuse infiltrative pattern this variant shows tubule or gland formation in much of the tumour. These tumours show the same tendency to multifocal involvement as classical lobular carcinoma and are not a variant of tubular carcinoma.

General features of lobular carcinoma in screen detected cancer

The overall growth pattern of lobular carcinoma

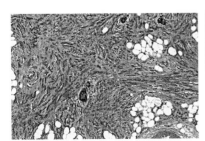
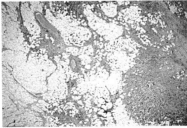
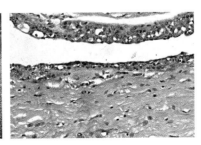

Fig. 16. Lobular carcinoma. Streaming or targetoid pattern. LP.

Fig. 17. Lobular carcinoma. Infiltrating edge with multifocal involvement. LP.

Fig. 18. Lobular carcinoma. Pagetoid spread in normal duct epithelium. HP.

Table V. Sizes of 395 invasive cancers from the Epping unit 1988-95.

Tumour size mm	1-10	10.1-15	15.1-20	20.1-50	Total
Total 1988-95	118	124	74	79	395
% Total	30%	31%	19%	20%	

combined with its lack of calcifications can make this a difficult tumour to detect mammographically. This is probably reflected in the larger average tumour diameter of 18.4 mm found in our series and the rather higher incidence in the "interval carcinomas" group" (Tables IV, V). The same features combined with the high incidence of multifocal invasive tumour may cause difficulty in patients treated by conservative surgery.

Tubular carcinoma

Forty-one of 427 patients with screen detected invasive cancers were found to have tubular carcinoma between 1987-95. The figure of 10% overall is higher than the incidence in symptomatic patients of 2%.[13]

Macroscopically these tumours are well circumscribed and firm to cut with a stellate cut surface. They are often small with an average macroscopic diameter in this series of 11.6 mm.

Microscopically the tumour is composed of quite well separated small regular glands which often appear angulated in a dense fibro-elastic stroma. The glands are composed of small regular cells one layer thick often with apocrine cytoplasmic luminal apical "snouts" (Figs 20, 21). Mitotic activity is low. Myoepithelial cells are not present around the tubules. Foci of cribriform differentiation (v.i.) are often present. At least 75%[3] to 90%[1] of the tumour should be composed of these tubular glands to allow the diagnosis although a substantial proportion (<50%) of cribriform carcinoma is allowed. With these criteria these tumours have an exceptionally good prognosis in symptomatic patients.[13]

Invasive cribriform carcinoma[14]

This variant of breast carcinoma is included with "other "carcinoma in the standard histopathology statistics issued by the NHSBSP. In my local database of 221 cases of invasive screen detected cancer between 1987-90 there were 7 cases of invasive cribriform carcinoma (3.2%).

The macroscopic features are unremarkable. Microscopically these tumours are composed of glandular masses with a lace-like appearance produced by bridges of cells 1-2 layers thick enclosing glandular spaces. The nuclear features are usually those of a low grade small cell tumour. Some mucin secretion is often present (Fig. 22).

Tubular (q.v.) differentiation is frequent and up to 50% still allows the diagnosis. However some carcinomas also show mixed lobular, colloid or ductal features and should be termed mixed carcinoma. The overall prognosis for pure cribriform carcinoma is excellent in symptomatic patients even when nodal metastases are present.[15]

Mucinous (colloid) carcinoma

Only 2 of 221 invasive carcinomas were classified as mucinous. The numbers are too small for any conclusions but this variety of low grade carcinoma does not appear to be more common in screen detected carcinoma.

The tumours are usually well circumscribed with a soft mucoid cut surface. Histologically low grade tumour cells in groups float free in pools of mucus (Fig. 23).

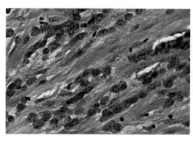

Fig. 19. Lobular carcinoma. Line-of-file infiltration by small regular cells. HP.

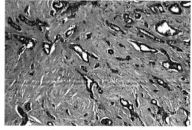

Fig. 20. Tubular carcinoma. Irregular tubules in fibrous stroma. MP.

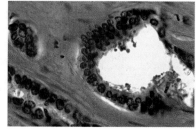

Fig. 21. Tubular carcinoma. Apical snouts in glands. HP.

At least 75% of the tumour should have this mucoid or colloid appearance to allow the diagnosis. In symptomatic cancers this variant has a better prognosis than ductal carcinoma NST.[16]

Papillary carcinoma[3]

This is typically found in elderly women but in this series 2 of 221 cases were diagnosed as papillary carcinoma.

Medullary carcinoma

This unusual and interesting tumour is defined in the WHO fascicle[2] as "a well circumscribed tumour composed of poorly differentiated cells with scant stroma and prominent lymphoid infiltration."

The definition has been much expanded.[3] The diagnostic criteria are strict and in practice neither I nor my colleagues make the diagnosis very often. Four cases were diagnosed as medullary carcinoma in the whole series of 427 screen detected cancers 1987 between 1995. Despite the predictions of colleagues the numbers diagnosed in the "interval" group of cancers (v.i.) are less.

Macroscopically these are sharply outlined firm tumours from 1-4 cm diameter.

Microscopically there must be a fairly to very dense lymphocytic infiltrate around tumour cells, a sharply defined rounded or pushing border and tumour is mainly composed of a syncytium of large anaplastic malignant cells. Mitoses are frequent (Figs. 24, 25).

Strict adherence to these criteria usually places putative medullary carcinomas in the category of Grade III ductal carcinoma (Fig. 26).

Atypical medullary carcinoma may be diagnosed even when all the diagnostic criteria are not met.[17] I am more willing to use this diagnosis than my colleagues.

In symptomatic breast cancer[18] medullary carcinoma is known to have a much better prognosis than expected from a high grade carcinoma.[18]

"Mixed" carcinoma of breast

Carcinoma with a mixed appearance is found not uncommonly in screen detected carcinoma. The tumour may consist of a mixture of virtually any of the types of carcinoma outlined previously and may be termed for example "mixed ductal and lobular carcinoma" or "mixed cribriform carcinoma". The term is particularly useful for a mixture of two low grade carcinomas which might otherwise have to be termed "ductal" (Fig. 27).

Eight of 221 tumours between 1987 and 1990 were thought to qualify for this diagnosis.

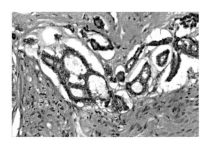

Fig. 22. Cribriform carcinoma. Perineural invasion by glands with intra-luminal bridges. HP.

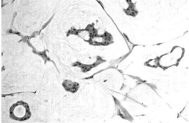

Fig. 23. Colloid carcinoma. Glandular groups free in pale staining mucin. HP.

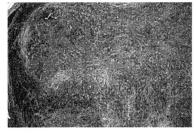

Fig. 24. Medullary carcinoma. LP view of tumour with lymphocytes and round edge.

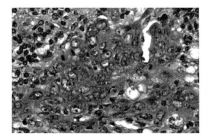

Fig. 25. Medullary carcinoma. Syncytial tumour cells with lymphocytic reaction. HP.

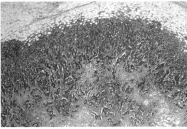

Fig. 26. Ductal carcinoma. Grade III mimicking LP appearance of medullary carcinoma.

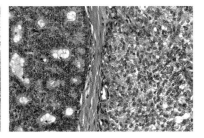

Fig. 27. Mixed carcinoma. Cribriform and solid lobular carcinoma in same field. HP.

Micro-invasive carcinoma of breast

This term is reserved for tumours with ≤1 mm invasion in the NHSBSP protocol.[1]

The topic is described in the chapter on DCIS. In our DGH population this was found in 3 of the 221 invasive cases between 1987-90 and even in screen detected carcinoma appears to be an uncommon phenomenon.

Paget's disease of nipple

Almost by definition Paget's disease would be expected to occur in the symptomatic patient. One case is known to have presented as an interval carcinoma. The intra-epidermal infiltrate of malignant cells is almost invariably associated in the breast with high grade (comedo) DCIS in the underlying breast (See chapter on DCIS).

Interval carcinoma

In a Breast Screening Programme an interval carcinoma is one that presents in the interval between routine mammographic screening.

Such tumours have been found in screening programmes performed at 1-2 yearly intervals[19] and it is to be expected that the NHSBSP with its 3-year screening interval would have a higher incidence of such tumours than programmes with a shorter screening interval.

These tumours occur in women who have been reassured by their screening centre that they are free from cancer and, particularly in and around larger metropolitan areas, it is very likely that they will ask for referral to a different hospital for treatment. In these circumstances finding cases can be very difficult.

The Epping team have tried very hard to find as many cases as possible. It may take 2-3 years after the treatment of the cancer before the screening centre is notified.

The existence of this group is one reason that the pathologists in Epping complete an NHSBSP form for every case of breast carcinoma since surgeons often appear unaware that a case clinically referred as a lump has had previous breast screening. One has often been told, by radiologists, that these must be tumours of high grade or lobular carcinoma which must have been mammographically undetectable or not present at the original screen.

The various subdivisions of interval cancer are analysed in the relevant chapter. Analysis of our interval cancers is currently in progress but a breakdown of the histological types in cases found so far is attached for interest (Table IV).

Prognostic factors

Tumour size, lymph node stage, histological grade and histological type are all recognised as having a significant influence on survival in patients with breast cancer.[20-22] 10-year survival figures are not yet available for the NHSBSP population and the figures given below are only indicative of differences that may exist between cancers detected at breast screening and those found in larger studies of breast cancer in unscreened populations.

Tumour size

Tumour size is one of the most significant prognostic indicators in patients with breast cancer. In general the smaller the tumour the better the long term prognosis.[23] In the absence of lymph node metastases the 10-year disease free interval for symptomatic T1N0 patients (tumour <20mm) is approximately 80% and for stage T1N0 tumours of 10 mm or less 90%.[24]

Size is expressed in the NHSBSP programme as the largest measurable diameter either in the specimen or as measured in the histological slide and recorded in the overall categories of :
≤ 10 mm, >10to≤ 15 mm, >15to≤20 mm, >20 to

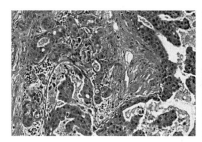

Fig. 28. Micro-invasive carcinoma. 1mm focus of mucin-secreting carcinoma (left) adjacent to micropapillary DCIS (right).

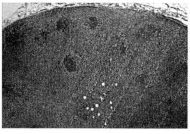

Fig. 29. Lymph node metastasis. Node almost replaced by metastatic lobular carcinoma with residual follicles. LP.

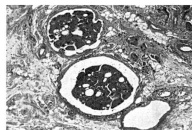

Fig. 30. Lymphatic invasion. MP.

Table VI. Lymph node metastases cases of invasive screen detected breast cancer 1987-90.

Lymph Nodes	Axillary dissection	Negative	1-3 Nodes	4 + Nodes
All Cases (n)	211	156	43	12
% of total		74%	20%	6%
Diam.≤10 mm (n)	27	25	2	0

Table VII. Histological grade of invasive cancers in Epping series.[1]

Tumour grade	I	II	III	Total (n)
Patients (n)	130	170	41	341
%	38%	50%	12%	100%

1. From available NHSBSP data.

50mm and > 50mm. No patient with a tumour larger than 50mm was found by the programme (Table V).

The NHSBSP's protocol strongly advises microscopic slide diameter measurement for any tumour of less than 15 mm on gross examination.

Lymph node metastasis

Lymph node metastasis is perhaps the single most important prognostic indicator demonstrating actual aggressive potential (Fig. 29). Within this group there appears to be a significant difference between patients with 1-3 nodes involved and those with 4 or more nodes involved (Table VI). Symptomatic patients at stage T1N1M0 (tumour < 20mm diam) have a 74% 10-year disease free survival if less than 3 nodes are involved versus a 50% 10-year survival if 4 or more nodes are involved.[24]

Eighty-one of 382 patients undergoing axillary node dissection in the Epping series of 400 patients between 1988-1994 showed metastases (21%).

There is some difference between the incidence of nodal metastases in the major histological groups in the screen detected cancers (see Table III).

Vascular/lymphatic invasion

Vascular and lymphatic invasion are recorded as one entity in the NHSBSP's data. In my experience demonstration of true vascular (venous) invasion in any breast carcinoma is uncommon and the data must usually be taken to imply lymphatic invasion.

Formalin-induced tissue shrinkage can produce pseudo spaces around tumour islands mimicking vascular space invasion. The pathologist must be satisfied that tumour emboli are present in a space lined by endothelium. The phenomenon is best demonstrated away from the main tumour (Fig. 30).

There is a significant incidence of local recurrence in patients with lymphatic invasion.[25]

Histological grade

Histological grade of tumours provides valuable prognostic data. With the majority of UK pathologists we use the method described by Elston & Ellis as modified from the original description of Bloom & Richardson.[26,27]

The NHSBSP pathology protocol[1] gives the most detailed and readily available practical guidance on recommended methods for application of the grading system. All tumours are graded in the range I- III with grade I tumours being well differentiated and grade III tumours poorly differentiated. Tumours are scored by separate semiquantitative observations of tubular (or glandular) differentiation, nuclear pleomorphism and mitotic rate in the range 1-3 for each feature. The three scores are added:
grade I score 3-5
grade II 6-7
grade III 8-9 (Figs.11-14) (Table VII).

Summary

The three major prognostic factors found in screen detected breast cancers all show features suggesting that as a group these tumours should have a better prognosis than cancers found in symptomatic patients. 60% of the 427 tumours were less than 15 mm diameter, 38% were grade I tumours and 21% overall showed lymph node metastasis. Combination of some of the factors makes for interesting comparisons, not only between populations with screen detected and symptomatic cancer, but also between the different types of cancer (see Table IV).

Conclusion

Participation in a Breast Screening Programme can be an enjoyable and stimulating experience for pathologists. This chapter has attempted to discuss methods and standards practicable in a district general Hospital setting and to discuss the pathology of the major tumours found in screen detected breast cancer in a local population.

References

1. Pathology Reporting in Breast Cancer Screening. 2nd Edition. National Coordinating Group for Breast Screening Pathology. NHSBSP Publications. April 1995
2. World Health Organisation. Histological typing of breast tumours. 2nd ed. International Histological Classification of Tumours No.2. Geneva. World Health Organization, 1981; 19
3. Atlas of Tumor Pathology (Third Series) Fascicle 7 Tumors of the Mammary Gland, P.P. Rosen & H.A.Oberman. American Registry of Pathology, AFIP, Washington DC, 1993
4. Page D.L. & Anderson T.J.: Diagnostic Histopathology of the Breast. Churchill Livingstone, 1987
5. Sloane JP Biopsy Pathology of the Breast. Chapman and Hall Medical 1988
6. Purushotham A.D., Macmillan R.D., George W.D.: Breast conserving surgery and tumour bed positivity in patients with breast cancer. Br. J. Surg. 1994; 81: 922-923
7. England D.W., Chan S.Y., Stonelake P.S., Lee M.J.R.: Assessment of excision margins following wide local excision for breast carcinoma using specimen scrape cytology and tumour bed biopsy. Eur. J. Surg. Oncol. 1994:20: 425-429
8. Wellings S.R., Jensen H.M., Marcum R.G.: An atlas of subgross pathology of the human breast. J. Nat . Cancer Institute 1975; 55: 231-273
9. Anderson T.J., Lamb J., Alexander F. et al.: Comparative pathology of prevalent and incident cancers detected by breast screening. Lancet 1986; 1: 519-522
10. Van Dongen J.A., Fentiman I.S., Harris J.R. et al.: In situ breast cancer: the EORTC consensus meeting. Lancet 1989: ii: 25- 27
11. Foote F.W. Jr., Stewart F.W.: A histological classification of carcinoma of the breast. Surgery 1946; bl 9: 74-99
12. Fisher E.R., Gregorio R.M., Redmond C., Fisher B.: Tubulolobular invasive breast carcinoma: a variant of lobular invasive carcinoma. Human Pathol. 1977; 8b: 679-683
13. Cooper H.S., Patchefsky A.S., Krall R.A.: Tubular carcinoma of the breast. Cancer 1978; 42: 2334-2342
14. Azzopardi J.C.: Problems in breast pathology. 1979; p241-274.
15. Page D.L., Dixon J.M., Anderson T.J., Lee D., Stewart H.J.: Invasive cribriform carcinoma of the breast. Histopathology 1983 ;7: 525-536
16. Melsmed M.R., Robbins G.F., Foote F.W. Jr.: Prognostic significance of gelatinous mammary carcinoma. Cancer 1961; 14: 699-704
17. Ridolfi R.L., Rosen P.P., Port A., et al.: Medullary carcinoma of breast. Cancer. 1977; 40: 1365-1385
18. Richardson R.W.: Medullary carcinoma of the breast: a distinctive tumour with a relatively good prognosis. Br. J. Cancer 1956; 10: 415-423
19. Von Rosen A., Erhardt K., Hellstrom L., Somell A., Auer G.: Assessment of malignancy potential in so called interval mammary carcinomas. Breast Cancer Res. Treat. 1985; 6: 221- 227
20. Rosen P.P., Groshen S., Saigo P.E., Kinne D.W., Hellman S.: Pathological prognostic factors in stage I (TINOM0) and stage II (TlNIM0) breast carcinoma. J. Clin. Oncol. 1989; 7; 1239-1251
21. Dixon J.M., Page D.L., Anderson T.J.: Long term survivors after breast cancer. Br. J. Surg. 1985; 72; 445-448
22. Pereira H., Pinder S.E., Dixon A.R., Elston C.W., Blamey R.W., Ellis I.O.: Pathological prognostic factors in breast cancer. Histopathology. 1995; 27.3; 219-226
23. Adair F., Berg J., Joubert L., Robbins G.F: Long term follow up of breast cancer patients: the 30 year report. Cancer 1974; 33: 1145-50
24. Rosen P.P., Groshen S., Saigo P.E., Kilme D.W., Hellman S.: A long term follow up of survival in stage I (TINOM0) and stage II (TINIM0) breast cancer. Clin. Oncol., 1989; 7: 355-66
25. Roses D.R. et al.: Pathological predictors of recurrence in stage I breast cancer. Am J. Clin. Pathol. 1982; 78: 817-820
26. Elston C.W., Ellis I.O.: Pathological prognostic factors in breast cancer. I The value of histological grade in breast cancer. Histopathology 1991; lg: 403- 410
27. Bloom H.J.G., Richardson W.W.: Histological grading and prognosis in breast cancer. Br. J. Cancer 1957; 11: 359-377

Cytological and histological correlation in breast cytopathology

P.A. Trott

Introduction

Although cytopathologists involved in breast fine needle aspiration cytodiagnosis are less concerned with histopathological classifications than with the diagnosis of malignancy, a thorough understanding of the histopathological appearances of breast disease is essential for correct cytological interpretation.[1]

This is partly because individual cells in benign lesions can have alarming appearances and also because of the heterogenous nature of breast carcinoma so that it is easy to imagine how a misdiagnosis of malignancy might be made.

Specificity and sensitivity

The cytological appearances of breast aspirates is related to the definitive histopathological appearances and the accuracy of the cytological diagnosis is compared in this way. By dividing all breast pathology into benign or malignant, the accuracy of the cytology can be determined. Unfortunately, the statistical methods of analysis of this information vary considerably in published papers and some reports, for example, take into account equivocal or suspicious diagnoses when assessing positive predictive value and others only include definitive or certainly positive diagnoses. It is therefore appropriate to list definitions of the terms used commonly in published material to evaluate the efficacy of breast aspiration cytodiagnosis.

Absolute sensitivity

This refers to the number of carcinomas unequivocally diagnosed, expressed as a proportion of the total number of carcinomas aspirated. In other words,

it is an expression of the ability of the test to give a positive result when cancer is present.

Complete sensitivity

Complete sensitivity is the number of carcinomas diagnosed positively including those with equivocal appearances, expressed as a proportion of the total number of carcinomas aspirated. This figure has particular relevance in stereotactic aspiration cytodiagnosis when detection rather than diagnosis is more important.

Specificity

Specificity is the number of correctly identified benign lesions expressed as a proportion of the total number of benign lesions aspirated. It is the corollary of sensitivity and demonstrates the ability to give a negative finding when cancer is absent.

Positive predictive value

Surgeons are particularly interested in the positive predictive value as it indicates the degree of confidence with which they can regard a positive cytology result.

When it is 100% the clinician will know categorically that a positive (C5) diagnosis of cancer has always meant malignancy and therefore probably always will.

If in the analysis it includes equivocal diagnoses then this should be made clear. A positive predictive value of an unequivocal positive result is the number of positive results less those that are falsely positive expressed as a proportion of the total number of true positive results.

False negative rate

The false negative rate is the number of falsely negative results expressed as a proportion of the total number of carcinomas aspirated.

Table I shows a list of comparative reporting data of seven large series. So far as it is possible the same data have been extracted from each paper and presented in tabular form and a similar statistical analysis has been undertaken. These are the calculations of the absolute and complete sensitivities, specificity and positive and negative predictive values. The largest series is from Franzen and Zajicek who reported on 3119 cases.[7] All the carcinomas were verified histologically and the specimens were taken by cytopathologists in the Cytology Clinic. Their results of 76% for absolute and 78% for complete sensitivity can be compared with those of the smaller series of Brown,[4] in which the aspirates were also performed by pathologists. Their sensitivity figures are also very high; indeed the highest figure of complete sensitivity of 94% is in the Brown series and indicates in statistical terms the advantages of the pathologist aspirating the tumour.

Many papers show a positive predictive value of 100% and others show a value in the high 90s. This indicates the level of the diagnostic threshold which should be geared towards only providing a diagnosis of carcinoma when this is certain. The phrase "the interpreter should feel at ease in making such a diagnosis"[9] aptly sums up the diagnostic pathologist's attitude in this regard. Giard and Hermans have highlighted the difficulties in attempting to compare the reported results of breast aspiration cytodiagnosis papers.[10] They reviewed 29 articles in which there were a total of 31,340 aspirations.

As well as sensitivity and specificity they included the likelihood ratios of four different results which included definitely malignant, suspicious, benign and unsatisfactory.

Their analysis showed striking differences between series in the diagnostic accuracy of aspiration cytodiagnosis. For example, patients with breast cancer had a chance of obtaining a "definitely malignant" cytological diagnosis with a positive predictive value ranging from 35% to 92%. It is hoped that with more training and experience the positive predictive value will rise universally.

False positive rate

So far as false positive reports are concerned Jatoi & Trott found four misdiagnoses of carcinoma in an analysis of 1104 cases of positive breast aspirates seen consecutively over a four-year period.[11] This is an incidence of 0.36% and represents a positive predictive value of 99.6%. The benign conditions that led to false positive diagnosis were radiation, granulomatous mastitis and fibro-adenoma.

Grading

Following the establishment and recognition that histopathological grading has prognostic value and is reproducible, attempts have been made to grade breast carcinoma in needle aspirates. Mouriquand[12] devised three grades in smears stained by the Papanicolaou technique using six parameters including cell pattern, naked nuclei, nuclear pleomorphism, nuclear size, chromasia and mitotic figures. This analysis was compared to the TNM stage of disease and appeared to have little advantage when this was taken into account. Ciatto[13] using the same method came to similar conclusions. There appeared to be rather more value in the method devised by Zajdela[14] who measured the nuclear size with a micrometer in Giemsa stained smears and related this to the stage of the disease. In the Netherlands techniques using image analysis morphometry have shown that sufficient division of cases can be achieved that correlates with histological diagnosis and survival.[15]

The advent of primary (neo-adjuvant) chemotherapy has prompted a need for cytological grading as a replacement for histological grading which may only become possible after therapy. A Nottingham scheme[16] relies on three cytological features which can easily be assessed in routinely prepared air dried Giemsa stained smears which includes the measurement of nuclear diameter compared to the diameter of a red blood cell, nuclear pleomorphism and abnormal nucleoli. Cases are divided into low grade and high grade tumours and the method is effective in the identification of high grade histological tumours (grade 3) but has poor discrimination for histological grades 1 and 2.

In Guildford, Robinson et al.[17] have established three cytological grades using several diagnostic parameters that includes extent of cell dissociation, cell size and uniformity and the appearance of nucleoli, the nuclear margin and chromatin. In an analysis of 28 invasive ductal carcinomas they showed that the grading matched well with conventional histological grading. These workers used wet-fixed smears stained by the Papanicolaou technique.

These observations are potentially extremely important because in patients undergoing primary chemo or endocrine therapy, the histological features relating to prognosis are compromised in that tumour size, and the lymph node status and histological grade are unknown before therapy is given.[18] Any clue to the biological nature of the tumour that can be derived before treatment from a cytological aspirate specimen may prove to be of great value.

The methods of evaluation have been outlined by Dowsett *et al.*[19] who described how the treatment of primary breast cancer by medical therapy prior to surgery has provided an opportunity to collect multiple samples of tumour using Tru-cut core biopsies and fine needle aspirates. The Tru-cut sample in which tissue architecture is retained provides a core of tissue which can be snap frozen for frozen section examination or embedded in paraffin wax. The needle aspirate sample[20] is obtained into 2ml of medium and cytocentrifuged in a Shandon cytospin using all twelve chambers. Thus twelve slides of cells are obtained from one needle aspirate sample. Studies of validation and precision have been carried out assessing ER and Ps2 showing that the results are comparable with conventional staining techniques using tissue frozen sections or histology slides. C-erB2, bc1-2, Ki67 and TGFBl have all been successfully demonstrated in these samples as well as oestrogen and progesterone receptor. Furthermore the residual suspension can be used for proliferation indices using flow cytometric analysis to measure DNA index and S Phase fraction. Although there

was difficulty in some cases obtaining a sufficiently cellular sample, aspiration cytology is comparatively painless and may be used sequentially to monitor response to treatment.

Correlation with Histological Types

Benign lesions

Breast cysts can be recognised in needle aspirates not only from the macroscopic appearance of fluid but also from the presence of foamy macrophages (Fig. 1) and apocrine cell clusters within the deposit.[21] Furthermore, the deposit from many cysts shows a diffuse granular appearance (Fig. 2) that can be mistaken for polymorphs. These are fine granules that may have originated from apocrine cells. Thus a cytopathologist can confidently diagnose a benign breast cyst.

Fibroadenomas have very characteristic appearances which consist of a combination of three features.[22] The epithelial sheets often spread in a "stag horn" shape, and large numbers of myo-epithelial cells both singly and in pairs (Fig. 3), are present between them. The third component is the recognition of the specialised stroma found in these lesions

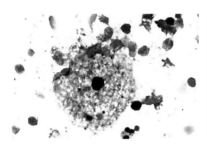

Fig. 1. Foamy macrophage from the spun deposit of breast cyst fluid. Giemsa × 100.

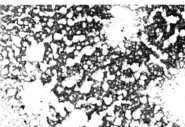

Fig. 2. Granular proteinaceous material from a benign cyst fluid. These appearances may be mistaken for polymorphs. Giemsa × 25.

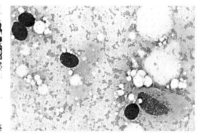

Fig. 3. Five nuclei from an aspirate from a fibro-adenoma. Four are myoepithelial nuclei the top left showing characteristic pair formation. A duct epithelial cell is present at bottom right. Giemsa × 100.

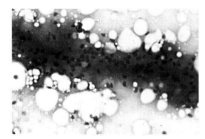

Fig. 4. Stroma aspirated from a fibro-adenoma staining a characteristic metachromatic purple colour. Giemsa × 25.

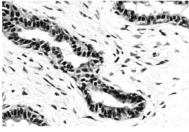

Fig. 5. Histological section from a fibro-adenoma showing epithelial clefts lined by hyperplastic cells. H & E × 40.

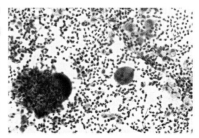

Fig. 6. Pus aspirated from a breast abscess. Note two multinucleated histiocytes. Pap stain × 25.

which stains pale pink with Giemsa (Fig. 4) . The identification of these three features, particularly in aspirates from lumps from young women, will provide an almost certain diagnosis of fibro-adenoma. It is important to note that fibro-adenomas are often misdiagnosed in needle aspirates as carcinoma. The reason for this is the extremely hyperplastic nature of the epithelial component (Fig. 5) which can be composed of pleomorphic irregular nuclei and include mitotic figures. The key to the diagnosis is the recognition of myoepithelial cells which are easily identified when they appear as pairs.

It is not possible and probably not useful to attempt to separate the other varieties of benign breast changes that can produce lumps and diffuse nodularity. There are reports of the description of the cytological appearances of radial scars[23] but these studies are retrospective and are directed more at research into the natural history of these lesions rather than the diagnostic ability of a needle aspirate. Aspirate samples containing a variety of inflammatory cells are often sent to the laboratory. These include sheets of polymorphs usually with cell debris and fibrinous streaks (frank pus) from a breast abscess (Fig. 6). This is a straightforward cytological diagnosis which has important clinical implications. If unsuspected a further sample can be taken and sent for microbiological analysis. Polymorphs and other inflammatory cells are commonly seen mixed with foam cells and apocrine cells in benign cyst fluids. These may indicate an inflammatory component to the lesion.

Chronic inflammation with or without multinucleated histiocytes (Fig. 7) is quite common and aspirates from granulomatous mastitis are often very cellular and the reactive fibroblasts can be mistaken for malignancy.[11] To avoid this the diagnosis should be considered especially in young women of child bearing age even without the tell-tale multinucleated histiocytes. Single epithelioid cells have a characteristic bean-shaped nucleus with a single nucleolus, and typical examples should be searched for in the slide. Occasionally exotic micro-organisms are aspirated including worms and ova in countries where these diseases are endemic.

Aspirates from intramammary lymph nodes (Fig. 8) consist mainly of mature lymphocytes but include occasional histiocytes, monocytes and macrophages. These lesions are usually present in the upper outer quadrant of the breast but may occur elsewhere and can present with a palpable lump, especially in women with small breasts. The cytological diagnosis is usually clear cut.

Malignant lesions

Between 70% and 80% of infiltrating ductal carcinoma is described as NOS (not otherwise specified). In these lesions there is a variety of infiltrating patterns but no sub-type other than grade is recognised. In these cases the cytopathology will be distinctive only in so far as the diagnostic criteria of carcinoma is concerned. Of the special sub-types of carcinoma, mucoid (mucinous) carcinoma is usually easily diagnosed in needle aspirates.[24]

In these lesions the mucin is recognised most easily in Giemsa preparations in which it stains a pale pink colour (Fig. 9). In the Papanicolaou stained slides it is not so easily seen and there may be difficulty in the diagnosis as the cells are usually small and not obviously "malignant". However, when mucin is identified there is seen to be a relationship between atypical small cells and the mucin in which the cells appear to line up in rows alongside the mucin. The histological diagnosis of mucoid carcinoma (Fig. 10) depends on 90% of the lesion being of this type and only those pure tumours have a good prognosis.[25] Furthermore, it should not be forgotten that some mucinous carcinomas are high grade lesions which will consist of clusters and single pleomorphic cells with a mucoid background.

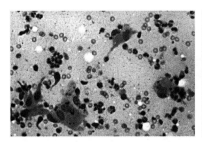

Fig. 7. Breast aspirate showing evidence of chronic inflammation. Several histiocytes are present with a background of lymphocytes and occasional polymorphs. Giemsa × 40.

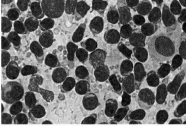

Fig. 8. Aspirate from an intramammary lymph node. Note the variety of mature and immature lymphoid cells. Giemsa × 100.

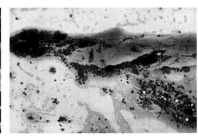

Fig. 9. Aspirate from a mucinous carcinoma. Note the purple staining extra-cellular mucus with carcinoma cells adjacent. Giemsa × 10.

Table I. Comparative reporting data.

| | | **References** | | | | | | |
		1	2	3	4	5	6*	7
Total number of cases	a	1671	793	1002	480	1283	3119	1181
Total with carcinoma	b	1539	228	356	276	689	1099	1014
Cytology positive	c	1031	158	295	219	481	832	500
Suspicious	d	335	26	40	9	88	30	372
Negative	e	166	31	21	6	48	206	142
Total without carcinoma	f	132	565	646	204	594	2020	167
Cytology positive	g	0	0	0	0	2	1	2
Suspicious	h	27	3	10	0	53	23	19
Negative	i	46	470	636	129	338	1464	146
Inadequate rate (%)		23	13	0	42	21	12	0
Absolute sensitivity (%)	$\frac{c}{b}$	0.67	0.69	0.83	0.79	0.69	0.76	0.49
Complete sensitivity (%)	$\frac{c+d}{b}$	0.89	0.81	0.94	0.83	0.83	0.78	0.86
Specificity (%)	$\frac{i}{f}$	0.35	0.83	0.98	0.63	0.57	0.72	0.87
Positive predictive value (%)	$\frac{c-g}{c}$	1.00	1.00	1.00	1.00	0.995	0.998	0.998

1. Eisenberg *et al.*[2] 2. Powles *et al.*[3]; 3. Brown *et al.*[4] 4. Smallwood *et al.*[5]; 5. Barrows *et al.*[6] 6. Franzen *et al.*,[7]; 7. Ciatto *et al.*[8]
* Includes cases of benign cysts.

Medullary carcinoma is rarer than mucoid carcinoma but can be distinctive in needle aspirate samples (Fig. 11). The large pleomorphic poorly differentiated carcinoma cells with prominent nucleoli are often seen singly and in fragmented clusters together with the lymphoid stroma in which plasma cells are identified. When these features are seen in samples which are occasionally cystic,[26] it is important to draw the possibility of medullary carcinoma to the notice of the clinician as these lesions can be mistaken for cysts radiologically because of their regular borders.

Papillary carcinomas are found usually deep to the nipple in post-menopausal women but they can occur in any part of the breast. The needle aspirates are often cystic and blood contaminated and the cells may be in papillary clusters (Fig. 12) and myoepithelial cells are absent. In practise identification is usually difficult and an equivocal diagnosis may be the only one possible.

Sarcoma

Malignant mesenchymal tumours of the breast are divided into those with an epithelial component

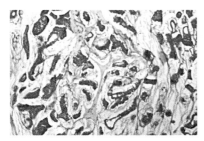

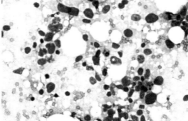

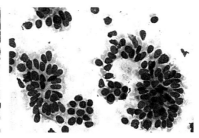

Fig. 10. Histological section of a mucinous carcinoma. Note islands of carcinoma floating in mucus. H & E × 25.

Fig. 11. Aspirate from a medullary carcinoma. Note scattered large carcinoma cells with prominent nucleoli. There is a background of lymphoid stroma in which a plasma cell is seen centrally. Giemsa × 40.

Fig. 12. Aspirate from an intracystic papillary carcinoma. The carcinoma cells appear palisaded in papillary clusters. Giemsa × 40.

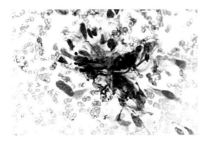
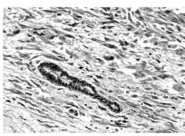

Fig. 13. Aspirate from a fibrosarcoma. The cells present a spindly appearance. Giemsa × 40.

Fig. 14. Histological section from a breast fibrosarcoma. An elongated breast duct is surrounded by a spindle cell malignant neoplasm. H & E × 40.

Fig. 15. Aspirate from an adenoid cystic carcinoma. Note blobs of pink staining mucin surrounded by small pleomorphic irregular cells. Giemsa × 40.

(malignant phyllodes tumour) and those without. Sarcomas without an epithelial component are less common and are usually fibrosarcomas. The diagnosis is made histologically after thorough sampling as sarcomatous metaplasia is common in carcinomas in which the epithelial components may be focal and widespread. Only in the absence of evidence of carcinoma can the diagnosis of sarcoma be made confidently and confirmation may be necessary using appropriate immunohistochemistry. Consequently, the cytodiagnosis of breast sarcoma (Figs. 13-14) is fraught with difficulties even when good quality samples containing spindle cells typical of sarcoma seen in other body sites are obtained.

The only situation where sarcoma can be confidently diagnosed in a breast aspirate is in recurrent sarcoma in which the primary tumour has been properly sampled and assessed histopathologically.

Lymphoma

Lymphoma of the breast usually occurs in association with known generalised lymphoma but occasionally primary breast lymphoma occurs or the breast is the site of the first presentation of more generalised disease. The majority of the cases are B cell non-Hodgkins lymphoma, although occasional reports of T cell lymphoma have appeared.[27] Cytodiagnosis is comparatively easy if the pathologist is aware of the condition. The usual disassociated round cells with scanty cytoplasm are seen with nuclear configurations with or without nucleoli. The appearances may be difficult to differentiate from small cell carcinoma in which the cells are also largely disassociated. However, careful hunting will reveal a few clusters of cells with an epithelial pattern.

Lymphomas of the breast are usually high grade but in doubtful cases immunocytochemical staining for lymphoid markers may be necessary.

There are many reports in the literature of the cytological appearances of rarer forms of breast malignancy, but these descriptions are unhelpful in prospective diagnosis. Adenoid cystic carcinoma (Fig. 15) appears similar to the lesions aspirated from the head and neck area so that it is important to remember the diagnosis when confronted with a case that is difficult to interpret and perhaps offer the diagnosis in the description. The main purpose of breast fine needle aspiration cytodiagnosis is to differentiate between a malignant and benign lesion. Many cytopathologists think this is hard enough without attempting refinements.

References

1. Trott P.A.: Breast Cytopathology: A Diagnostic Atlas. London, Chapman & Hall, 1996
2. Eisenberg A.J.: Preoperative aspiration cytology of breast tumours. Ada Cytologica, 1986; 30: 135-46
3. Powles T.J., Trott P.A., Cherryman, G.: Fine needle aspiration cytodiagnosis as a prerequisite for primary medical treatment of breast cancer. Cytopathology, 1991; 2: 7-12
4. Brown L.A., Coghill S.B., Powis S.A.J.: Audit of diagnostic accuracy of FNA cytology specimens taken by the histopathologist in a symptomatic breast clinic. Cytopathology, 1991; 2, 1-7
5. Smallwood J., Herbert A., Guyer, P.: Accuracy of aspiration cytology in the diagnosis of breast disease. Br. J. Surg., 1985; 72: 841-843
6. Barrows G.H., Anderson T.J., Lamb J.L., Dixon, J.M.: Fine needle aspiration of breast cancer. Cancer, 1986; 58, 1493-1498
7. Franzen S.L., Zajicek, J.: Aspiration biopsy in diagnosis of palpable lesions of the breast. Critical review of 3479 consecutive biopsies. Acta Radiol., 1968; 7, 241-262
9. The Royal College of Pathologists Working Group. Guidelines for Cytology Procedures and Reporting in Breast cancer Screening. NHSBSP No 22 (revised 1993)
10. Giard R.W.M., Herman J.O.: The value of aspiration cytologic examination of the breast: a statistical review of the medical literature. Cancer, 1992; 69, 2104-2111
11. Jatoi I., Trott P.A.: False positive reporting in breast fine needle aspiration cytology: incidence and causes. Breast, 1996; 5: 270-273
12. Mouriquand J., Gozlan-Fior M., Villemain D., et al.: Value of Cytoprognostic classification in breast carcinomas. J. Clin. Pathol., 1986; 39: 489-496
13. Ciatto S., Cecchiani S., Grazzini G.: Positive predictive value of fine needle aspiration cytology of breast lesions. Acta Cytol. 1989; 33, 894-898

14. Zajdela A., DeLaRiva L., Ghossein N.: The relation of prognosis to the nuclear diameter of breast cancer cells obtained by cytologic aspirations. Acta Cytol., 1984; 23: 75-80

15. Van Driest P.J, Baak J.P.A.: The morphometric prognostic index is the strongest prognosticator in premenopausal lymph node negative and lymph node positive breast cancer patients. Human Pathology, 1991; 22: 326-330

16. Hunt, C.M., Ellis, I.O., Elston, C.W. *et al.*: Cytological grading of breast carcinoma - a feasible proposition? Cytopathology, 1990; 1: 287-295

17. Robinson I.A., McKee Grace, Nicholson A., D'Arcy J., Jackson P.A., Cook M.G., Kissin M.W.: Prognostic value of cytological grading of fine-needle aspirates from breast carcinomas. Lancet, 1994; 343: 947-949

18. Trott P.A.: Pathological assessment in patients receiving primary medical therapy for breast cancer. Cytopathology., 1996; 7, 75-77

19. M. Dowsett, S.R.D Johnston, S. Detre, J. Salter, S. Humphries, G. Saccani-Jotti, I.E. Smith, K. MacLennn, P.A. Trott: Cytological evaluation of biological variables in breast cancer patients undergoing primary medical treatment. Elsevier Science BV 1994, 329-336

20. I.N. Fernando, T.J. Powles, M. Dowsett, S. Ashley, L. McRobert, J. Titley, M.G. Ormerod, N. Sacks, M.C. Nicolson, A. Nash, H.T. Ford, S.M. Allan, P.A. Trott: Determining factors which predict response to primary medical therapy in breast cancer using a single fine needle aspirate with immunocytochemical staining and flow cytometry. Virchows Archiv., 1995, 426: 155-161

21. Ciatto S., Cariaggi P., Bulgaresi P.: The value of routine cytologic examination of breast cyst fluids. Acta Cytol., 1997; 31, 301-4

22. Trott, P.A.: Aspiration cytodiagnosis of the breast. Diagn. Oncol., 1991; 1: 79-87

23. Lamb J., McGoogan E.: Fine needle aspiration cytology of breast carcinoma of tubular type and in radial scar/complex sclerosing lesions. Cytopathology, 1994; 5: 17-26

24. Stanley M.W., Tani E.M., Skoog, L.: Mucinous breast carcinoma and mixed mucinous infiltrating ductal carcinoma: A comparative cytologic study. Diagn. Cytopathol., 1989; 5: 134-138

25. Clayton F.: Pure mucinous carcinomas of breast; Morphologic features and prognostic correlates. Human Path., 1986; 17: 34-38

26. Howell, L.P. and Kline, T.S.: Medullary carcinoma of the breast; a rare cytologic finding in cyst fluid aspirates. Cancer, 1990; 65: 277-282

27. Peltinato G., Manivel J.C., Petrella G., De Chiara A.: Primary multilobated T-cell lymphoma of the breast diagnosed by fine needle aspiration cytology and immunocytochemistry. Acta Cytol., 1991; 35: 294-299

Radio-pathological correlations

S. Ciatto, D. Ambrogetti, S. Bianchi

The appearance of breast lesions at mammography is strictly correlated with the macro- and microscopic pathological features. A description of such correlations may help in understanding the limits of mammography in the differential diagnosis of breast carcinoma and the occurence of radiological false negative/benign or false positive reports.

Radio-pathological correlations which may justify radiological false negative/benign reports

Invasive lobular carcinoma

This histological type may present diagnostic difficulties at radiological examination and is currently reported to be associated with a high rate of false negative reports at mammography. The explanation of such a finding depends on the peculiar growth pattern of the typical invasive lobular carcinoma variant, which is characterized by small cells diffusely infiltrating the mammary stroma, sometimes with no tendency to form a well defined mass as it produces a poor desmoplastic reaction (Fig. 1). Such a growth pattern may result in some abnormality at palpation, such as an indeterminate area of increased consistency, but does not contribute to form a radiological opacity; mammography is often completely normal, especially if a dense parenchymal pattern is present (Fig. 2). The evidence at sonography is also often negative, or sometimes a vague non-specific hypoechoic area is appreciated, which allows no reliable diagnostic conclusion.

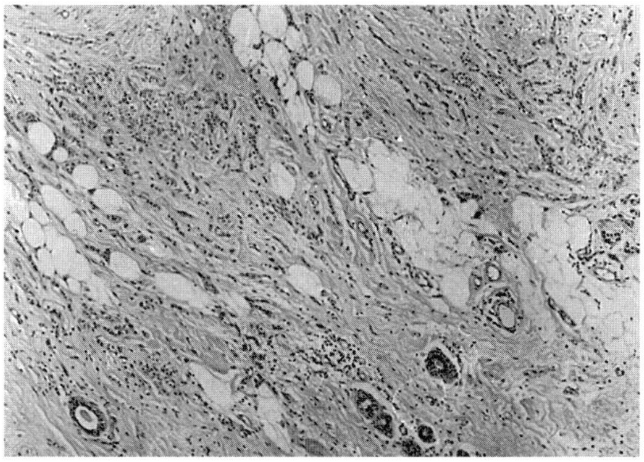

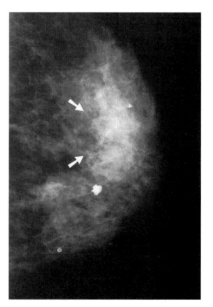

Fig. 1. Invasive lobular carcinoma. Histology: classical variant - the tumour cells infiltrate the mammary stroma with a linear growth pattern, entrapping normal structures. The desmoplastic reaction is absent (H.E. × 100).

Fig. 2. Invasive lobular carcinoma. Mammography: a 2 cm, palpable lesion in the upper central quadrant (arrows) is not associated with any mammographic abnormality.

The diffuse growth pattern of the classic variant of invasive lobular carcinoma may also justify a lower accuracy of cytology, mostly due to the difficulty of aiming the needle at the lesion either freehand or guided.

Medullary carcinoma

This histological type often presents as a sharp, regular, rounded mass with well circumscribed margins (Fig. 3), which are evident also at mammography (Fig. 4) and sonography (Fig. 5). This radiopathological pattern is typical of medullary carcinoma but may be associated also with other non-medullary invasive carcinomas (*e.g.* mucinous), whenever a "pushing" rather than an "infiltrating" growth pattern is present. A similar appearance may occur also with breast localization of malignant lymphoma (Fig. 6). Radiological diagnosis of carcinoma is impossible at mammography. Although carcinomas with regular margins are round in shape, whereas fibro-adenomas are mostly oval-shaped with the major axis parallel to the skin surface, such a difference is not constant and reliable. Suspicion may arise when the lesion is reported for the first time in women over 60 years of age (fibroadenomas are often typically calcified), especially if a negative previous mammogram is available. The accuracy of fine needle aspiration cytology is not influenced by tumour morphology in this case and routine aspiration of isolated solid lesions with regular margins at their first appearance is recommended, particularly in post-menopausal women.

Non-comedo intraductal carcinoma

Microcalcifications are often associated with breast cancer and their typical appearance (linear, branching, casting, grouped in an isolated cluster) is well known, being typically associated with comedo intraductal or invasive carcinomas. Unfortunately, microcalcifications associated with carcinoma may also have a less suspicious appearance (punctate, crystalline, granular, sparse), which occurs typically with non-comedo intraductal carcinoma (Fig. 7). At histological examination (Fig. 8) these calcifications appear as calcium deposits in lumina of micropapillary or cribriform ductal carcinoma *in situ*. Differential diagnosis on a radiological basis is very difficult and poor specificity (high benign/ malignant biopsy ratio) is generally associated with the effort of maximum sensitivity in these cases. Even the prediction of non-comedo intraductal carcinoma on a radiological basis is unreliable.[1] Sonography is of no help in this case as most microcalcifications are not visualized.[2]

Radio-pathological correlations which may justify radiological false positive reports

Radial scar

Radial scar of the breast was described more than 50 years ago but became the object of renewed interest after a report by Linell *et al*[3] in 1980. A number of synonyms have been used in the recent

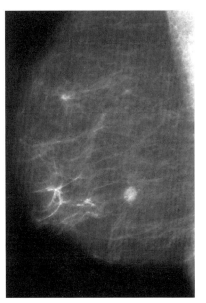

Fig. 4. Invasive medullary carcinoma. Mammography. An 8 mm, non-palpable lesion in the lower central quadrant is evident as a rounded mass with sharp margins, virtually indistinguishable from a cyst or fibro-adenoma.

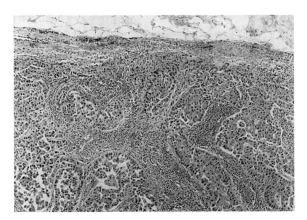

Fig. 3. Invasive medullary carcinoma. Histology. The lesion is well defined with pushing sharp margins (H.E. × 40).

literature to indicate this lesion (sclero-elastotic lesion, proliferation centre of Aschoff, infiltrating epitheliosis, non-encapsulated sclerosing lesion, indurative mastopathy). It has a spiculated cancer-like appearance at mammography, and although some typical signs foretelling its benign nature have been described,[4,5] such as the absence of central opacity, or the presence of a radiolucent central area, and of long thin spicules radiating from the central lesion (Fig. 9), they are not fully reliable and surgical biopsy is currently recommended. A typical radiological appearance, a negative cytological report, and the fact that the lesion is relatively large and superficial but still not palpable may justify careful surveillance in selected cases.[6]

At histological examination diagnosis is not simple. At low magnification the lesion strikes for its stellate or radial arrangement, with a central nucleus dominated by fibro-elastosis and hyalinization. At high magnification, haphazardly distributed and distorted, entrapped tubular structures with irregular angulated contours are evident (Fig. 10). The latter finding may justify some diagnostic difficulties at microscopic examination in differentiating radial scar from tubular carcinoma.

Sclerosing adenosis

Sclerosing adenosis is a lobular proliferation of both epithelial and myo-epithelial cells, in which the acinus appears distorted and with pseudo-infiltrative margins. Ductules exhibit elongation and obstruction of their lumen due to compression by the prominent or hyperplastic myoepithelial cell layer (Fig. 11).

At mammography (Fig.12) sclerosing adenosis may appear as an asymmetrical density with poorly defined or definitely irregular margins and cancer is suspected in these cases. Suspicion may be reduced by the absence of clinical and sonographic findings, or by a negative cytological report, but open biopsy is recommended in most cases.

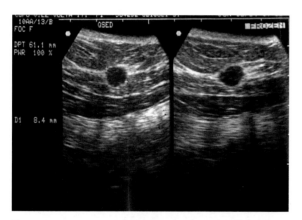

Fig. 5. Invasive medullary carcinoma. Sonography. A 8 mm, non-palpable lesion appears with regular margins, a feature which might be consistent with benign fibroadenoma.

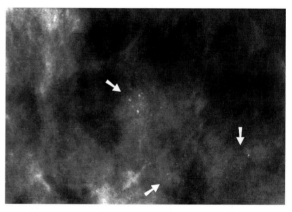

Fig. 7. Non-comedo intraductal (cribriform) carcinoma. Mammography. Sparse granular and punctate microcalcifications (arrows) are the only radiological evidence.

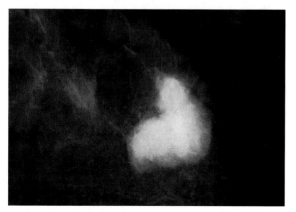

Fig. 6. Malignant non-Hodgkin lymphoma. Mammography. Rounded mass with sharp lobulated margins is visible.

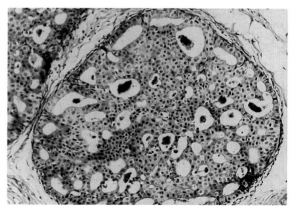

Fig. 8. Non-comedo intraductal carcinoma. Histology. Fine granular calcifications are evident within the lumina of intraductal carcinoma, cribriform variant (H.E., × 250).

Benign calcifications

Microcalcifications are often visible at mammography in normal breasts. Although benign microcalcifications usually have a typical appearance (punctate, anular, tea-cup-like, diffuse, sparse, and bilateral), sometimes they may assume a granular crystalline appearance, being circumscribed to a limited area (Fig. 13).

Histological examination (Fig. 14) shows benign microcalcifications within normal lobules, cysts, or stroma. In this case differential diagnosis with carcinoma (*e.g.* non-comedo intraductal type) may be very difficult, and when the decision about recommending open biopsy or not is based only on the radiological appearance, a high benign/malignant biopsy ratio is expected. The recent adoption of stereotaxic fine needle aspiration cytology as a part of the routine assessment of non-palpable lesions represents a great help, and the benign/malignant biopsy ratio in presence of microcalcifications with a questionable/probably benign appearance has been definitively reduced, with no appreciable impact on cancer detection rates.

Asymmetrical parenchymal densities

The radiological density of cancer is equal to that of normal breast parenchyma, and cancers may be depicted at mammography as asymmetrical densities with non-stellate poorly defined margins. Such mammographic abnormalities may be easily suspected in older women, especially if they occur in fibro-adipose breasts, or if they were not present in a previous available mammogram, but differential diagnosis between a scattered asymmetric area of breast parenchyma (Fig. 15) and breast cancer (Fig. 15a) may be difficult in a normally dense pre-menopausal breast.

In past years such cases were often sent for open biopsy and histological diagnosis did usually confirm the presence of an island of normal breast parenchyma in most cases (Fig. 16).

Since sonography has been introduced in the assessment of breast lesions the need for histological confirmation of such mammographic abnormalities has been dramatically reduced as areas of breast parenchyma are easily recognized as they appear as hyper-echoic areas on the hypo-echoic background of the surrounding fat (Fig. 17a). Only hypo-echoic

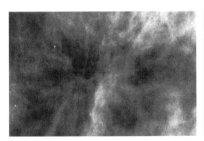

Fig. 9. Radial scar. Mammography. Typical appearance of a large stellate lesion with a radiolucent centre and thin elongated radiating spicules.

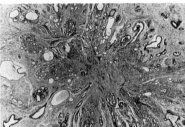

Fig. 10. Radial scar. Histology. The typical stellate arrangement with entrapped tubular structures in the central fibro-elastotic zone is evident (H.E., × 40).

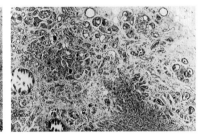

Fig. 11. Sclerosing adenosis. Histology. Lobular proliferation due to an increased number of acini shows compressed and elongated tubules (H.E., × 100).

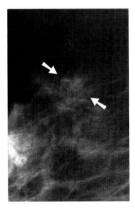

Fig. 12. Sclerosing adenosis. Mammography (arrows) evidences an irregular opacity with a distorted appearance.

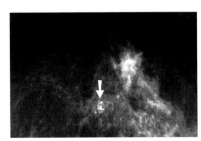

Fig. 13. Benign calcifications. Mammography. Isolated cluster of granular crystalline microcalcifications (arrow).

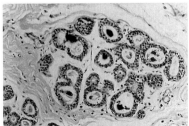

Fig. 14. Benign calcifications. Histology. Fine granular microcalcifications are evident in the ductules of a normal lobule. (H.E., ×250).

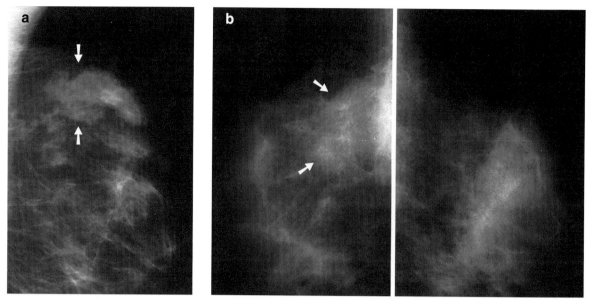

Fig. 15. **a)** Asymmetrical pseudo-nodular area of normal breast parenchyma. Mammography. An asymmetric density (arrows) stands out from the fatty background. The margins of the lesion are poorly defined but not frankly irregular. **b)** Breast cancer. Mammography. The lesion (**arrows**) appears as an asymmetric density with poorly defined borders, quite similar to the surrounding areas of normal breast parenchyma.

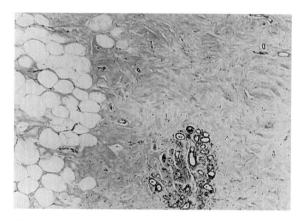

Fig. 16. Asymmetrical pseudo-nodular area of normal breast parenchyma. Histology. A microcystic atrophic lobule is surrounded by fibrosis and fat tissue (H.E., × 100).

lesions (Fig. 17b) are worth further investigation and the benign/malignant biopsy ratio is thus reduced.

Spicules of cancer lesions erroneously interpreted as malignant

Breast cancer is often depicted at mammography as a nodular density with radiating spicules (Fig. 18), a pattern which is typical of tubular carcinoma. In these cases it is questionable whether the spicules should be assumed as an expression of cancer invasion or not. In fact, in some cases, the radiating spicules are accounted for by simple desmoplastic reaction (Fig. 19).

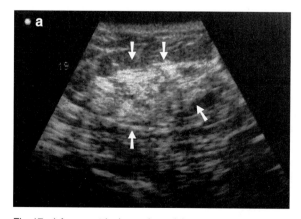
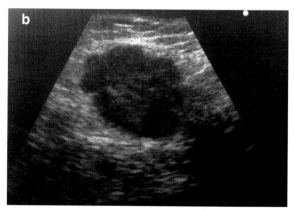

Fig. 17. **a)** Asymmetrical pseudo-nodular area of normal breast parenchyma. Sonography. A frankly hyper-echoic area, consistent with breast parenchyma, is evident within a hypo-echoic fatty context (arrows). **b)** Breast cancer. Sonography. A circumscribed hypo-echoic pseudo-nodular solid lesion is evident with respect to the surrounding parenchyma.

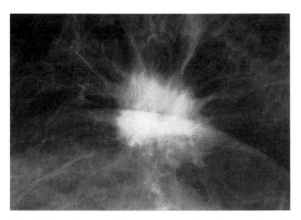

Fig. 18. Breast cancer. Mammography. Irregular opacity with thin elongated radiating spicules. Tumour size, including or not spicules, varies from 30 to 55 mm.

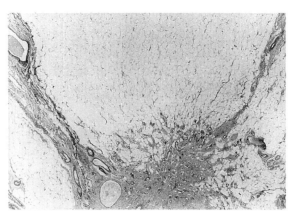

Fig. 19. Breast cancer. Histology. Spicules radiating from the lesion, without evidence of neoplastic invasion, are caused by desmoplastic reaction and fibrous tissue (H.E., × 40).

It is evident that radiological measurement of tumour size may be quite different depending on how spicules are considered, and it is evident that pathological tumour size is much more reliable for clinical purposes.

The examples of radio-pathological correlation here presented confirm that, in a number of instances, mammography is not fully reliable for the differential diagnosis of cancer. Nevertheless, this limit is intrinsic to the method: a false negative/benign or a false positive mammographic report in such cases is not a matter of interpretation but may be ascribed to the fact that some benign lesions simulate cancer and vice versa, as shown by the histopathological features which are consistent with and justify mammographic findings.

Such mammographic errors cannot be overcome by modifying the criteria of radiological suspicion as this would alter the overall accuracy of mammography to unacceptable levels. Such errors must be accepted as unavoidable but may be corrected by adopting a multimodal diagnostic approach, that is using sonography and cytology as an adjunct to clinical and mammographic examination whenever a minimal suspicion of cancer is present.

References

1. Ciatto S., Bianchi S., Vezzosi V.: Mammographic appearance of microcalcifications as a predictor of intraductal carcinoma hystologic subtype. Eur. Radiol., 1994; 4: 23-26
2. Ciatto S., Catarzi S., Morrone D., Rosselli Del Turco M.: Fine needle aspiration cytology of nonpalpable breast lesions: US versus stereotaxic guidance. Radiology, 1993; 188: 195-198
3. Linell F., Ljungberg O., Andersson I.: Breast carcinoma: aspects of early stages, progression and related problems. Acta Pathol. Microbiol. Immunol. Scand., 1980; 272 (suppl): 199-217
4. Tabar L., Dean P.B.: *Teaching atlas of mammography*. New York, Thieme-Stratton, 1985; 87-136
5. Mitnick J.S., Vazquez M.F., Harris M.N., Roses D.F.: Differentiation of radial scar from scirrhous carcinoma of the breast: mammographic-pathologic correlation. Radiology, 1989; 173: 697-700
6. Ciatto S., Morrone D., Catarzi S., Rosselli Del Turco M., Bianchi S., Ambrogetti D., Cariddi A.: Radial scars of the breast: review of 38 consecutive mammographic diagnoses. Radiology, 1993; 187: 757-760

Surgical treatment of minimal breast cancer

R.M. Simmons, M.P. Osborne

Introduction

The term "minimal breast cancer" was established in the late 1960s to include lobular neoplasia (lobular carcinoma *in situ*), ductal carcinoma *in situ*, and invasive breast cancer less than 0.5 cm in diameter. Further revisions of the definition of this entity by the American College of Surgeons, the National Cancer Institute, and the American Cancer Society have defined minimal breast cancer as any non-infiltrating breast carcinoma (ductal carcinoma *in situ* and lobular neoplasia) and invasive breast cancer less than 1 cm in diameter[1] (Fig. 1).

As physicians, it is important that we are familiar with this group of breast lesions because these are becoming more commonly diagnosed with the increasing sophistication of mammography, and the public awareness of breast cancer screening. Several decades ago, *in situ* carcinomas represented only 1.4% of all breast cancers, whereas presently this figure has risen to 18%.[2] The Breast Cancer Detection Demonstration Project in a nation wide screening project found pre-invasive and invasive cancers less than 1 cm in diameter to represent 38% of positive breast biopsies[3,4] (Fig. 2).

It has become evident that this grouping is in some ways rather arbitrary. It includes three pathologic entities that are quite distinct, behaving very differently clinically, and deserving very different treatment.[2] For this reason, each will be discussed separately, with its respective characteristics and appropriate treatment options.

Lobular neoplasia (LN) (lobular carcinoma *in situ*)

Lobular neoplasia (LN) is a proliferation of the epithelial cells in the terminal lobular unit. This proliferation often progresses to fill the acini (Fig. 3).

This pathological entity was first described in a classic article by Foote and Stewart in 1940.[5] Lobular neoplasia is frequently multifocal, multicentric, and bilateral.[5,6] Multicentricity has been noted in 42.9 per cent to 90 per cent of specimens studied.[7]

Lobular neoplasia is associated with an increased frequency of subsequent invasive carcinoma. Lobular neoplasia is often seen in mastectomy specimens associated with invasive cancer.[8-10] Conversely, in patients who are diagnosed with LN on biopsy and choose to have a mastectomy, 4-6% of these mastectomy specimens contain foci of invasive cancer.[9,11]

Women with LN treated with local excision have an incidence of developing subsequent invasive cancers that is nine times the average relative risk.[3] Approximately one third of these women will develop a subsequent invasive carcinoma.[9] This subsequent cancer is usually ductal, not lobular invasive cancer. LN is typically detected in patients who are an average of 5-15 years younger than those who develop invasive breast cancer.[11]

The probability of developing invasive cancer is equal for the contralateral and the ipsilateral breast.[9,12,13]

With lobular neoplasia treated with local excision, the incidence of ipsilateral invasive breast cancer at 10 years was 15%, at 15 years was 27%, and at 20 years was 35%.[14] Similar results were found by Walt *et al.*, with a 14.8% incidence of invasive cancer in a follow up period of 96 months.[15] The contralateral incidence at 10 years was 10%, at 15 years was 15%, and at 20 years was 25 %[14] (Table I).

The interval to development of invasive breast cancer, with the ipsilateral breast, ranged from 2 to 31 years, with 32% occurring after 20 years. Similarly, the contralateral interval, ranging from 3 to 30 years, with 44% occurring at more than 20 years.[16] Thirty-eight per cent of the patients who eventually developed invasive breast cancer had no evidence of disease until more than 20 years after initial diagno-

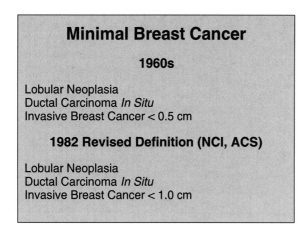

Fig. 1. Previous and current definitions of minimal breast cancer

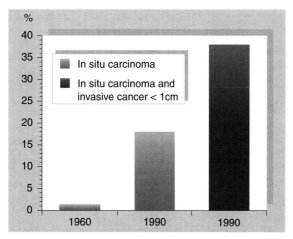

Fig. 2. Incidence of minimal breast cancer.

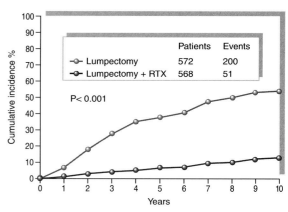

Fig. 3. Lobular neoplasia (photograph courtesy of Dr. Syed Hoda, NYH-CMC)

Table I. Risk of development of invasive breast cancer after diagnosis of LCIS.[14]

	Ipsilateral Breast	Contralateral Breast
10 years	15%	10%
15 years	27%	15%
20 years	35%	25%

sis.[17] The incidence of future invasive breast cancer after the diagnosis of LN did not vary with the age of the patient at the time of the initial LN diagnosis.[12]

Many of the characteristics of LN support the belief that LN is a marker for increased risk, not a true pre-invasive entity. These include that the subsequent invasive cancer is usually a different histological type (ductal not lobular), the long time interval to development of invasive cancer, and the equal incidence in either breast of subsequent cancer.

Lobular neoplasia is clinically asymptomatic in the majority of cases. It is often found incidentally on breast biopsy for benign breast disease or mastectomy for other detectable breast pathology.

The recommended treatment of patients with lobular neoplasia is close observation with examinations by a physician 3-4 times a year and annual mammography. Routine biopsy of the contralateral breast in a "blind" random fashion is not generally recommended. A positive biopsy is not statistically likely and a negative biopsy does not reduce the risk

of future development of invasive cancer in the contralateral breast. Axillary lymph node dissection is not justified in LN.[18]

Bilateral total prophylactic mastectomies with immediate reconstruction is a possible option for selected patients. Appropriate patients for consideration include those at a further increased risk because of a strong family history of breast cancer. Another group of patients that may be candidates are those who suffer extreme psychological distress from the diagnosis of LN and its consequent increased risk of future development of breast cancer. Before such a radical surgical treatment is contemplated, the patient and her partner should be given the opportunity to discuss realistically the potential outcome of such surgery with a plastic surgeon and a psychologist (Fig. 4).

Ductal carcinoma *in situ* (DCIS)

Ductal carcinoma *in situ* (intraductal carcinoma, DCIS) is frequently present in breasts containing simultaneous invasive cancer.[19,20] Ductal carcinoma *in situ* is often multifocal (additional disease within the same quadrant but at least 2 cm from the initial lesion),[20-22] as well as multicentric (additional disease in a different quadrant of the breast as the initial

Lobular Neoplasia
Treatment Options

- Close observation (physical examination every 3-4 months, mammograms annually)

- Contralateral breast biopsy not recommended

- Axillary node dissection not recommended

- Bilateral prophylactic mastectomy (rarely recommended)

Fig. 4. Treatment options of lobular neoplasia.

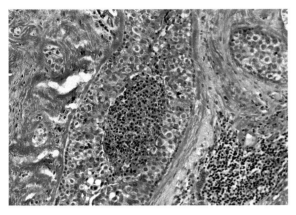

Fig. 5. Ductal Carcinoma *in situ* (photograph courtesy of Dr. Syed Hoda, NYH-CMC)

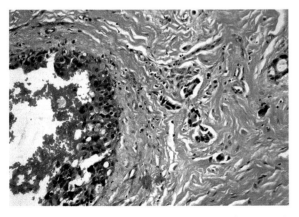

Fig. 6. Ductal carcinoma *in situ* with microinvasion (photograph courtesy of Dr. Syed Hoda, NYH-CMC)

lesion). The rate of multicentricity is 33% to 39%, and the multifocality rate is 41%.[21-23] There is also a 22% risk of bilaterality.

A diagnosis of DCIS is accompanied by an increased risk, both of synchronous and metachronous

contralateral breast cancer. The risk of synchronous contralateral breast cancer in a patient diagnosed with DCIS is 10-15%. This is the same as the synchronous contralateral risk for a patient with an invasive breast cancer.[18]

Ductal carcinoma *in situ* is generally divided into two main histologic categories: comedo and non-comedo. Comedo carcinomas are the most common type of DCIS. Non-comedo type includes papillary, micropapillary, cribriform, and solid forms. The comedo type ducts often have expressible cores of soft necrotic material. This central plug of necrotic material resembles a comedo, thus originated the name "comedo carcinoma" for this form of ductal carcinoma *in situ* (Fig. 5).

Distinguishing between the different subtypes of DCIS is important because there is evidence of differences in clinical behaviour. Some studies show that comedo type DCIS is more likely to recur than non-comedo type DCIS,[24] with 8% *versus* 1% recurrence rate respectively at 5 years.[25] Other studies fail to show a statistical difference in the recurrence of comedo and non-comedo, unless comedo type is combined with a nuclear grade 3 classification. Also, the time to local recurrence was also found to be shorter with comedo, nuclear grade 3 tumours, with the mean time to recurrence of 42 months versus 80 months.[26]

Comedo subtype tumours are more likely to have positive margins with a segmental resection, thus an incomplete resection[25] (Table II). Solid and cribriform DCIS are rarely multicentric, whereas micropapillary is often multicentric[27,28] (Table III).

The appropriate treatment of DCIS with micro-invasion, a subtype of DCIS, is a controversial topic. Ductal carcinoma *in situ* with micro-invasion is defined as an area of focal invasion 1 mm or less in diameter[25] (Fig. 6). It is unclear whether it should be treated as DCIS or as a small invasive tumour.

Micro-invasion is more common with comedo than non-comedo DCIS.[25,28] It is also more likely to be multicentric than other histologic types of DCIS[27] (Tables IV-V). The larger the size of the DCIS

Table II. Intraductal carcinoma: histologic subtype and biopsy margins.[25]

Histologic subtype	Clear	Biopsy margins involved	Not done	Total cases
Comedo	49	50	6	105
Cribriform	29	14	0	43
Micropapillary	8	14	1	23
Papillary	7	7	1	15
Solid	16	6	0	22
Total	109	91	8	208

tumour, the more likely it is to have a component of micro-invasion[25] or associated occult invasion (Table VI). In a series by Lagios, no occult invasion was found with mastectomy specimens for DCIS less than 25 mm in diameter, whereas with lesions greater than 55 mm, 50% had occult invasion.[29]

It is generally agreed that unresected DCIS significantly increases the risk of subsequent invasive carcinoma in the range of 30-50% at 10 years in the ipsilateral breast.[19] The average interval from diagnosis of DCIS to the development of invasive breast cancer is 9.7 years in patients treated with biopsy alone.[30,31] The fact that these recurrences are almost exclusively ductal, always within the same breast, and often (96%) within the same quadrant supports the concept that DCIS is a direct precursor of invasive ductal carcinoma.[2]

DCIS has become an increasingly common diagnosis, usually associated with mammographic microcalcifications. When no microcalcifications are present, ductal carcinoma *in situ* is often an incidental finding on pathologic examination. However, when extensive and involving large volumes of breast tissue, DCIS may be palpable.[32]

The standard treatment for DCIS has historically been total mastectomy. This approach is justified by the substantial risk of future development of invasive breast cancer if not resected, and the potential multicentric and multifocal nature of this entity.[18] The data suggest that in DCIS greater than 5 cm in diameter, diffuse microcalcifications associated with DCIS, and in multicentric lesions, total mastectomy is the preferred method of treatment. Other reasons to recommend a mastectomy for DCIS include any contra-indication to radiation therapy (*i.e.* pregnancy, prior radiation, collagen-vascular disease). It is important to assure negative histological margins on resection of the DCIS, and if this cannot be done, a mastectomy is the preferred method of treatment (Fig. 7). Recurrence after treatment of DCIS with total mastectomy is less than 1%.[33]

Another option for treatment of DCIS includes wide local excision with radiation. The studies to

Duct Carcinoma *In Situ*
Indications for Total Mastectomy

- Previous RT to breast or other contra-indication (scleroderma, pregnancy, non-compliant patient, etc.)

- DCIS diameter > 5 cm

- Diffuse microcalcifications

- Multicentric foci

- Male patient

- Inability to obtain free margins

Fig. 7. Duct Carcinoma *In Situ* (reprinted with permission of publisher).[53]

Table IV. Histologic findings *vs* micro-invasion in DCIS*.[27]

Histologic Findings	Not Micro-invasive		Micro-invasive		
	No.	(%)	No.	(%)	Total
Comedo carcinoma	9	(47)	10	(53)	19
Cribriform	5	(100)	0	(0)	5
Papillary	11	(92)	1	(8)	12
Solid	6	(86)	1	(14)	7
Micropapillary	6	(86)	1	(14)	7
Total	37	(74)	13	(26)	50

*DCIS indicates ductal carcinoma *in situ*.

Table V. Characteristics of DCIS histologic subtypes.

Comedo
    often multicentric and micro-invasion

Papillary
    often multicentric, rarely micro-invasion

Solid, Cribiform
    rarely multicentric or micro-invasion

Table III. Histologic findings *vs* multicentricity in DCIS*.[27]

Histologic Findings	Not Multicentric		Multicentric		
	No.	(%)	No.	(%)	Total
Comedo-carcinoma	11	(58)	8	(42)	19
Cribriform	5	(100)	0	(0)	5
Papillary	8	(67)	4	(33)	12
Solid	7	(100)	0	(0)	7
Micropapillary	1	(14)	6	(86)	7
Total	32	(64)	18	(36)	50

* DCIS indicates ductal carcinoma *in situ*.

Table VI. Intraductal carcinoma: tumour size and no. of patients with micro-invasion.[25]

Size (cm)	No. of cases	No. patients with micro-invasion	Percent (%)
Up to 0.5	33	1	3
0.6-1.0	49	3	6
1.1-2.0	50	9	18
2.1-4.9	46	8	17
5.0 or greater	30	7	23
Total	208	28	13

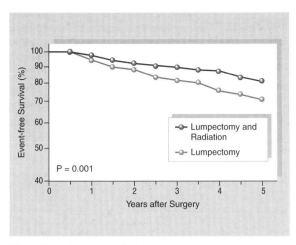

Fig. 8. Event-free survival of women treated by lumpectomy or lumpectomy and radiation therapy (reprinted with permission of publisher).[36]

Duct Carcinoma *In Situ*
Patient Selection Criteria for Wide Excision

- Occult duct carcinoma *in situ* detected by mammographic microcalcifications

- Focus 25 mm or less in maximum extent confirmed histologically

- Negative histologic margins

- Postoperative mammographic examination confirms no residual microcalcifications

- Breast favourable for clinical and mammographic evaluation

- Patient capable of understanding protocol and sharing risk

Fig. 9. (reprinted with permission of publisher).[29]

date show no statistically significant difference in survival with mastectomy and lumpectomy with radiation therapy.

In a study by Cutuli *et al.*, the local recurrence rate for DCIS was compared with treatment of modified radical mastectomy and breast conservation. At 55 months the local recurrence rate of the radical mastectomy group was 3%, and the local recurrence rate of the conservative treatment group was 9%, which was not statistically significant.[34]

The addition of radiation treatment to wide local excision in patients with DCIS is the standard of treatment. A retrospective analysis of the NSABP B-06 trial evaluated the treatment of DCIS by lumpectomy alone versus lumpectomy plus radiation. Women treated with lumpectomy alone had a 23% recurrence, whereas, only 7% of those who received radiation in addition to surgical excision had a local recurrence in a period up to 53 months.[35]

Because of the issues raised with the B-06 study on DCIS, the NSABP conducted a separate study, the B-17 study, which randomized women with DCIS into those to receive excision and radiation versus surgical excision only. The results of this study showed that those who had radiation in addition to surgical excision of the DCIS had a statistically significant lower local recurrence rate[36] (Fig. 8). These results were confirmed with other studies in which DCIS treated with biopsy alone, 28%-39% developed infiltrating breast cancer in the same breast.[22,37-39]

The local recurrences with DCIS consist of 50% non-invasive and 50% invasive carcinomas.[11,36] It is important to recognize that the majority of local recurrences with DCIS are within the same quadrant as the initial tumour and usually at the original biopsy site, which implies inadequate resection of the initial tumour.[18]

There is some evidence that excision alone is adequate in selected cases of DCIS. The criteria specified by Lagios for candidates to undergo excision alone without radiation include mammographically detected microcalcifications less than 25 mm, or those detected as an incidental finding, negative resection margins, and negative post-biopsy mammogram. Lagios *et al*, found a 10% ten year local recurrence in DCIS treated with local excision without irradiation in selected cases[29] (Fig. 9). A subsequent study showed that in DCIS found incidentally or by mammographically detectable microcalcifications, and meeting the criteria established by Lagios, the recurrence for resection alone was similar, at 15% in 47 months mean follow-up.[40] No patients recurred in the group where DCIS was diagnosed incidentally during a biopsy for a separate mammographic or palpable lesion. Of note, however, none of these patients had comedo type DCIS. In the patients that did recur, all but one had comedo type DCIS, implying that this is a main indicator of recurrence, and that non-comedo DCIS may be added to the criteria of resection without radiation. These results have been confirmed by other studies where those with a comedo-type of pathology had a 19% recurrence at 87 months, whereas none of the patients with a papillary or cribriform type had a local recurrence.[29]

In patients with DCIS an axillary node dissection is not generally recommended. The rate of positive axillary lymph nodes in DCIS without micro-invasion is less than 1%.[22,41-43] If a mastectomy is performed it is reasonable to do a low level I axillary dissection at the time of mastectomy with little or no added morbidity.[18] There is some support for a low level I axillary dissection for patients with palpable comedo type DCIS because of the increased association of micro-invasion and occult invasion.[27,44]

Axillary dissection in patients with DCIS and micro-invasion is controversial. In patients with micro-invasion, axillary node dissection may be justified. In a series by Silverstein et. al., invasive cancers less than 5 mm in diameter, there was a node positivity rate of 3%.[45] Other series have found positive axillary node dissection in up to 27% of patients with micro-invasion[28,42,46-49] (Table VII).

Minimal invasive breast cancer

Minimal invasive breast cancers are defined as less than 1 cm in diameter. These cancers are typically detected by mammography with 52.6% being detected by mammography alone, and only 8.4% diagnosed by physical examination alone.[1]

The prognosis for these small cancers is generally excellent. The overall survival at seven years in tumours less than 5 mm is 94%, and 87% in tumours 5-10 mm.[50]

The two surgical options for minimal invasive cancers of the breast are modified radical mastectomy and breast conserving surgery. It is generally accepted that an axillary dissection and radiation treatment of the breast should be included with breast conserving surgery. Axillary dissection is controversial in invasive cancers less than 5 mm in diameter, and those of special types, such as tubular carcinoma, where the likelihood of axillary involvement is small.

It has been shown in the NSABP B-06 clinical trial that mastectomy and breast conserving surgery for small invasive tumors of the breast have equal survival rates.[51] Veronesi et al., compared the removal of a quarter of the breast (quadrantectomy), axillary dissection, and radiation (QUART) to radical mastectomy with tumours less than two centimeters and no palpable axillary lymph nodes. At nineteen years follow up, there was no difference in the overall survival rates of these two groups. Further comparison of axillary dissection and radiation therapy with tumorectomy (TART) versus quadrantectomy (QUART) showed no difference in survival at 7 years.[52]

There are certain contra-indications to breast conservation which do not allow acceptable local-regional control. Some of these contra-indications include previous radiation treatment, pregnancy, extensive microcalcifications, and the inability to

Table VII. Duct carcinoma in situ with Micro-invasion and positive axillary lymph nodes.

Silverstein et al.[46]	3%
Schuh et al.[47]	5%
Patchefsky et al.[29]	10%
Kinne et al.[43]	20%
Rosner et al.[48]	27%

Invasive Cancer
Indications for Mastectomy

- Tumour > 5 cm

- Pregnancy

- Prior irradiation or other contra-indication to RT (scleroderma, non-compliant patient, etc.)

- Male patient

- Two ipsilateral tumours in different quadrants

- Diffuse mammographic calcifications

- Inability to obtain adequate tumour-free margins

- Local recurrence after breast-conserving therapy

- Occult cancer presenting as axillary metastases

Fig. 10. (reprinted with permission of publisher).[53]

achieve tumour-free margins. The presence of two or more separate tumours, unless within the same quadrant of the breast, is also a contradiction to breast conservation[53] (Fig. 10).

Because of the multicentricity of breast cancer, radiation of the remaining breast with breast conserving surgery is critical.[54] In the NSABP B-06 trial, total mastectomy was compared with lumpectomy and axillary dissection with and without radiotherapy. Lumpectomy followed by irradiation showed similar results in diseases free survival (DFS) and overall survival to mastectomy. The results of this study show local recurrence rates are significantly higher in patients treated by lumpectomy without radiation therapy, with a 12% local recurrence rate in those irradiated and 53% in those not receiving radiation at ten years.[51] A benefit was found both in node negative and node positive patients. Overall survival is not influenced in these groups[50,51,55] (Fig. 11).

The issue of axillary dissection on women with a small invasive or micro-invasive breast carcinoma remains controversial. Although the likelihood of axillary nodal involvement increases with the size of

Table VIII. Nodal positivity for various T categories.[45]

Category	No. of patients	No. of positive dissections (%)	P value
Tis (DCIS)	189	0 (0)	0.015
T1a	96	3 (3)	0.0007
T1b	156	27 (17)	0.0006
T1c	357	115 (32)	0.0015
T2	330	145 (44)	0.0014
T3	92	55 (60)	

DCIS: duct carcinoma *in situ.*

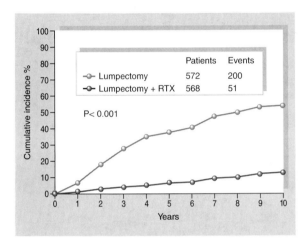

Fig. 11. Cumulative incidence of ipsilateral breast tumour recurrence at 10 years' follow up in patients treated by lumpectomy alone (L) or by lumpectomy and breast irradiation (L + RTX) (reprinted with permission of publisher).[51]

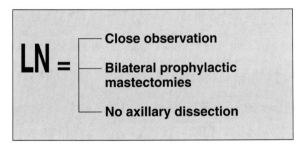

Fig. 12. Treatment options for lobular neoplasia.

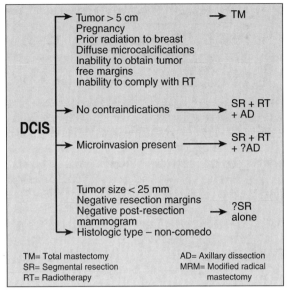

Fig. 13. Treatment options for ductal carcinoma *in situ.*

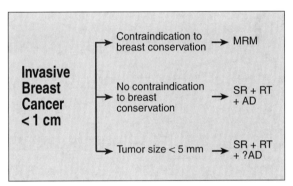

Fig. 14. Treatment option for invasive breast cancer <1 cm.

the primary tumour, the possibility of axillary nodal involvement in small breast carcinoma is not insignificant. In invasive tumours measuring less than 1 cm in diameter, the axillary nodes are positive in 16-23%.[1,45,56] Silverstein *et al.* evaluated axillary metastasis in breast cancers less than 1 cm and found in tumours between 5 mm and 1 cm a 17% positivity rate, and in tumours less than 5 mm only a 3% positivity rate (Table VIII).

Invasive tumours, less than 1 cm in diameter, with negative axillary nodes, have a 5 year survival rate that does not differ significantly from that of patients in the same series with DCIS, 70.3% and 74.3% respectively. This was significantly different from the survival in patients with tumours less than 1 cm, with positive nodes, which was 53.0%.[1]

In addition to size, the presence of lymphatic invasion (LVI) is associated with positive axillary lymph nodes. In patients with tumours smaller than 1 cm and no LVI only 9% had axillary nodal involvement of tumour.[57]

There is much debate among clinicians as to when the likelihood of having a positive axillary dissection is so small as to justify not performing it. In this group of women with very small tumours, treatment with chemotherapy is dictated by nodal status. There was a significant survival advantage in the patients with tumours less than 1 cm who had axillary dissection.[58] Failure to perform axillary dissection in these patients would result in significant understaging, altered treatment recommendations, and possible increased chance of recurrence. It seems reasonable to perform axillary node dissections on these patients with small tumours especially if LVI is present.

Conclusion

"Minimal breast cancer" is an increasingly important clinical problem. Although grouped together, lobular neoplasia, ductal carcinoma *in situ*, and invasive breast cancers less than 1 cm should be considered as very different pathological entities. Each, due to its specific characteristics and behaviour, should be treated in its respective appropriate methods (Figs. 12-14).

References

1. Hartmann W.H.: Minimal breast Cancer. Cancer, 1984; 53: 681-684
2. Frykberg E.R., Masood S., Copeland E.M., Bland K.I.: Ductal Carcinoma *in situ* of the Breast. Surgery, Gynecology and Obstetrics, 1993; 177: 425-440
3. Rosen P.P., Braun D.W., Kinne D.W.: The Clinical Significance of Pre-invasive Breast Carcinoma. Cancer, 1980; 46: 919-925
4. Ward B.A., McKhann C.F., Ravikumar T.S.: Ten-Year Follow-Up of Breast Carcinoma *In Situ* in Connecticut. Archives Surgery, 1992; 127: 1392-1395
5. Foote F.W., Stewart F.W.: Lobular Carcinoma *in Situ*. American Journal of Pathology, 1940; 17: 491-496
6. Haagensen C.D., Lane N., Bodian C.: Coexisting lobular neoplasia and Carcinoma of the Breast. Cancer, 51: 1468-1482, 83
7. Neilsen M., Jensen J., Andersen J.: Precancerous and Cancerous Breast Lesions During Lifetime and At Autopsy. Cancer, 1984; 54: 612-615
8. Haagensen C.D., Lane N., Lattes R., Bodian C.: Lobular Neoplasia (so-called Lobular Carcinoma *in situ*) of the Breast. Cancer, 1978; 42: 737-769
9. Hutter R.V.: The management of Patients with Lobular carcinoma *in situ* of the breast. Cancer, 1984; 53: 798-802
10. Kern W.h., Brooks R.N.: Atypical Epithelial Hyperplasia associated with Breast Cancer and Fibrocystic Disease. Cancer, 1969; 24: 668-675
11. Graham M.D., Lakhani S., Gazet J.C.: Breast conserving surgery in the management of insitu breast carcinoma. European Journal of Surgical Oncology, 1991; 17: 258-264
12. Anderson, J.A.: Lobular Carcinoma *in situ* of the Breast. Cancer, 1977; 39: 2597-2602
13. Rosen, P.P.: Lobular Carcinoma *in Situ*: Recent Clinicopathologic Studies at Memorial Hospital. Path. Res. Pract., 1980; 166: 430-455
14. McDivitt R.W.: *In Situ* Lobular Carcinoma. JAMA, 1986; 201: 82-86
15. Walt A.J., Simon M., Swanson G.M.: The Continuing Dilemma of Lobular Carcinoma *In Situ*. Archives Surgery, 1992; 127: 904-909
16. Musio F., Mozingo D., Otchy D.P.: Multiple Giant Fibroadenoma. The American Surgeon, 1991; 438-441
17. Rosen P.P., Lieberman P.H., Braun D.W., Kosloff C., Adair F.: Lobular Carcinoma *in situ* of the breast; Detailed analysis of 99 patients with average follow-up of 24 years. American Journal of Surgical Pathology, 1978; 2: 225-251
18. Bland K.I., Frykberg E.R.: Selective Management of *In Situ* Carcinoma of the Breast. Breast Diseases, 1992; 3: 11-21
19. Page D.L., Dupont W.D., Rogers L.W., Rados M.S.: Atypical Hyperplastic Lesions of the Female Breast: A Long-term Follow-up Study, 1985; Cancer, 55: 2698-2708
20. Wellings S.R., Marcum R.G.: An Atlas of Subgross Pathology of the human Breast with special Reference to Possible Precancerous Lesions. Journal of the National Cancer Institute, 1975; 55: 231-273
21. Lagios M.D., Westdahl P.R., Margolin F.R., Rose M.R.: Ductal Carcinoma *In Situ*; Relationship of Extent of Noninvasive Disease to the Frequency of Occult Invasion, Multicentricity, Lymph Node Metastases, and Short-Term Treatment Failures, 1982; Cancer, 50: 1309-1314
22. Silverstein M.J., Cohlan, B.F. Gierson, E.D. Furnandki, M. Colburn, W.J. Lewindky, B.S. Waisman J.R.: Duct Carcinoma *in situ*: 227 cases without microinvasion. European Jornal of Cancer, 1992; 28: 630-634
23. Ciatto S., Cecchini, S. Iossa, A. Grazzini, G. Bravetti, P. Del Turco M.R., Cataliotti L., Cardona G., Bianchi S.: Prognosis of nonpalpable infiltrating carcinoma of the breast. Surgery, Gynecology, and Obstetrics, 1990; 170: 61-64
24. Fisher E.R., Leeming R., Anderson S., Redmond C., Fisher B.: Conservative Management of Intraductal Carcinoma (DCIS) of the Breast. Journal of Surgical Oncology, 1991; 47: 139-147
25. Silverstein M.J., Waisman J.R., Gamagami P., Gierson E.D., Colburn W.J., Rosser R.J., Gordon P.S., Lewinsky B.S., Fingerhut, A.: Intraductal Carcinoma of the Breast (208 cases); clinical factors influencing treatment choice. Cancer, 1990; 66: 102-108
26. Solin L.J., Yeh I., Kurtz J., Fourquet A., Recht A., Kuske R., McCormick B., Cross M.A., Schultz D.J., Amalric, R., LiVolsi V.A., Kowalyshyn M.J., Torhorst J., Jacquemier J., Westermann C.D., Mazoujian G., Zafrani B., Rosen P.P., Goodman R.L., Fowble, B.L.: Ductal Carcinoma *In Situ* of the Breast Treated with breast-conserving Surgery and Definitive Irradiation. Cancer, 1993; 71: 2532-2542
27. Schwartz G.F., Patchefsky A.S., Finkelstein S.D., Prestipino A., Feig S.A., Singer J.S.: Nonpalpable *In Situ* Ductal Carcinoma of the Breast; Predictors of multicentricity and microinvasion and implications for treatment. Archives Surgery, 1989; 124: 29-32
28. Patchefsky A.S., Schwartz G.F., Finkelstein S.D., Prestipino A., Sohn S.E., Singer J.S., Feig S.A.: Heterogeneity of Intraductal Carcinoma of the Breast. Cancer, 1989; 63: 731-741
29. Lagios M.D., Margolin F.R., Westdahl P.R., Rose M.R.: Mammographically Detected Duct Carcinoma *In Situ*. Cancer, 1989; 63: 618-624
30. Rosen P.P., Braun D.W., Lyngholm B., Urban J.A., Kinne D.W.: Lobular Carcinoma *in situ* of the Breast: Preliminary Results of Treatment by Ipsilateral Mastectomy and Contralateral Breast Biopsy. Cancer, 1981; 47: 813-819
31. Betsill W.L., Rosen P.P., Lieberman P.H., Robbins G.F.: Intraductal Carcinoma: long-term follow-up after treatment be biopsy alone. JAMA, 239: 1863-1867, 1978
32. Simmons R.M., Serafin D., McCarty K.S. Jr.: Pathologic Considerations in the High-Risk Breast Patient. Clinics in Plastic Surgery, 1988; 15: 655-665
33. Ashikari R., Hajdu S.I., Robbins G.F.: Intraductal Carcinoma of the Breast. Cancer, 1971; 28: 1182-1187
34. Cutuli B., Teissier E., Piat J.M., Janser J., Renaud R., Rodier J., Jung G.: Radical Surgery and Conservative Treatment of Ductal Carcinoma insitu of the breast. European Jornal of Cancer, 1992; 28: 649-654
35. Fisher E.R., Sass R., Fisher B., Wickerham D.L., Paik S.M.: Pathologic Findings from the National Surgical Adjuvant Breast Project (Protocol 6) Intraductal Carcinoma (DCIS). Cancer, 1986; 57: 197-208
36. Fisher B., Costantino J., Redmond C., Fisher E., Margolese R., Dimitrov N., Wolmark N., Wickerham D.L., Deutsch M., Ore L., Mamounas E., Poller W., Kavanah M.: Lumpectomy compared with lumpectomy and radiation therapy for the treatment of intraductal breast cancer. NEJM, 1993; 328: 1581-1586

37. Aitken, D.R., Minton, J.P.: Complications associated with mastectomy. unknown, 1994

38. Page D.L., Dupont W.D., Rogers L.W., Landenberger M.: Intraductal Carcinoma of the Breast: Follow up after biopsy only 1982; Cancer, 49: 751-758

39. Gallagher W.J., Koerner F.C., Wood W.C.: Treatment of Intraductal Carcinoma With Limited Surgery: Long Term Follow-up. Journal of Clinical Oncology, 1989; 7: 376-380

40. Schwartz G.F., Finkel G.C., Garcia, J.C., Patchefsky A.S.: Subclinical Ductal Carcinoma *in situ* of the breast. Cancer, 1992; 70: 2468-2474

41. Silverstein M.J., Gierson E.D., Colburn W.J., Rosser R.J., Waisman J.R., Gamagami, P.: Axillary Lymphadenectomy for Intraductal carcinoma of the breast. Surgery, Gynecology, Obstetrics, 1991; 172: 211-214

42. Kinne D.W., Petrek J.A., Osborne M.P., Fracchia A.A., DePalo A.A., Rosen, P.P.: Breast Carcinoma *in Situ*. Archives Surgery, 1989; 124: 33-36

43. Van Dongan J.A., Holland R., Peterse J.L., Fentiman I.S., Lagios M.D., Millis R.R., Recht A.: Ductal Carcinoma in-situ of the Breast; Second EORTC Consensus Meeting. European Jornal of Cancer, 1992; 28: 626-629

44. Gump F.E., Jicha, D.L., Ozello, L.: Ductal Carcinoma *in situ* (DCIS): a revised concept. Surgery, 1987; 102: 790-795

45. Silverstein M.J., Gierson E.D., Waisman J.R., Senofsky, G.M., Colburn W.J., Gamagami P.: Axillary Lymph Node Dissection for T1a Breast Cancer, Is it indicated? Cancer, 1994; 73: 664-667

46. Schuh M.E., Nemoto T., Penetrante R., Rosner D., Dao T.L.: Intraductal Carcinoma; analysis of presentation, pathologic findings, and outcome of disease. Archives Surgery, 1986; 121: 1303-1307

47. Rosner D., Lane W.W., Penetrante R.: Ductal Carcinoma *In situ* With Microinvasion; A curable entity using surgery alone without need for adjuvant therapy. Cancer, 1991; 67: 1498-1503

48. Kopald K.H., Hiatt J.R., Irving C., Giuliano A.E.: The Pathology of Nonpalpable Breast Cancer. The American Surgeon, 1990; 56: 782-787

49. Clark G.M., Wenger C.R., Beardslee S., Owens M.A., Pounds G., Oldaker T., Vendely P., Pandian M.R., Harrington D., McGuire W.L.: How to Integrate Steroid Hormone Receptor, Flow Cytometric, and Other Prognostic Information in Regard to Primary Breast Cancer. Cancer, 1993; 71: 2157-62

50. Amos E.H.: Conservative Surgery and Radiation Therapy in Early Breast Cancer: Ten year experience at the West Florida Cancer Institute. Southern Medical Journal, 1993; 86: 513-517,

51. Fisher B., Anderson S.: Conservative Surgery for the Management of Invasive and Noninvasive Carcinoma of the Breast: NSABP Trials. World Journal of Surgery, 1994; 18: 63-69

52. Veronesi U., Luini A., Galimberti V., Zurrida, S.: Conservation Approaches for the management of Stage I/II Carcinoma of the Breast: Milan Cancer Institute Trials. World Journal of Surgery, 1994; 18: 70-75

53. Osborne M.P., Borgen P.I.: Role of Mastectomy in Breast Cancer. Surgical Clinics of North America, 1990; 70: 1023-1046

54. Simmons R.M., Daly J.M.: Can Radiation Therapy Following "Lumpectomy" for Invasive Breast Cancer Be Safely Omitted? Correspondence Society of Surgeons, 1994; 17: 7-8,

55. Fisher B., Redmond C., Poisson R., Margolese R., Wolmark N., Wickerham D.L., Fisher E.R., Deutsch M., Caplan R., Pilch Y., Glass A., Shibata H., Lerner H., Terz J., Sidorovich, L.: Eight-Year Results of a Randomized Clinical Trial Comparing Total Mastectomy and Lumpectomy with or without irradiation in the Treatment of Breast Cancer. NEJM, 1989; 320: 822-828

56. Margolis D.S., McMillen M.A., Hashmi H., Wasson D.W., MacArthur J.D.: Aggressive Axillary Evaluation and Adjuvant therapy for nonpalpable carcinoma of the breast. Surgery, Gynecology, and Obstetrics, 1992; 174: 109-113

57. Chadha M., Chabon A.B., Freidmann, P., Vikram B.: Predictors of Axillary Lymph Node Metastases in Patients with T1 Breast Cancer. Cancer, 1994; 73: 350-353

58. Cabanes P.A., Salmon R.J., Vilcoq J.R., Durand J.C., Fourquet A., Gautier C., Asselain B.: Value of axillary dissection in addition to lumpectomy and radiotherapy in early breast cancer. Lancet, 1992; 339: 1245-1248

The management of the axilla

M. Greco, N. Cascinelli

Introduction

Axillary dissection has been considered an integral part of breast cancer treatment for more than 100 years and is routinely carried out in all breast cancer patients. Even after the introduction of breast conserving treatments into clinical practice, axillary dissection remained a permanent part of breast cancer care with only some little debate on the extent to which it should be performed in patients with small breast cancer.

The role of axillary surgery in the management of breast cancer has to be related to four different objectives:
1. to remove local disease;
2. to prevent recurrence;
3. to stage breast cancer;
4. to plan adjuvant treatments.

The Halstedian concept of the initial spread of breast cancer through lymphatics to axillary nodes, which are very likely sites of metastatic deposits and possible sources of tertiary spread, is the cultural basis of the curative intention of axillary surgery. The extent of the dissection is related to the necessity of a complete removal of local disease and of prevention of local recurrence. The relatively recent concept that breast cancer is a systemic disease from the beginning confirmed the importance of axillary dissection for staging and prognostic purposes in order to plan adjuvant systemic treatments. Furthermore, many clinical trials, especially in medical oncology, require an accurate stage and prognostic assessment of the disease on the basis of the current TNM classification system. The rigidity of this classification, the unreliability of pre-operative imaging techniques so far available, disagreement on the prognostic value in clinical practice of the different tumour characteristics and the classical indication for adju-

vant treatments on the basis of nodal status and number of nodes involved, are all factors which make axillary surgery inevitable.

Extent of axillary surgery

The above-mentioned objectives of axillary surgery can be obtained by different technical modalities that reflect a distinct cultural approach. The most widely adopted surgical options are:
1. axillary sampling;
2. low axillary dissection (first and second level);
3. full axillary clearance (first, second and third level).

The choice of the best option is related to the cost-benefit balance between the maximum information obtainable, without unacceptable damage to the patient. It is a matter of fact that there is a significant, though not severe, morbidity associated to a radical axillary clearance. This involves lymphoedema of the arm, stiffness of the shoulder, damage to the intercostal brachial nerve leaving anaesthesia and paraesthesia of the upper arm and the rare but ever possible complication of surgical damage to the long thoracic and thoracodorsal nerves. The more aggressive the axillary dissection, the more likely it is to result in these morbidities. At the same time, the higher up the axilla the surgeon explores, the less likely he is to find involved nodes. This suggests there must be a point of diminishing returns when the morbidity of the procedure exceeds the benefit of possible additional gain for local control or staging. At the other extreme, an inadequate axillary dissection might leave the surgeon with the dilemma of positive lymph nodes at the highest point of his dissection. Axillary sampling and low axillary dissection may result in many circumstances insufficient to stage the disease properly and inadequate to obtain local control in case of positivity. The surgeon then may be forced to ask the radiotherapist to intervene with high risk of lymphoedema of the arm and the possible risk of brachial plexus neuropathy because of the combination of surgery and radiotherapy.

The choice of optimal axillary surgery cannot rely on pre-operative procedures. Physical examination is misleading in about 30% of cases and imaging techniques are not completely reliable at the moment and their cost is prohibitive. Some Authors explored the possibility of deciding the best treatment during axillary surgery by using intra-operative staging procedures. This means collecting information on the stage of the disease as the first part of an operation and changing treatment plan on the basis of information collected. The methods proposed for intra-operative staging are Apex Biopsy and Sentinel Node Biopsy.

Apex biopsy is a subclavicular node biopsy carried out as a first step of axillary surgery. This procedure was developed in the Netherlands Cancer Institute and has been considered routine in operable breast cancer since the late 50s.[1] The apex biopsy is reported to be tumour-positive in 4% of TNM stage I patients, in 17% of TNM stage II patients and in 40% of TNM stage IIIA patients. The outcome of the apex biopsy is used to decide on the final therapy choice. The main objective of this procedure is to avoid unnecessary surgical dissection of the third axillary level in node-negative patients.

Sentinel node biopsy is used to select patients for treatment of the regional lymph nodes. This procedure was originally described for melanoma by Morton et al. in 1992.[2] At the moment the value of this technique is under investigation in several cancer centres to validate the hypothesis that dissemination of cancer cells first occurs to the lymph node located at the opposite end of the lymphatic vessel draining the primary tumour. This node is called the "sentinel node" and can be revealed by injection of patent blue dye and/or radioisotopes in the tumour at the beginning of the operation. In case of involvement of this node, axillary dissection is performed.

Both these procedures need further validations in terms of reliability and reproducibility and a definitive answer will probably be produced by a clinical trial.

Currently the optimal extent of axillary surgery is still controversial and it should probably be more often related to patient and tumour characteristics than happens in daily clinical practice. A definite rule in this field cannot be given and different treatments could be optimal for each individual patient.

On the other hand, the extent and distribution of axillary node involvement in breast cancer is less controversial and can usefully be adopted in selecting treatment for the individual patient.

In a retrospective study carried out at the National Cancer Institute in Milan, the extent of axillary involvement in 1446 node-positive cases of breast cancer was evaluated.[3] All these patients were submitted to full dissection including all three axillary levels regardless of size and site of the tumour and age of the patient.

The results of this study showed that:
1. the spread of breast cancer to the axilla follows a regular pattern: the rate of skip metastases is very low (1.3%);
2. the probability of invasion of the second and/or the third levels appears related to the number of lymph nodes involved at the first level (Table I) and, globally, if the first level is invaded, the risk of nodal involvement at the higher levels is consistent (54%);
3. the risk of metastases at the third level, in cases with metastatic involvement of the first and second levels, is also correlated to tumour size;
4. the prognostic significance of a complete dissection is much more accurate and reliable than that of a partial one, also because the involvement of the apex of the axilla has severe prognostic implications and can change treatment plans.

All this information is useful for surgeons who believe it is sufficient to remove only the lymph nodes of the first level for staging purposes. In case of positivity of the first level, the high risk of residual disease imposes further axillary treatment, considering that recurrence beyond the pectoralis minor muscle or at the apex of the axilla is very difficult to detect and may rapidly invade the nerves of the brachial plexus.

In the light of these findings, full axillary clearance appears preferable compared to other surgical options on condition that morbid sequelae are incidental and not permanent. This objective can only be reached if axillary dissection is regarded in every hospital as a surgical operation which requires surgical skill and diligence. No surgeon, however skilled, should carry out axillary dissection if he or she cannot

Table I. Number of metastatic nodes found: percentage of cases with metastatic involvement.

At level I number of nodes	At level II and/or III percentage
One	12.1
Two	19.5
Three	37.5
Four	40.3
More than four	83.9

provide patients with a course of post-operative physiotherapy beginning the first day after the operation.

The problem of the clinically negative axilla

The recent history of breast cancer management reports many attempts to simplify loco-regional treatment, especially when the risk of regional lymph node metastases or local failure may be low.

Attempts to reduce surgery involving the breast and the axilla are in line with the above-mentioned trend. The biological knowledge to avoid axillary dissection in selected patients comes firstly from the National Surgical Adjuvant Breast Program (NSABP) in the B-04 protocol published in 1977.[4] This prospective clinical trial established the fact that lymph node metastases are "indicators, but not governors"[5] of survival and that survival is identical when clinically comparing node-negative patients who had the axilla treated by either dissection or radiation, or who went untreated and received axillary surgery only in case of relapse. In the same year, preliminary results were published of a multicentre prospective trial carried out in the United Kingdom (Cancer Research Campaign trial) which included patients who were clinically node positive as well as clinically node negative and were randomised in two ways: mastectomy alone *versus* mastectomy plus radiotherapy to regional lymphatic fields. The CRC trial reached the conclusion that "untreated axillary nodes do not appear to act as a source of tertiary spread" and that "delayed (therapeutic) radiotherapy may achieve the same objective as immediate post-operative radiotherapy".[6]

If this is so, the arising question is whether or not, from a strictly therapeutic point-of-view, axillary dissection could safely be avoided in clinically node negative patients when accurate staging purposes can be considered of second choice. The real question is not a dichotomy between treatment *versus* neglect, but prophylactic therapy to the axilla *versus* selective therapy when evidence of progressive disease emerges.

In current clinical practice, screening mammography and educational programmes have increased the number of small invasive breast cancers detected, particularly in patients aged 50 years or more.[7]

These earlier-stage breast cancers result from the discovery of smaller cancers with fewer axillary nodal metastases. Even though it is likely that a smaller tumour does not necessarily mean earlier cancer, and that these smaller tumours might only be garden-variety breast cancers, it is also likely that these can be a less lethal variant. The involvement of axillary nodes is directly and significantly correlated to tumour size,[8-11] while the role of other histopathological features, like degrees of differentiation, or endocrine receptor status, is controversial. Many recent reports suggest that tumours of 5 mm or smaller in diameter may have an extremely low incidence of lymph node metastases (about 3%) and for cancers up to 1 cm, the incidence of axillary involvement is calculated between 10 and 13%. The real extent of lymph node metastases in very early breast cancer is still controversial. Nevertheless, in recent years many claims have been put forward to avoid useless surgical procedures in selected subgroups of patients at low risk of axillary involvement. Attempts to further simplify therapy by avoiding general anaesthesia for axillary dissection may enable breast cancer treatment to become an entirely outpatient procedure. When a variety of tumour prognostic factors, besides axillary nodal involvement, is used for selection of patients to adjuvant treatment, the importance of axillary dissection for staging purposes will be reduced.

The crucial point is to identify sub-groups of patients for which axillary dissection can safely be avoided. The definition of "safety" in cancer management should involve both cost-benefit and risk-benefit ratios in terms of accepting slight increases in non-lethal, relatively inconsequential, or extremely low-incidence recurrences in some patients for the sake of avoiding treatment morbidity and excessive cost for the overwhelming majority of patients when treatment effects are relatively small The simplification and reduction of the morbidity of therapy, together with an increase in its efficacy, are worthy goals of contemporary cancer management.

Regarding the question of whether or not it can be safe to leave loco-regional nodes untreated, the experience achieved with nodes of the internal mammary chain, generally left untreated in clinical practice, can provide important information. In a series of patients studied at the Istituto Nazionale Tumori in Milan, randomly allocated to treatment as part of a multicentre clinical trial, no difference in overall survival and local failure was observed in the sub-set of patients who did not receive any treatment to internal mammary nodes.[12]

In clinically negative patients, axillary dissection is generally carried out so as to allow the selection of patients for adjuvant treatment on the basis of nodal involvement. Furthermore, some clinical trials have recently proved the prognostic importance of micrometastases found in the axillary nodes. In general, those patients with pathologically negative axillae do not undergo an adjuvant treatment, while those with pathologically involved axillae undergo either adjuvant cytotoxic chemotherapy or adjuvant hormone therapy. For years nodal status was the sole criterion used for the referral of patients to medical oncologists for additional treatment. More recently a number of randomised clinical trials have shown the value of adjuvant systemic therapy, either hormone or cytotoxic, regardless of the status of the axillary nodes. Currently decisions regarding adjuvant systemic therapy are being increasingly based upon other factors such as tumour size, age of the patient, menopausal and hormone receptor status, tumour cell proliferation, nuclear grading and other pathological features of the primary tumour. The prognostic power of many biological determinants of the tumour is under investigation so as to identify breast cancer patients at high risk of recurrence regardless of nodal involvement. Different authors recently reported the possibility of evaluating the risk of axillary node involvement on the basis of tumour characteristics. One of the most promising studies in this respect comes from the Istituto Nazionale Tumori in Milan, where a series of 813 patients surgically treated from 1968 to 1969 for infiltrating breast carcinoma, were studied to establish a new prognostic score based solely on parameters of the primary tumour as an alternative to axillary surgery in assessing prognosis. In this study the importance of laminine-receptor and c-erbB-2 over-expression was stressed together with tumour size and staging as prognostic factors.[13]

Thus, clinicians may become less dependent on pathological axillary nodal status for decision making in the management of breast cancer patients and women have become dubious about the need to accept the morbid sequelae of a not indispensable axillary dissection. Outside a clinical trial, the necessity of axillary dissection may be questioned if systemic therapy has already been defined, based on other clinical and pathological factors. This is particularly relevant for post-menopausal, oestrogen receptor-positive patients for whom the current standard of care would be tamoxifen therapy regardless of the status of axillary nodes.

The same argument is more controversial for pre-menopausal patients, although in these patients the pathological features of the primary cancer are very often sufficient to refer them to medical treatments and do not need any confirmation by the pathological examination of the axillary nodes. It is a matter of fact that node negative pre-menopausal patients are increasingly treated with adjuvant therapy on a basis which differs from nodal status. Furthermore, the ever more extensive use of adjuvant treatments and the recent introduction into clinical practice of pre-operative chemo- and hormone-therapy, even for operable breast cancer, has progressively reduced the need for the accurate anatomical staging of the

disease which axillary dissection can provide. The rigid, anatomical TNM staging system is now inadequate for the modern purposes of breast cancer management and should shortly be substituted by a new one based on both biological and pathological findings of the primary tumour.[14]

From this perspective, axillary dissection is on its way toward losing much of its value as a staging procedure.

In conclusion, outside a protocol setting, where the patient and the treating physician will remain uninfluenced by the pathological status of the lymph nodes with respect to systemic therapy, there are no compulsory reasons to carry out an axillary dissection in patients with clinically negative axillae.

If it can be accepted that axillary dissection may be optional in clinically negative patients, the problem emerging is whether or not they should be treated by radiotherapy instead of surgery to avoid local failure in the axillae. Clinical trials and retrospective studies have proved that irradiation of the axilla or of the lower part of the axilla can reduce the number of local recurrences within the limits of an acceptable risk. The estimated value of this risk is between 3% and 8% at five years for small tumours with minimal morbidity for the patients. The alternative is no treatment at all at axillary level and surgery (full dissection) or radiotherapy in cases of progressive disease. The CRC trial showed that delayed radiotherapy may achieve the same objectives as immediate post-operative radiotherapy and at the same time a large percentage of women may be spared the discomfort and anxiety associated with radiotherapy. It seems that these words can also be properly applied to surgery, and that a "wait and see" policy at axillary level can be safely proposed, as proved by Fisher in the B-04 protocol. A full axillary dissection in cases of progressive disease has advantages in comparison with radiotherapy because it is radical (with almost no recurrences even in the presence of consistent axillary involvement) and reliable for staging and prognostic purposes, as well as in respect of additional treatments.

References

1. Van Slooten E.A., Hampe J.F.: Indicatiestelling voor de behandeling van mammacarcinoom; bepaling van de operabiliteit door proefexcisie van de subclaviGulaire klieren. Jaarbeok van Kankeronderzoek Kankerbestrijding. 1958; 8: 64 (first report of his series, summary in English)
2. Morton D.L., Wen D.R., Wong J.H. et al.: Technical details of intraoperative lymphatic mapping for early stage melanoma. Arch. Surg., 1992; 127: 392-399
3. Veronesi U., Luini A., Galimberti V.: Extent of metastatic

axillary involvement in 1446 cases of breast cancer. Eur. J. Surg. Onc., 1990; 16: 127-133

4. Fisher B., Montague E., Redmond C.: Comparison of radical mastectomy with alternative treatments for primary breast cancer. A first report of results from a prospective randomized clinical trial. Cancer, 1977, 39: 2827-2839

5. Cady B.: Lymph node metastases. Indicators, but not governors of survival. Arch. Surg., 1984, 119: 1067-1072

6. Baum M., Coyle P.J.: Simple mastectomy for early breast cancer and the behaviour of the untreated axillary nodes. Bull du Cancer 1977, 64: 603-610

7. Cady B., Stone M.D., Wayne J.: New therapeutic possibilities in primary invasive breast cancer. Ann. of Surg. 1993, 218: 338-349

8. Ponten J., Holmberg L., Trichopoulos D.: Biology and natural history of breast cancer. Int. J. Cancer 1990, Supplement 5: 5-21

9. Atkinson E.N., Brown B.W., Montague E.D.: Tumor volume, nodal status and metastasis in breast cancer in women. JNCI 1986, 76: 171-178

10. Carter C.L., Allen C., Henson D.E.: Relation of tumor size, lymph node status, and survival in 24,740 breast cancer cases. Cancer 1989, 63: 181-187

11. Reger V., Beito G., Jolly Pc.: Factors affecting the incidence of lymph node metastases in small cancers of the breast. Am. J. Surg. 1989, 157: 501-502

12. Veronesi U., Cascinelli N., Greco M., *et al.*: Prognosis of breast cancer patients after mastectomy and dissection of internal mammary nodes. Ann. Surg. 1985, 202: 702-707

13. Menard S., Bufalino R., Rilke F., Cascinelli N., *et al.*: Prognosis based on primary breast carcinoma instead of pathological nodal status. Br. J. Cancer 1994, 70: 709-712

14. Yarnold J., Dixon J.M., Greco M.: Consensus document of staging for breast cancer. The Breast 1994, 3: 238-240

The importance of resection margins in conservative surgery

L. Cataliotti, V. Distante, S. Bianchi

Conservative surgery of breast cancer is now widely accepted for small size tumours. With the introduction of limited surgery, new problems have been created for both pathologists and surgeons.

From the oncological point of view one of the most important considerations is how much tissue should be removed to obtain a complete resection of the tumour without compromising the cosmetic results. Holland et al.[1] showed that by removing only one centimetre of apparently uninvolved tissue around the tumour, neoplastic foci are present in 59% of the cases. This percentage drops to 17% if the size of uninvolved tissue removed around the tumour is 3 cm. On the other hand, because conservative surgery is usually followed by radiation therapy which should control the possible presence of both multifocal and residual tumour, the surgical treatment does not need to be very radical; the excision of the tumour, without considering the possible presence of neoplastic foci in the residual breast, could be acceptable. Nevertheless several studies have demonstrated that patients with negative resection margins after conservative surgery have the lowest percentage of local recurrence.[2-5] Actually, although many years have passed since conservative surgery was introduced and the first randomized trials were done, it is still difficult to assess which type of surgery is most effective and to what extent positive resection margins affect the risk of local recurrence when conservative surgery is combined with radiation therapy. There are many reasons for this uncertainty such as type of surgery, technical difficulties of pathological assessment of margins, lack of a uniformly accepted definition of margin involvement and type of tumour growth.

Type of surgery

Tumourectomy is the removal of the tumour with free gross margins; wide excision is when the clear margins vary from 1 to 2 cm; quadrantectomy is the removal of a wide segment of tissue with skin and pectoral fascia. The true differences among these surgical treatments are however not clear-cut and often tumourectomy, as well as quadrantectomy, are reported as wide excision.

This is the reason why the results of several studies are difficult to interpret and the role of margin involvement in local control of the disease is not clear. Veronesi[6] found positive margins after tumourectomy in 16% of patients while this percentage rose to 47% in the report from Schnitt et al.[5] and to 57% in that of Schmidt-Ullrich.[7]

As stated by Fisher and Anderson[8] when cytological examination is positive, the surgeon must try to excise the tumour with negative margins. Re-excision is usually performed when the margins are positive, close to the tumour or unknown;[9] however residual tumour is found in 30 to 80% of cases[7,10] so when different experiences are compared, it is difficult to evaluate the role that certain factors have in the final results.

A clearer description of the surgical treatment would be useful for an accurate interpretation of the results. When the wide excision is more like a lump consisting of the tumour wrapped by a variably thick layer of parenchyma and/or fat, the orientation is undoubtedly more complex and the presence of markers is essential for a correct exchange of information between the surgeon and the pathologist. In this case the possible resection margins are six: superior, inferior, medial, lateral, anterior (skin) posterior (fascia) (Fig. 1). They are further identified according to the position of the cancer in the breast.

The excision of a radial specimen with the skin and the fascia reduces the real margins to four, two of which are fairly distant from the tumour and two of which are closer. Of the two distant margins the distal is rarely positive whereas the proximal, close to the nipple, sometimes may show a neoplastic intraductal

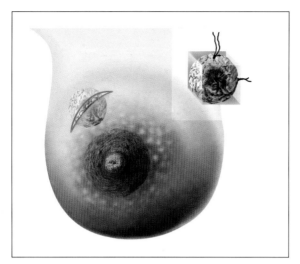

Fig. 1. When the wide excision is more like a lump the surgeon, must mark the anterior (skin), medial (nipple) and superior margins. Different coloured or different length stitches can be used.

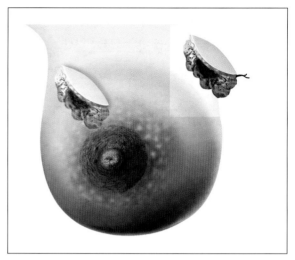

Fig. 2. In the radial excision the surgeon must mark only the margin close to the nipple to orientate the specimen.

growth. However, the two lateral margins remain those which are at greatest risk of neoplastic involvement.

In this type of operation it is easier for the pathologist to orientate the lump as it is a segment of tissue which rests on the fascia and is partially covered by the skin (Fig. 2).

Technical difficulties in margin evaluation

As stated previously, close co-operation between

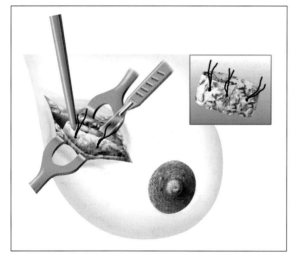

Fig. 3. If the surgeon has to widen the excision he must indicate the margin of the re-excision close to the tumour.

the surgeon and the pathologist is essential and the latter must have all the necessary information about clinical, mammographic and cytological findings and the site of the lesion in the breast. The intact specimen with suture-markers should be submitted to the pathologist; the surgeon should not cut the specimen. If the surgeon were to find it necessary to widen the excision, he must indicate the location of the new excision with respect to the previously removed specimen (Fig. 3). A good method is to design how the surgeon performed the operation and in what part of the excision he re-excised the margins.

Correct surgical practice implies that the pathologist should receive the specimen with information on whether there was a palpable or non-palpable tumour. If the lesion is non-palpable the specimen must be accompanied by an X-ray.

It should be remembered that it is more difficult to obtain a regular margin around the tumour during excision of non-palpable lesions and that it is important, if necessary, to re-excise immediately after the X-ray of the specimen is assessed[11] (Fig. 4).

On the contrary, the X-ray of the specimen in palpable lesions for the evaluation of margins is questionable.[12]

The current lack of surgical quality control makes it difficult to determine if the above mentioned guidelines have been followed, and therefore the interpretation of the data deriving from the evaluation of the margins reported in the literature is particularly uncertain.

In addition to the surgical problems and the management of the specimen, there is a technical problem

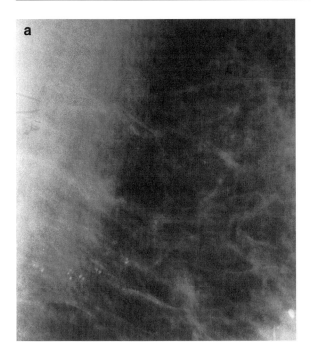

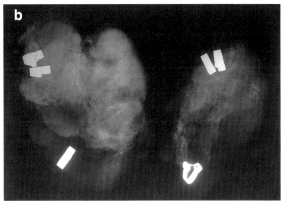

Fig. 4. **a.** Mammography shows suspect microcalcifications.
b. 1. The X-ray of the specimen,
with clock wise markers,
shows the microcalcifications
in the margin.
2.The X-ray of the re-excision specimen
shows the residual microcalcifications
with a wide clear margin.

which is exclusively histopathological. Until some years ago the pathological assessment of margins was not done routinely, as correctly mentioned by some authors,[5] and there was not, and perhaps there still is not, a uniform technique in the pathological assessment of margins.

There are many methods proposed to assess resection margins;[1,13] marking margins with Indian ink is widely used at present. This procedure, however, is not without difficulties as observed by Schnitt and Connolly.[14] Ink has the tendency to seep into defects of the irregular surface of the specimen, making it difficult to define the true surgical resection margins on microscopic examination. On the other hand, sampling errors may occur in all methods and, above all, there are no generally accepted guidelines for the sampling of margins and the methods for specimen sectioning. Also, the extent of sampling varies widely among different authors.

Fisher *et al.*[15] propose orientating the specimen with suture-markers and sectioning it in different planes to obtain a representative sampling of the tumour and various margins of resection (Fig. 5).

Another method, proposed by Carter,[16] involves inking the surface of the specimen, peeling off the margins in their entirety and embedding the inked surface for sectioning. Histologic sections are then cut parallel to the inked surface. The margin is considered positive if tumour is seen anywhere on the sections (Fig. 6).

Connolly and Schnitt[17] propose two different methods depending on the size of the excised speci-

men. For small specimens (3 cm or less in greatest diameter) the margin of excision is inked and the specimen is "bread loafed" into 3 to 4 mm sections. Tissue submitted for histologic examination includes the tumour with the surrounding grossly uninvolved breast tissue to demonstrate its relationship to the margins of excision (Fig. 7). For larger specimens (larger than 3 cm in greatest dimension) a single incision through the centre of the tumour is made, to assess the relationship between the lesion and the margins. Consequently, representative portions of the inferior, superior, anterior, posterior, medial and lateral margins are shaved from the specimen and embedded with the inked surface down (Fig. 8).

Veronesi *et al.*[18] have assessed the possibility of finding tumour cells in cell suspension by scraping the surface of the surgical resection margins. The sensitivity they observed with this method sometimes proved to be greater than at histological examination. Other authors[19] used cytological examination for margin assessment and concluded that this method can usefully complement the use of frozen section. With this method, 97.7% of accuracy has been found correlating histology and cytology.[20]

A controversial issue is the use of frozen section for margin assessment. Its aim is to reduce the number of re-excisions. Connolly and Schnitt[17] do not consider this method useful when gross examination is negative, due to the high number of errors; they carry it out only on specific request by the surgeons. On the other hand, when comparing results relating to frozen section and permanent histologic

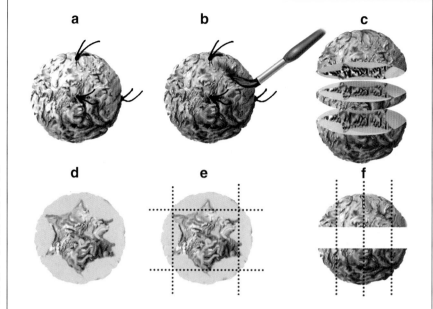

Fig. 5. **a**. Mark with stitches the superior, anterior, lateral or medial margins, to provide a proper orientation;
b. Coat surface of the specimen with Indian ink;
c-d. Section the specimen transversely to visualise the tumour.
e-f. Take blocks of margins and tumour both in transversal and sagittal sections.

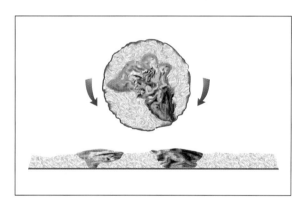

Fig. 6. The margin is peeled off and submitted for sectioning with the inked surface down.

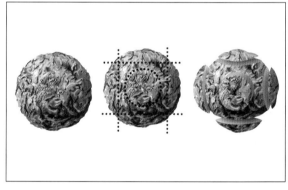

Fig. 8. For larger specimens, representative areas of margins are sampled and embedded with the inked surface down.

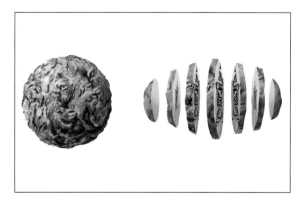

Fig. 7. In small excisions, after inking, the specimen it is cut at 3 to 4 mm intervals and the sections are embedded to demonstrate the relationship of the tumour to the margins.

sections, Cox et al.[19] observed 77% sensitivity and 100% specificity for frozen section. Sauter et al.[21] studied frozen section of re-excision margins and observed a sensitivity above 85% and 96% specificity. These authors are clearly in favour of frozen section for margin assessment (ideally 6: lateral, medial, superior, inferior, anterior, posterior) since this procedure made re-excision unnecessary in 32% of the cases.

Definition of margin involvement

The most important problem, however, is the lack of a generally accepted definition of how close the tumour should be to the surgical resection margins for them to be considered positive. This could indicate that the tumour is either present at the surface of the section or within an arbitrary distance from the surface itself.

In the absence of an objective definition, a margin should be considered positive when the tumour is present at the surface of the specimen; if not, it is important to give the exact distance between the tumour and the resection margin.

Schnitt et al.[5] consider margins positive when the tumour (in situ, invasive or both) is present at one or more margins (Fig. 9), close when the tumour is at a distance of 1 mm or less from the edge (Fig. 10) and negative when such distance is over a millimetre.

Patients with positive margins are further divided into two subgroups, focally positive (cancer present at the margins in three or fewer low-power microscopic fields using a 4 x objective) and more than focally positive (cancer present at the margins in more than three low-power fields).

We believe, however, that for each case other pathological parameters should also be taken into consideration in order to evaluate the margins accurately.

The situation is in fact more complex: first, the tumour may show a well circumscribed or an infiltrative pattern of growth; second, the possible presence of extensive involvement of peritumoural lymphatic vessels makes it impossible to establish the adequacy of the surgery even if the margins are clear.

On the other hand, the presence of tumour at the margins is not always indicative of residual tumour in the rest of the breast.[22]

In the experience of Frazier et al.,[23] mastectomy and margin re-excision after previous wide excision have shown residual tumour in 52.5% of cases if the margins were positive, in 32.1% if the tumour was close to the margin, and in 26.3% if the margins were negative.

Sauter et al.[21] carried out re-excision of margins when at first operation the margins were positive, close or unknown. They observed that in 33% of the cases the margins were positive or close to the tumour again but, above all, they found that this occurred more frequently when margins were unknown (42% vs 27%) at first operation.

Silverstein et al.[10] performed mastectomy or re-excision after biopsy for DCIS. They observed the presence of residual DCIS in 76% of the patients with positive margins and in 43% of the patients with negative margins. These data are important and confirm unreliability of margin investigation with reference to surgical radicality, even for cases with negative margins. This is also demonstrated by the results of NSABP B06 Trial[24] in which patients with negative margins, treated only with conservative surgery for invasive carcinoma, presented local recurrences in 40% of the cases.

Schnitt et al.[5] on the other hand, reported that negative margins reduce local recurrence in patients treated with radiotherapy. The percentage of local recurrence at 5 years was in fact 0% in patients with negative margins and 21% in those with margins more than focally positive. These authors also observed in these two groups a difference in the appearance of distant metastases – 14% and 32% respectively – even though in the group of patients with

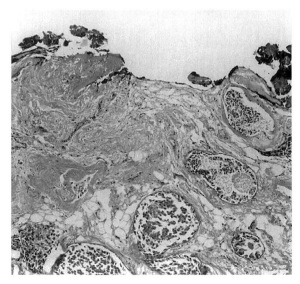

Fig. 9. In situ ductal carcinoma extending to inked margin of excision.

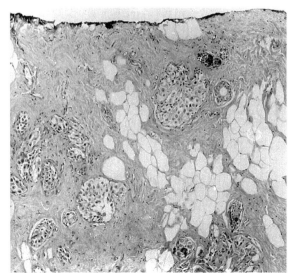

Fig. 10. Infiltrating ductal carcinoma in which tumour cells are at a distance less than 1 mm from inked margin of excision.

positive margins, the number of those with positive lymph nodes was higher. According to the Authors, margin involvement may reveal tumour with a more aggressive biological behaviour.

It seems clear at this point that despite all the described difficulties and limitations of pathological margin assessment, the surgeon's aim should be a surgical excision with clear margins.[4,6,8,25]

Type of tumour growth

Most breast cancers show an infiltrative pattern of growth which may be associated with the presence of extensive intraductal component (EIC). In these cases evaluation of margins may be particularly complex.

Less frequently, a tumour has a well defined growth pattern without EIC, which makes margin assessment easier. The presence of multifocality in the excised specimen, observed in 30% of cases,[26] contributes to making the work of the pathologist more difficult.

Gross examination of the margins during surgery can give preliminary information concerning the radicality of the excision.

Misinterpretations are frequent particularly in the case of invasive lobular carcinoma since tumour cells diffusely infiltrate the mammary stroma without forming lumps and sometimes only a change in consistency of the parenchyma can give rise to suspicion. Sauter et al.[21] reported a sensitivity value of 44% and a specificity value of 94% for gross examination of margins.

Risk factors of positive margins

Positive margins are only one of the risk factors of local recurrence though the majority of these factors are also responsible for involvement of margins. Some of them can be considered pre-operatively. In our experience, the age of the patient (< 40 vs > 40: 13.4% vs 7.6% p=0.03) and the tumour size (pT2 vs pT1; 11.5% vs 7.3% p=0.04), particularly if related to breast volume, influences the frequency of positive margins. Important elements are also the mammographic findings: the presence of microcalcifications with or without a mass is highly indicative of risk of insufficient excision with respect to other globally considered findings (12.9% vs 6.6% p=0.001); this observation is not confirmed by other authors.[4] Gluck et al.[27] advise post-operative mammography to evaluate the adequacy of the excision in patients whose tumours are associated with microcalcifications, especially in the presence of DCIS.

With regard to pathological data, the extensive intraductal component (EIC) and multifocality are the most important factors in predicting margin involvement and local recurrence.[28,29] These are, however, "a posteriori" elements which do not affect the initial surgical treatment. Schnitt et al.[5] found that 40% of patients with EIC had positive margins vs. 17% of those without EIC; 24.2% vs 3.3% (p=0.001) in our experience. The same authors observed that the presence or absence of EIC influences the local recurrence at 5 years as follows: 20% and 7% respectively. When EIC and positive margins are associated, the percentage increases to 50% but it is 0% when margins are negative.

According to Dixon[4] EIC and margin involvement are interrelated but have an independent significance in predicting local recurrence. Schnitt et al.[5] conclude that conservative therapy is advisable both when margins are negative, even if an EIC is present, and when margins are only focally positive in the absence of EIC. Re-excision or mastectomy are indicated when margins are more than focally positive or focally positive with EIC.

Their final consideration, which is agreed upon by most of the authors, is an answer to the question concerning the type of treatment which should be performed in the presence of margin involvement by tumour proliferation. In our experience, however, the indication for mastectomy in those cases with more than focally positive margins has proved to be unjustified in 25% of the cases where no residual tumour was found.

In conclusion:

- The aim of conservative surgery is to remove the tumour with clear margins.
- It seems to be a well-defined concept that a margin should be considered positive when the tumour is present at the edge of the specimen. Less clear is the definition in borderline cases even though what Schnitt et al.[5] proposed is particularly interesting and could lead to an universally accepted definition.
- Close co-operation is necessary between the surgeon and the pathologist and a standardised technique of margin assessment is mandatory; in spite of this, the risk of false negative margins is a real one.
- It is possible to find residual tumour foci in the breast although margins are negative, but radiotherapy has the task of further reducing the chance of local recurrence.
- The young age of the patient, the tumour size and particularly microcalcifications at mammography call for particular caution in performing conservative surgery as the risk of positive margins is particularly high.

- How much uninvolved tissue should be removed to reduce the percentage of recurrences is difficult to define but probably it should not be less than 15 mm.
- The presence of EIC and multifocality are two pathological elements of positive margin risk.
- Re-excision or mastectomy are indicated when margins are more than focally positive or focally positive with EIC.

References

1. Holland R., Velking S.H.J., Mravunac M., Hendricks J.H.C.L.: Histologic multifocality of TIS, T1-2 breast carcinomas: implications for clinical trials of breast conserving surgery. Cancer, 1985; 56: 979-990
2. Solin L., Fowble B., Schultz D., Goodman R.: The significance of the pathology margins of the tumor excision on the outcome of patients treated with definitive irradiation for early stage breast cancer. Int. J. Radiat. Oncol. Biol. Phys., 1991; 21: 279-287
3. Anscher M.S., Jones P., Prosnitz L.R., Blackstock W., Hebert M. et al.: Local failure and margin status in early-stage breast carcinoma treated with conservation surgery and radiation therapy. Ann. Surg., 1993; 218: 22-28
4. Dixon J.M.: Histological factors predicting breast recurrence following breast conserving therapy. Breast, 1993; 2: 197
5. Schnitt S.J., Abner A., Gelman R., Connolly J.L., Recht A. et al.: The relationship between microscopic margins of resection and the risk of local recurrence in patients with breast cancer treated with breast-conserving surgery and radiation therapy. Cancer, 1994; 74: 1746-1751
6. Veronesi U.: How important is the assessment of resection margins in conservative surgery for breast cancer. Cancer 1994; 74: 1660-1661
7. Schmidt-Ullrich R.K., Wazer D.E., Di Petrillo T., Marchant D.J. et al.: Breast conservation therapy for early stage breast carcinoma with outstanding 10-year locoregional control rates: a case for aggressive therapy to the tumor bearing quadrant. Int. J. Radiat. Oncol. Biol. Phys., 1993; 27: 545-552
8. Fisher B., Anderson S.: Conservative surgery for the management of invasive and non invasive carcinoma of the breast: NSABP trials. World J. Surg., 1994; 18: 63-69
9. Gwin J.L., Eisenberg B.L., Hoffman J.P., Ottery F.D., Boraas M., Solin L.J.: Incidence of gross and microscopic carcinoma in specimens from patients with breast cancer after re-excision lumpectomy. Ann. Surg., 1993; 218:729-734
10. Silverstein M.J., Gierson E.D., Colburn W.J., Cope L.M., Purmanski M. et al.: Can intraductal breast carcinoma be excised completely by local excision? Cancer, 1994; 73: 2985-2989
11. Dixon J.M., Ravi Sekar O., Walsh J., Paterson D., Anderson T.J.: Specimen-orientated radiography helps define excision margins of malignant lesions detected by breast screening. Br. J. Surg., 1993; 80: 1001-1002
12. Aitken R.A., Going J.J., Chetty U.: Assessment of surgical excision during breast conservation surgery by intra-operative two dimensional specimen radiology. Br. J. Surg., 1990; 77: 322-323
13. Anderson T.J.: Breast cancer screening: principles and practicalities for histopathologists. In: Recent advances in histopathology. Edinburgh, Churchill Livingstone, 1989; 14: 43-61
14. Schnitt S.J., Connolly J.L.: Processing and evaluation of breast excision specimens. A clinically oriented approach. Am. J. Clin. Pathol., 1992; 98: 125-137
15. Fisher E.R., Sass R., Fisher B., Gregorio R., Brown R. et al.: Pathologic findings from the National Surgical Adjuvant Breast Project (Protocol 6). II. Relation of local recurrence to multicentricity. Cancer, 1986; 57: 1717-1724
16. Carter D.: Margins of "lumpectomy" for breast cancer. Hum.Pathol., 1986; 17: 330-332
17. Connolly J.L., Schnitt S.J.: Evaluation of breast biopsy specimens in patients considered for treatment by conservative surgery and radiation therapy for early breast cancer. Path. Ann., 1988; 23: 1-23
18. Veronesi U., Farante G., Galimberti U., Greco M., Luini A. et al.: Evaluation of resection margins after breast conservative surgery with monoclonal antibodies. Eur. J. Surg. Oncol., 1991; 17: 338-341
19. Cox C.E., Ku N.N., Reintgen D.S., Greenberg H.M., Nicosia S.V. et al.: Touch preparation cytology of breast lumpectomy margins with histologic correlation. Arch. Surg., 1991; 126: 490-493
20. Ku N.N.K., Cox C.E., Reintgen D.S., Greenberg H.M., Nicosia S.V.: Cytology of lumpectomy specimens. Acta Cytol., 1991; 35: 417-421
21. Sauter E.R., Hoffman J.P., Ottery F.D., Kowalyshyn M.J. et al.: Is frozen section analysis of reexcision lumpectomy margins worthwhile? Cancer, 1994; 73: 2607-2612
22. Singer J.A.: Residual breast cancer at a distance from the primary tumor, Am. Surg., 1993; 59: 435-437
23. Frazier T.G., Wong R.W.Y., Rose D.: Implications of accurate pathologic margins in the treatment of primary breast cancer. Arch. Surg., 1989; 124: 37-38
24. Fisher E., Anderson S., Redmond C., Fisher B.: Ipsilateral breast tumor recurrence and survival following lumpectomy and irradiation: pathological findings from NSABP protocol B-06 Semin. Surg. Oncol. 1992; 8: 161-166
25. Sibbering D.M., Galea M.H., Morgan D.A.L. et al.: Safe criteria breast conservation without radical excision. Breast, 1993; 2:198
26. Dawson P.J.: What is new in our understanding of multifocal breast cancer? Path.Res.Pract., 1993; 189: 111-116
27. Gluck B.S., Dershaw D.D., Liberman L., Deutch B.M.: Microcalcifications on postoperative mammograms as an indicator of adequacy of tumor excision. Radiology, 1993; 188: 469-472
28. Holland R., Connolly J.L., Gelman R. et al.: The presence of an extensive intraductal component following a limited excision correlates with prominent residual disease in the remainder of the breast. J. Clin. Oncol., 1990; 8: 113-118
29. Campbell I.D., Theaker J.M., Royle G.T. et al.: Impact of an extensive in situ component on the presence of residual disease in screening detected breast cancer. J.R.Soc.Med. 1991; 84: 652-656

Adjuvant therapy of breast cancer

N. Davidson, A. Patel

Screening for breast cancer has led to an increase in the detection of early breast cancer with more cases being feasible for breast conservation surgery and adjuvant treatment with local radiotherapy and in selected cases additional systemic therapy. Here we shall endeavour to review the current consensus regarding adjuvant radiotherapy and adjuvant systemic therapy in the management of early breast cancer.

Local radiotherapy in breast conserving surgery

Screen detected invasive breast cancer is often amenable to breast conserving surgery followed by local radiotherapy. The recent overview of the randomised trials on the effects of radiotherapy and surgery in early breast cancer[1] studied nine trials of mastectomy versus breast conserving surgery and radiotherapy with no apparent difference in total mortality (22.9% vs 22.9%). Data on recurrence patterns was available in six of these studies and there was no significant difference between the two groups.

The recent re-analysis of the NSABP protocol B-16[2] in various cohorts comparing mastectomy with lumpectomy with or without radiotherapy found no significant difference in overall survival between the various cohorts and treatment groups. In addition, there was no significant difference in the disease free survival and distant disease free survival.

There was a significant difference in the incidence of ipsilateral breast tumour recurrence between the two conservative surgery arms of this trial. The cumulative incidence of ipsilateral breast tumour recurrence was 35% in the group treated by lumpectomy alone compared to 10% in those treated by lumpectomy and breast irradiation (p<0.001). In patients with node negative cancer, the cumulative incidence of ipsilateral breast tumour recurrence was

32% and 12% respectively (p<0.001) and in those with node positive cancer the cumulative incidence of ipsilateral breast tumour recurrence was 41% and 5% respectively (p<0.001). Both these recent publications have emphasised the value of radiotherapy in the treatment of early breast cancer.

Although the impact on survival of locally recurrent breast carcinomas after conservative therapy is unclear, such recurrence defeats the major goal of conservative surgery. In addition, local recurrence leading to a subsequent mastectomy after conservative management causes a severe psychological blow to the patient. Therefore it is essential that the possibility of local recurrence be minimised with careful attention to patient selection and treatment.

Radiotherapy technique

The radiation oncologist must optimize techniques and doses of radiotherapy in order to minimize the risk of local recurrence, achieve excellent cosmetic results and avoid both short and long term complications. The entire breast must be treated and the dose to the breast should be in the range of 4500cGys to 5000cGys given at 200cGys per day for 5 days each week. Shorter fractionation treatment regimes though more acceptable to the patient often carry greater long term complications. Doses higher than 5000cGys (delivered in daily treatments over 5 weeks) cause significant breast reaction and fibrosis. The need for a radiation boost to the primary site lies in the fact that many patients have microscopic residual cancer in the breast tissue surrounding the primary tumour[3] and most of the local recurrences are in the vicinity of the primary tumour.[4] However the morbidity of a boost of moderate size and dose is small. The boost dose is usually 1000cGys to 1500cGys, thus increasing the tumour bed dose to 6000 to 6500cGys. The boost can be given with either external beam radiotherapy (x-rays or electrons) or interstitial implantation.

The cosmetic results after treatment with conservative management and radiotherapy are important. Overall cosmetic results decline during the first three years after treatment and then remain stable. Several factors are associated with poor cosmetic outcome; large breast size, large tumour size, extensive surgical resection, large radiotherapy fractions, use of low energy radiation beams, use of iridium – 192 implant and chemotherapy given concurrently with radiation.[5,6]

The use of routine radiotherapy to regional lymph nodes is controversial. Axillary dissection yields information concerning the prognosis and the risk of involvement of the internal mammary and supra-clavicular regions. Axillary dissection also helps to define the role and type of adjuvant systemic therapy. Radiotherapy treatment to the breast alone after axillary dissection is acceptable in all cases. However it is reasonable to treat axillary, supra-clavicular fossa and/or internal mammary nodal areas in selected high risk patients. If axillary dissection has not been performed then it is reasonable to treat the axilla with radiotherapy.

The role of radiotherapy after mastectomy is controversial. The use of post-operative radiotherapy clearly decreases the risk of local or regional recurrence but it is not certain whether this will ultimately improve the survival rate. Multiple randomised prospective studies comparing patients treated with mastectomy only or with mastectomy and radiotherapy have not shown any significant survival advantage. However, these studies did not employ adjuvant systemic therapy. An advantage in disease-free survival and overall survival for patients who receive both radiotherapy and systemic treatment after mastectomy has been shown in more recent studies.[7,8] A possible explanation to those results which appear to contradict Fisher's theory is that poor local control of the disease might cancel the benefit of systemic treatment.[9] Therefore, at present it seems reasonable to use radiotherapy after mastectomy in patients who have a very high risk of local-regional failure, such as those with locally advanced disease.

Systemic adjuvant therapy

1985 NIH Consensus Conference[10]

This conference concluded that:
1. For pre-menopausal women with positive axillary nodes, regardless of hormone receptor status, treatment with combination chemotherapy should be standard care.
2. Tamoxifen should be the treatment of choice for

post-menopausal women with node positive receptor positive disease.
3. Chemotherapy could be considered for postmenopausal women with node positive receptor negative disease.
4. Adjuvant therapy was not generally recommended for node negative breast cancer, although its administration to certain high risk groups could be considered.

1990 NIH Consensus Conference[11]

This focused primarily on node negative breast cancer and concluded that:
1. Patients should be made aware of the risk of recurrence without adjuvant therapy, the expected reduction in risk with adjuvant therapy, toxic effects of therapy and their impact on quality of life as part of the decision-making process.
2. In view of the excellent prognosis of node negative patients with tumours less than, or equal to 1 cm, treatment was not recommended outside of clinical trials.
3. Adjuvant therapy should consist of either combination chemotherapy or tamoxifen 20 mg/day for two years.

Early Breast Cancer Trialists Collaborative Group overview[12,13]

In this study with a world-wide collaboration, information was sought and centrally checked on mortality and recurrence for each woman in any randomised study that began before 1985 of any aspect of systemic adjuvant therapy for breast cancer. Data was available for about 75,000 women in 133 trials involving 31,000 recurrences and 24,000 deaths.

This included 30,000 women in tamoxifen trials, 3,000 in ovarian ablation trials, 11,000 in polychemotherapy trials, 15,000 in other chemotherapy comparisons and 6,000 in immunotherapy trials.

Results of tamoxifen

The review showed that tamoxifen improved the survival at 10 years by 6.2% for patients of all ages on tamoxifen, compared to those not on tamoxifen (58.8% vs 52.6%). The recurrence free survival was also better by 6.6% in the tamoxifen group (51.2% vs 44.7%). The benefits in recurrence free survival were in the first 5 years and the gains were not significantly increased or decreased over the next 5 years.

The benefit in overall survival continued to accrue over 10 years. When data was analysed with respect to nodal status, the benefit of tamoxifen was seen in both groups but was greater in node positive patients.

When data was analysed by menopausal status and age, there was a difference between women under 50 and those over 50. Though the effect of Tamoxifen was much greater in those over 50 than in those under 50 years of age, it was significantly beneficial even in those under 50 years of age. Within the age groups, menopausal status did not influence outcome of disease. The directly randomised comparisons of different tamoxifen durations (2 vs 5 years or longer) show[14] that 5 years treatment is better than 2 years; however there seem to be no further benefit after 5 years. Additionally, tamoxifen reduced the risk of contralateral breast cancer by 39% and the risk of non-breast cancer death by 12%. Recently the benefit of tamoxifen in oestrogen negative tumours has been denied.[15]

Results of ovarian ablation

Ovarian ablation improved recurrence free survival (52.9% vs 42.3%) and overall survival (58.5% vs 48.3%) significantly at 15 years. The effect was significant in both node negative and node positive, but much greater in those with positive nodes. The effects of ovarian ablation seemed to be somewhat smaller in the presence than in the absence of cytotoxic chemotherapy, but this apparent interaction was not statistically significant and even in the presence of cytotoxic chemotherapy, ovarian ablation still significantly reduced both recurrence and mortality.

Results of chemotherapy

Adjuvant polychemotherapy in this study improved the recurrence free survival and overall survival at 10 years significantly (44.0% vs 35.6% and 51.3% vs 45.0%). The benefits in recurrence free survival were in the first five years and the gains were not significantly increased over the next 5 years. The benefit in overall survival continues to accrue over ten years. When data was analysed with respect to nodal status, the benefit of chemotherapy was seen in both groups but was greater in node positive patients. For recurrence free survival there is a statistically significant trend towards the effects of polychemotherapy being greater at younger than at older ages. For overall survival the general pattern resembles that for recurrence-free survival and the trend towards greater effect among younger women is again significant, though less than for recurrence free survival. Menopausal status did not influence outcome within the age groups. Polychemotherapy courses of

longer duration (mean 15 months) when compared with those over shorter duration (mean 6 months) were of no additional benefit. The update of this data in 1995 (unpublished) generally confirms all the previous views with no significant change in the absolute figures; it reiterates the 30% reduction in odds of local recurrence and 25% reduction in odds of death with adjuvant chemo-endocrine treatment.

1992 St. Gallen Conference[16]

The treatment recommendations of the 1992 St. Gallen conference for individuals who are not on clinical trials are summarized below:

Node negative

Minimal/low risk:
Patients with
1. non-invasive tumours;
2. small invasive tumours detected by mammography or by microscopic examination of tissue removed because of benign breast disease or because of *in situ* breast carcinoma and
3. tubular, colloid and papillary tumour types are included in this category.

For these patients observation without adjuvant therapy is the current recommendation.

Good risk:
Patients with
1. ER positive tumours larger than 1 cm, but less than or equal to 2 cm and low nuclear grade, are included in this category.

All women, irrespective of age and menopausal status, falling into this category, are treated with adjuvant tamoxifen only.

High risk:
Patients with
1. ER negative tumours larger than or equal to 1 cm
2. ER positive tumours larger than 2 cm and
3. nuclear grade 3 tumours are included in this category.

All patients in this category should receive some form of adjuvant therapy. In this category all premenopausal receptor negative patients receive adjuvant chemotherapy. Pre-menopausal receptor positive patients receive chemotherapy alone, or chemotherapy plus concurrent tamoxifen or chemotherapy followed sequentially by tamoxifen. In this node negative high risk category post-menopausal receptor positive patients receive tamoxifen. The addition of chemotherapy is a reasonable option for this subgroup of patients. For post-menopausal patients who are receptor negative, adjuvant chemotherapy is indicated as standard treatment.

Node positive

All patients with node positive breast cancer should receive some form of adjuvant therapy. For pre-menopausal node positive patients who are either hormone receptor positive or negative, adjuvant chemotherapy is the standard treatment. Tamoxifen can be added to receptor positive patients.

For post-menopausal node positive receptor positive patients, Tamoxifen is the standard treatment. There is increasing evidence of the added benefit of chemotherapy when given in addition to tamoxifen for this subgroup of patients. For post-menopausal node positive oestrogen receptor negative patients, the standard treatment is adjuvant chemotherapy.

Controversies

Pre-menopausal women

Adjuvant chemotherapy *versus* ovarian ablation

The findings of the Early Breast Cancer Trialists Collaborative Group overview has renewed interest in ovarian ablation.

The Scottish Cancer Trials Breast Group and the ICRF Breast Unit of Guy's Hospital,[17] randomised 332 pre-menopausal node positive women to either ovarian ablation or CMF for six months. Each regimen was given alone or combined with long term prednisolone therapy. After a median follow up of 5.9 years there were no statistically significant differences in the event free survival or overall survival in the two groups. When patient outcome was analysed in relation to the concentration of oestrogen receptor in the tumour, there was a statistically significant interaction, such that ovarian ablation was associated with improved survival in patients with ER concentration 20 fmols/mg protein or more and CMF was more beneficial for patients with values less than 20 fmols/mg protein. Further trials are required to appreciate the role of ovarian ablation in view of the findings of the Early Breast Cancer Trialists overview.

Adjuvant chemotherapy *vs* tamoxifen *vs* chemotherapy + tamoxifen

The findings of the Breast Cancer Trialists Collaborative overview,[12-13] showed the efficacy of Tamoxifen in pre-menopausal women, though not to as great an extent as in post-menopausal women. At the same time it showed that Tamoxifen does not add substantially to the benefits of chemotherapy in pre-menopausal women. This has prompted interest in randomised studies assessing the efficacy of Tamoxifen in pre-menopausal women either alone or in combination with chemotherapy.[18-20]

The Breast Cancer Adjuvant Chemo Hormone Therapy Co-operative Group,[18] randomised 504 node positives, ER positive women to chemotherapy or Tamoxifen or both. In pre-menopausal women, no significant difference among treatment was disclosed by univariate analysis, either in terms of disease free survival or overall survival. A trend close to significance was shown by multivariate analysis, favouring patients receiving combined treatment with chemotherapy and Tamoxifen in relation to relapse free survival. The results with Tamoxifen alone or chemotherapy alone were virtually identical.

The findings of the Gynaecological Adjuvant Breast Group,[19] were in contrast to this study. Two hundred and seventy-six low risk patients (one to three involved nodes ER or PR positive) were randomised after mastectomy to receive Tamoxifen 30mg/day orally for two years or CMF intravenously for six cycles. Overall, there was no statistically significant difference between the two groups. However, in the subset of 119 patients, less than or equal to 49 years of age, CMF was significantly superior to tamoxifen in regard to disease-free and overall survival. This same study also reported on 471 high risk patients (greater than or equal to four involved nodes) who were randomised to receive doxorubicin and cyclophosphamide alone or with tamoxifen. In the subset of 212 patients less than or equal to 49 years of age, addition of tamoxifen to chemotherapy did not improve results for disease free or overall survival.

The NSABP trial B-09,[20] which randomised 1,891 patients with primary operable breast cancer and positive axillary nodes to receive chemotherapy with or without tamoxifen, also failed to demonstrate any benefit in those less than or equal to 49 years of age. The benefit of combining chemotherapy and tamoxifen was almost restricted to those greater than or equal to 50 years and with greater than or equal to four nodes. Several other studies have shown that additions of chemotherapy to tamoxifen consistently resulted in superior treatment outcome compared with adjuvant tamoxifen alone in post menopausal women with ER positive tumours.[21-24] To account for the disparity in outcome among pre-menopausal and post-menopausal women following combination chemo-endocrine therapy, it is suggested that tamoxifen alters the metabolism of chemotherapeutic agents, reducing their effectiveness.[25]

In vitro studies,[26-27] have suggested that the cytotoxic effect of chemotherapeutic drugs is decreased by tamoxifen unfavourably altering tumour cell kinetics. The answer to this disparity lies in clinical trials comparing sequential and concurrent administration of chemotherapy and tamoxifen.

Post-menopausal Women

Tamoxifen *vs* tamoxifen + chemotherapy

The National Surgical Adjuvant Breast and Bowel Project B-16[21] compared adjuvant chemotherapy and Tamoxifen with tamoxifen alone in the treatment of node positive breast cancer patients aged 50 years and older with tamoxifen responsive tumours. This study of 1,124 eligible patients showed a distinct advantage for patients given chemotherapy and Tamoxifen compared to those given Tamoxifen alone. Disease free survival at 3 years was significantly better in the chemotherapy and tamoxifen group compared to tamoxifen alone.

There was no difference in the overall survival but a study period of 3 years is probably inadequate to ascertain the true impact of combination chemo-endocrine therapy. Other studies[22-24] have also shown better disease free survival in post-menopausal women, given combination chemotherapy and tamoxifen therapy compared to tamoxifen alone.

References

1. Early Breast Cancer Trialists Collaborative Group: Effects of Radiotherapy and Surgery in Early Breast Cancer - An Overview of the Randomised Trials. N. Eng. J. Med. 1995; 333: 1444-1455
2. Fisher B. Anderson S. Redmond C.K. *et al.*: Reanalysis and Results after 12 years of follow-up in a randomised clinical trial comparing total mastectomy with lumpectomy with or without irradiation in the treatment of breast cancer. N. Eng. J. Med., 1995; 333: 1456-1461
3. Holland R., Veling S.H.J., Mravunac M. *et al.*: Histologic multifocality of Tis, Tl-2 breast carcinomas: Implication for clinical trials of breast conserving treatment. Cancer, 1985; 56: 979-990
4. Recht A., Silen W., Schnett S.J. *et al.*: Time course of local recurrence following conservative surgery and radiotherapy for early stage breast cancer. Int. J. Radiat. Oncol. Biol. Phys.1988; 15: 255-261
5. Gore S.M., Come S.E., Criem K. *et al.*: Influence of sequencing of chemotherapy and radiation therapy in node negative breast cancer patients treated by conservative surgery and radiation therapy. In: Salmon S.E. (Ed.): *Adjuvant therapy of cancer.* Orlando, Grune and Stratton, 1987; 365-373
6. Abner A., Recht A., Vicini F. *et al.*: Cosmetic results after conservation surgery, chemotherapy and radiation therapy for early breast cancer.(abstr) Int. J. Radiat. Oncol. Biol. Phys. 1990; 19 (Suppl. 1): 174
7. Ragaz J., Jackson S.M., Plenderleith I.H. *et al.*: Adjuvant radiotherapy and chemotherapy in node positive premenopausal women with breast cancer. N. Eng. J. Med., 1997; 337: 956-962
8. Overgaard M., Hansen P.S., Overgaard J. *et al.*: Postoperative radiotherapy in high risk premenopausal women with breast cancer who receive adjuvant chemotherapy. N. Eng. J. Med., 1997; 337: 949-955
9. Querci della Rovere G., Daniels I.R.: Local treatment for breast cancer. The breast, 1998; 7: in press
10. Consensus Conference: Adjuvant chemotherapy for breast cancer. JAMA, 1985; 254: 3461-3463
11. NIH Consensus Conference: Treatment of early stage breast cancer. JAMA 1991; 265: 391-395
12. Early Breast Cancer Trialists Collaborative Group: Systemic Treatment of early breast cancer by hormonal, cytotoxic or immune therapy: 133 randomised trials involving 31,000 recurrences and 24,000 deaths among 75,000 women. Lancet, 1992; 339: 1-15
13. Early Breast Cancer Trialists Collaborative Group: Systemic Treatment of early breast cancer by hormonal, cytotoxic or immune therapy: 133 randomised trials involving 31,000 recurrences and 24,000 deaths among 75,000 women. Lancet, 1992; 339: 72-85
14. Fisher B., Dingam J., Brian J. *et al.*: Five versus more than five years of Tamoxifen therapy for breast cancer patients with negative lymph nodes and estrogen receptor positive tumours. J. Nat. Canc. Inst. 1996; 88: 1529-1541
15. Early breast cancer trialist collaborative group. Tamoxifen for early breast cancer: an overview of the randomised trials. Lancet, 1998; 351: 1451-1467
16. Glick J.H., Gelber R.D., Goldhirsch A., Senn H-J.: Adjuvant therapy of primary breast cancer: closing summary. Rec. Res. in Cancer Res., 1993; 127: 289-300
17. Scottish Cancer Trials Breast Group, ICRF: Breast unit of Guy's Hospital, London. Adjuvant ovarian ablation versus CMF chemotherapy in premenopausal women with pathological stage II breast carcinoma: The Scottish trial. Lancet, 1993; 341: 1293-1298
18. Boccardo F., Rubagotti A., Bruzzi P. *et al.*: for the Breast Cancer Adjuvant ChemoHormone Therapy Co-operative Group: Chemotherapy vs Tamoxifen vs Chemotherapy plus Tamoxifen in node positive, estrogen receptor positive breast cancer patients. Results of a multicentre Italian study. J. Clin. Oncol., 1990; 8: 1310-1320
19. Kaufmann M., Jonat W., Abel U., *et al.*: Adjuvant randomised trials of doxorubicinl cyclophosphamide *versus* doxorubicin/ cyclophosphamide/tamoxifen and CMF chemotherapy *versus* tamoxifen in women with node positive breast cancer. J. Clin. Oncol., 1993; 11: 454-460
20. Fisher B., Redmond C., Brown A., *et al.*: Adjuvant chemotherapy with and without Tamoxifen in the treatment of primary breast cancer: 5 year results from the National Surgical Adjuvant Breast and Bowel Project Trial. J. Clin. Oncol., 1986; 4: 459-471
21. Fisher B., Redmond C., Legault-Poisson S., *et al.*: Post-operative chemotherapy and Tamoxifen compared with Tamoxifen alone in the treatment of positive node breast cancer patients with aged 50 years and older with tumours responsive to Tamoxifen: Results from the National Surgical Adjuvant Breast and Bowel Project B-16. J. Clin. Oncol., 1990; 8: 1005-1018
22. Pearson O.H., Hubay C.A., Gordon N.H.: Endocrine versus endocrine plus five drug chemotherapy in postmenopausal women with stage II oestrogen receptor positive breast cancer. Cancer, 1989; 64: 1819-1823
23. Goldhirsch A., Gelber R.D.: Adjuvant chemoendocrine therapy or endocrine therapy alone for postmenopausal patient: Ludwig studies III and IV. In: Senn H., Goldhirsch A., Gelber R.D., Osterwalder B. (Eds.): *Recent Results in Cancer Research - Adjuvant Therapy of Primary Breast Cancer*, Berlin, Springer-Verlag, 1989; pp. 153-162
24. Early Breast Cancer Trialists Collaborative Group. Effects of adjuvant Tamoxifen and of Cytotoxic Therapy on Mortality in Early Breast Cancer. N. Eng. J. Med., 1988; 319: 1681-1692
25. Fisher B., Redmond C., Brown A., et al.: Influence of tumour oestrogen and progesterone receptor levels on the response to Tamoxifen and chemotherapy in primary breast cancer. J. Clin. Oncol., 1993; 1: 227-241
26. Osborne C.K, Kitten L., Arteaja C.L.: Antagonism by chemotherapy induced cytotoxically for human breast cancer cells by antiestrogens. J. Clin. Oncol., 1989; 7: 710-717
27. Hug V., Hortobagyi G.N., Drewinko B., Finders M.: Tamoxifen citrate counteracts the anti-tumour effects of cytotoxic drugs in vitro. J. Clin. Oncol., 1985; 3: 1672-1677

Local recurrence after breast conservation

M.W. Kissin

Introduction

The primary goal for the National Health Service Breast Screening Project in the United Kingdom (NHSBSP) is a 25% reduction in mortality by the year 2000. The principle method for achieving this target is the development of integrated breast teams capable of expert diagnosis and treatment. High rates of cancer detection will only be translated into improved cure rates if treatment plans adhere to optimum therapeutic guidelines. Treatment to obtain cure is based on a need to achieve local and systemic control. A recent report from the Early Breast Cancer Trialists Collaborative Group (EBCTCG) has concentrated on the effects of radiotherapy and surgery on mortality and recurrence.[1]

This overview of 58 randomised trials concludes that the extent of surgery and the use of radiotherapy has no adverse influence on a ten year survival. In other words, breast conserving surgery with or without radiotherapy is equivalent to mastectomy with or without radiotherapy.

In contrast, however, radiotherapy produced a highly significant three fold reduction in the local recurrence rate from 19.6% to 6.7%. Women with screen detected cancer are more likely to have small impalpable tumours compared to symptomatic patients and are, therefore, often good candidates for breast preservation.

Indeed, their own perception is often that early detection must logically translate into less aggressive treatment. Not only do they seek to avoid mastectomy (for cultural reasons) but also radiotherapy (adverse media attention), seeing both such avoidances as the tangible perk for attending for screening. For these several reasons, the psychological side effects of local recurrence in the retained breast may be more devastating to the screened group of patients who may well have impalpable disease compared to their symptomatic counterparts.

In this chapter, I will discuss the mechanisms contributing to local recurrence, its detection, prevention and treatment and an assessment of the cost within the framework of the NHSBSP. The conservation trials from the NSABP and Milan, and breast preserving protocols from Nottingham will be discussed in detail together with case histories of patients who have suffered from local recurrence.

Pathogenesis of local recurrence (LR)

The precise cause of local recurrence remains a perplexing oncological problem. The traditional concept is that local recurrence represents a failure of technique rather than of biology. The ipsilateral breast tumour recurrence rate (IBTR) after breast conservation seems to correlate with the extent of excision and the use of radiotherapy. Nonetheless, the majority of patients treated by lumpectomy alone do not suffer from IBTR. Thus even in the by now infamous NSABP B-06 Trial, the IBTR 12 years after lumpectomy alone is only 35%. In other words, 65% remained free of further breast disease.[2]

Same quadrant local recurrence

Residual disease

This may be related to inadequate resection of the primary or its surrounding multifocal disease. This is true for both invasive and non-invasive components. Same quadrant LR occurs relatively early. In the B-06 Trial, Fisher found that the rate of IBTR was always highest in the first three years irrespective of therapy.[3] The overall rate in the trial with lumpectomy alone is roughly equivalent to the extent of residual disease found within 2 cm of the resection margin in the bench studies of Holland *et al.*, which lie at around 20-40%.[4] This figure also correlates with the incidence of further tumour detected close to the surgical cavity by multiple tumour bed biopsies.[5]

Scar phenomenon

Another factor contributing to IBTR relates to the breast scar itself. Local recurrence may be related to the direct consequences of interference with the tumour micro-environment. Reid et al. have recently reviewed the role of cytokines and growth factors in promoting local recurrence after breast conservation.[6] Breast-conserving surgery may liberate tumour cells into the excision cavity or disseminate tumour cells into the blood stream. Blood-borne cancer cells may again lodge in the site of the scar within the breast due to scar neovascularisation. Experimental studies suggest that persisting cancer cells are more likely to develop into locally clinical evident disease if stimulated by the release of growth factors and cytokines into the healing wound. It is possible that clinical examination, mammography, cytology and core biopsy techniques all could liberate cells from the primary into the tumour micro-environment and lymphovenous support system. This mechanism gives notional credence to the popular conception that surgery could make the situation worse. Peri-operative strategies to neutralise tumour cell and growth factor interaction should help maximise local control and prevent this scar phenomenon.

Other quadrant local recurrence

This is less common and occurs later than other types of ipsilateral breast recurrence. It accounts for less than 20% of all cases of local recurrence and represents the development of a new primary in a breast at risk. It can be defined as cancer occurring in the treated breast more than 2 cm away from the scar.

Risk factors for local recurrence

Variations in the reported local recurrence rates after beast conservation are related to several clinical and histological factors. These include the completeness of excision, the presence of extensive intraduct disease, lymphovenous invasion, tumour type, grade, size, young age and adjuvant therapy.

Involved margins

The majority of studies of breast conservation therapy have looked at the relationship between the presence of tumour margins and local recurrence. Five out of 13 trials report a strong statistical association with the relative risk of 3 to 5. A further 5 show an excess risk with positive margins ranging from 1.5 to 3. Three studies failed to show an association between margins and local recurrence, and in each of these cases higher doses of radiotherapy were given which may account for the lack of effect. In order to avoid a breast-preserving procedure with a positive margin, the surgeon should aim to remove a minimum of 1 cm of macroscopically normal breast around the cancer.

This should be confirmed by biplanar intra-operative specimen radiography for all cases both palpable and impalpable. Where the radiological appearances show tumour encroaching close to a margin further tissue could then be taken at that same operation. At the pathological assessment, 5 mm of clear tissue around a tumour is a minimum acceptable distance for safe breast conservation. Even then there may be a high incidence of tumour in the vicinity of the tumour bed. MacMillan et al. found 38% of 264 patients having breast-conserving surgery had residual tumour in their cavity shavings and bed biopsies.[5] In their series half of these contained invasive disease. In contrast Rubin et al. reported 9% tumour bed positivity in a series of 135 but three quarters of these had non-invasive change.[7]

Extensive intraduct component (EIC)

EIC is defined as a tumour with more than 25% intraduct component associated within the invasive component and also with DCIS in the surrounding otherwise normal breast. Local recurrence rates as high as 21% are found when EIC is present compared to 6% if EIC negative. The majority of trials have found EIC to be a significant risk factor. Holland's data showed not only the EIC positive tumours had a greater incidence of tumour in the surrounding breast but also that this was predominantly further DCIS rather than more invasive cancer.[4] The significance of EIC is that attempted breast conservation for these cases may leave further DCIS present in the surrounding tumour bed and radiotherapy may not be able to prevent its subsequent growth and progression to invasive transformation. The relative risk of local recurrence after removal of an EIC positive tumour is 3 to 5 times.

Vascular invasion (VI)

Vascular or lymphatic infiltration is associated with an increase risk of local recurrence of 1.8 to three times. The relevance of vascular invasion has only been appreciated recently and has been generally under-reported. It now forms part of the standard pathological data-set.

The importance of vascular invasion was brought to the fore by the Nottingham group who found it to be the most significant factor contributing to their high local recurrence rate of 21% out of 263 patients treated by lumpectomy and radiotherapy.[8] Vascular invasion is thought to be particularly important as far as local recurrences within the first three years is concerned.

Tumour type and grade

It was initially thought that infiltrating lobular cancer was itself a risk factor for local recurrence due to its multicentric tendency. Studies have now shown that local recurrence rates with lobular cancer are comparable to ductal cancer and the finding of lobular cancer should no longer be regarded as a contra-indication for breast preservation. The importance of grade is variable from trial to trial but it seems that grade 1 cancers have a slightly lower recurrence rate than grades 2 and 3.

Size

Local recurrence rates also appear to be related to the size of the primary. The recurrence rates in the control group of the NSABP B-06 Trial is considerably higher than that in the corresponding group of the Milan Trial. This could be explained by the fact that the former allowed breast conservation for cancers up to 4 cm in size compared to 2.5 cm in size for the latter trial. The size issue also interrelates strongly with the cosmetic outcome.

Age

Young age has also generally been found to correlate with an increased risk of local recurrence particularly for patients younger than thirty-five years. However, young age has been reported to be associated with multicentricity, multifocality, vascular invasion, EIC and high grade and, therefore, it may not be an independent risk factor. Nonetheless, as local recurrence tends to be a steady phenomenon with an eventual risk of 1% per annum, younger patients should be advised very carefully about breast conserving therapy as they have more years at risk from both local recurrence and the treatments used to prevent local recurrence.[9]

Adjuvant therapy

Most patients having breast conservation will also be receiving adjuvant chemotherapy and or tamoxifen. Clarke and Martinez report a reduction of the local recurrence rate from 17% to 5% in pre-menopausal patients receiving adjuvant chemotherapy.[10] Similar findings in the B-06 trial showed a reduction of local recurrence in node positive patients from 4% compared to node negative (9%). There may, therefore, be a synergistic effect of radiotherapy and chemotherapy on the local control rate. Results from a Scottish trial of conservation plus optimum adjuvant strategy versus the same treatment plus the addition of radiotherapy show that radiotherapy still had an important role to play in reducing local recurrence even in the face of optimum adjuvant strategy.[11] Here the local recurrence rate was reduced from 28% to 5% and this demonstrates that adjuvant systemic therapy alone is no replacement for adequate radiotherapy.

Incidence and significance

In order to determine the incidence of local recurrence after breast conservation and to ponder on its significance, four treatment protocols are considered in detail. The first is the NSABP B-06 randomised control trial from America. The second are the Milan randomised control trials. The third consists of observational studies of a policy of breast conservation in Nottingham. Finally there is consideration of local recurrence after DCIS in the NSABP B-17 trial and other considerations specific to DCIS.

NSABP B-06

This hallmark multicentre collaborative randomised trial recruited patients from 1976 to 1984. Just under 2000 women from 89 centres were randomised either to have mastectomy, a lumpectomy, or lumpectomy and radiotherapy. The major findings were reported initially in 1985 and then subsequently in 1989 and 1995.[2,3,12] The overall findings have remained remarkably consistent with time. There appears to be no difference in the overall survival and distant disease free survival between the three different treatment arms. At 8 years follow-up, overall survival was running at 71% for all groups and at 12 years was 62% for all groups. Similarly, distant disease free survival at 8 years was approximately 63%, and at 12 years 50%. There was however, a significant difference in the local recurrence rate in patients having breast conservation who were treated with or without radiotherapy. At 8 years the local recurrence after the use of radiotherapy was 10% and that has remained stable out to 12 years. At 8 years in patients treated without radiotherapy the local recurrence rate was running at 39% falling to 35% at 12 years due to competing influences. These differences are highly significant. The overall message of this trial is clear. Breast-conserving surgery and mastectomy have equivalent overall survival results and breast-conserving surgery plus radiotherapy reduces the likelihood of local recurrence. However the subsidiary conclusion is that local recurrence after breast conservation without radiotherapy does not have any detrimental effect on overall survival.

Fisher et al.[3] have pondered the meaning of these findings. They concluded that local recurrence is a marker of future distant recurrence. In other words, those patients who have got local recurrence after breast preservation without radiotherapy were those patients who were also destined to get distant failure as well. The use of radiotherapy in these patients prevents the manifestation of the local recurrence at a time when distant recurrence is starting to develop. Thus in their trial, IBTR is a risk factor for distant recurrence with a relative risk of 3.4 times.

The use of adjuvant chemotherapy for lymph node positive patients in this trial also enabled observations to be made regarding the local recurrence rate with or without chemotherapy. At the 12 year analysis in the lumpectomy and radiotherapy group of patients, the overall local recurrence rate was 10%, but in node negative patients it was 12% and in node positive patients it was only 5%. Opposite differences were found in patients treated by breast preservation alone. Here the overall local recurrence rate of 12 years was 35% with a 32% rate in node negative patients and a 41% rate in node positive patients. These figures suggest that local irradiation has a synergistic effect with chemotherapy on the prevalence of local recurrence.

Several excellent points have come out from these studies. There is long follow up and there are important observations on the role of adjuvant therapy. It must be borne in mind that the patient cohort was for patients with tumours up to 4 cm in diameter. There have however been several problems associated with interpretations of the data from this trial. First of all, one questions the quality control that can be exercised in such a study where up to 90 different centres were randomising patients. Concerns about the data quality have surfaced recently from one of the Montreal contributors (322 cases) where some local data manipulations seem to have occurred. Re-analysis excluding these patients has not altered the overall findings. There is also the problem that if patients randomised to have breast conservation had

positive margins, they then went on to have a mastectomy but were analysed as if they had breast conservation. It must be remembered that at the time that this trial was devised, there was no data to suggest that the safety margin of resection was a crucial factor in the development of local recurrence. Nonetheless the high incidence of local recurrence in this trial must be matched up with the surgical procedure which was of lumpectomy rather than of wide local excision with meticulous attention to margin details.

Milan Trials of Conservation

Under the guidance of Umberto Veronesi, a series of methodical trials has been carried out in Milan, testing various aspects of breast-preserving procedures. In the first trial, a Halsted radical mastectomy was compared to a breast quadrantectomy plus radiotherapy. After 18 years of follow up there was no significant difference in overall survival, and there was only a 3% local recurrence rate after the breast-preserving procedure (QUART) compared to a 1% local recurrence after radical mastectomy. With these findings the question that was posed was, is this excellent series of results due to the wide margins of safety involved in resecting a quadrant of breast rather than lumpectomy, or is it due to the addition of radiotherapy? This led to the second Milan trial where QUART was compared to local excision plus radiotherapy (TART).

This was for tumours up to 2.5 cm in maximum dimension. After 6 years of follow up there was no difference in overall survival, but there was increased local recurrence after TART which was approximately twice the frequency than after QUART. The cosmetic result was slightly better after TART, but local control was obviously inferior. In the third Milan trial, QUART has been compared to the same surgical procedure without radiotherapy (QUAD). In this protocol radiotherapy was given for local recurrence in the group of patients who had not been randomised to receive it initially. The 3-year findings in this trial were again of no significant difference in overall survival, but increased local recurrence after QUAD. Thus it seems radiotherapy protects against local recurrence especially in younger groups of patients.

The overall recommendation from Milan is that quadrantectomy plus radiotherapy is a satisfactory treatment for the pre-menopausal patients to balance reasonable cosmesis with a low risk of local recurrence. For the post-menopausal patient a quadrantectomy alone may be sufficient. A fourth Milan Trial is looking at the role of neo-adjuvant chemotherapy as part of the strategy to decrease the local recurrence rate (C-TART). Shrinkage of the primary tumour may allow a much more cosmetic procedure to be performed, and also decrease the need for radiotherapy as well.

Within the third Milan Trial after 39 months of median follow up Veronesi reported a local recurrence rate of 8.8% after surgery alone, *versus* 0.3% after surgery and radiotherapy. Wherever possible local recurrence was treated by a further breast conserving procedure plus radiotherapy.[13]

In 1995 the Milan group reported on more than 2200 QUART procedures.[14] The follow up was 8.5 years and there was a total of 119 true local recurrences as the first event, and 32 recurrences of a new primary in the ipsilateral breast distant to the original scar. This compares with a total of 110 contralateral cancers during the same period of follow up. The rate of local recurrence was approximately 1% per annum. The risk of local recurrence was related to young age under 45 years of age, and size of tumour more than 20 mm.

It was also decreased if adjuvant therapy was given because of node positivity. As in many other series local recurrence was also related to extensive intraduct component. They also found that in patients suffering from local recurrence, there was an increased risk of distant recurrence, especially if the local recurrence had occurred early during the follow up. They concluded that the relationship between local recurrence and distant recurrence is complex and that the prognostic factors governing its occurrence and significance may be different from those of the primary tumour. The 5 year survival with patients with local recurrence was 70%.

The question remains why the local recurrence rate in this series of patients is so different from that of the NSABP studies. The main difference between the two groups of patients is that in the American series tumours up to 4 cm were investigated, whereas in Milan it was up to 2.5 cm. Furthermore the margins of safety around a quadrantectomy surgical procedure are far in excess compared to those after lumpectomy. Finally the quality of data and surgical technique is far more likely to be strict in a study from a single institution.

Taken together the studies of NSABP and Milan demonstrate that local recurrence is a marker for distant failure and also that inadequate local therapy will lead to a higher rate of local recurrence. The overall local recurrence rate of 5% in QUART procedures has to be taken as the gold standard for everyday practice. Whilst a quadrant resection of the breast may lead to an inferior cosmetic result, the way around this may be to take out a mirror image amount of tissue from the contralateral breast so that symmetry can be achieved.

Studies from Nottingham

Between 1979 and 1986, 263 patients were given breast-conserving therapy in Nottingham.[8] Tumours up to 5 cm were included and no systemic therapy was given. The surgery consisted of macroscopic excision and is therefore equivalent to a NSABP style lumpectomy. Surgery was followed by radiotherapy. When patients were followed up to median follow up period of 3 years, a high local recurrence rate of 21% was observed. 33 out 56 cases had local recurrence alone and 18 out of 56 had uncontrolled local recurrence, many of these cases appearing within the first year. Patients suffering from diffuse uncontrolled local recurrence without distant disease were often salvaged by a mastectomy but they had a significant reduction in the quality of their life with increased amounts of anxiety and depression solely because of the development of their local recurrence. Further analysis of this study showed that there were several independent factors that were predictors of local recurrence. These were vascular invasion, tumour size, age, and lymph node stage. Grade and the extent of DCIS were not independent significant factors. Interestingly the completeness of resection margin did not come out as a significant prognostic marker of local recurrence, but this was probably due to the fact that the margin status was often not recorded. The overall findings here were very much in keeping with the NSABP group. The level of local recurrence was deemed to be unacceptable and therefore a change of policy was initiated. The upper limit for breast conservation was changed to 3 cm, a safety margin of 5 mm of clear tissue around the tumour was deemed necessary and a resection of the cavity margin performed if appropriate. If there was vascular invasion and the patient was under the age of 50, breast conservation was not advised for tumours of greater than 1 cm.

Between 1988 and 1992, 275 women had breast conservation satisfying these new criteria. This was again followed by radiotherapy. Only 3.3% developed local recurrence with a median follow up of 4 years. Furthermore, there have been no cases of uncontrolled local recurrence. These figures are much more in keeping with the Milan series of QUART, and have demonstrated that a change in policy in Nottingham has been successful in reducing the local recurrence rate.[15]

Local recurrence after breast-conserving surgery for DCIS

With the emergence of large numbers of patients with localised DCIS found through the breast screening project, there is an urgent need to know what is their optimum therapy. Many patients previously presenting with DCIS would have been treated very successfully by mastectomy but it is thought that such ablative surgery is not necessary for many patients with biologically non-aggressive disease. Several trials are underway both in the United Kingdom, other European Countries and America to try and determine whether surgery alone, surgery plus radiotherapy, or surgery plus radiotherapy and Tamoxifen represents the optimum treatment to keep the breast free of further disease. The only trial to have reported results so far is the NSABP B-17 trial from America. 790 patients have been randomised to receive surgery alone (lumpectomy), or surgery plus radiotherapy.[16] Patients were accrued from 1985 to 1990 and only 573 of the original cohort were deemed to be suitable for further study as in many of the others the pathological diagnosis of DCIS was not fully satisfied. After 7 years median follow up, 14% of patients treated by surgery alone have developed further tumour in the same breast. This compares to only 5% in those patients treated by surgery and radiotherapy. The number of patients with DCIS alone in their recurrent tumour was reduced from 26 to 11 by the addition of radiation, and those with invasive disease from 12 to 4. Only two histological features were predictive for local recurrence, and these were the presence of comedo necrosis and uncertain or involved lumpectomy margin.

Whilst this study provides interesting information regarding the risk of local recurrence after treatment of DCIS, it suffers from the same disadvantages of the NSABP B-06 trial for invasive disease. This relates to not enough attention being paid to safety margins around tumour resection. Unfortunately there are similar deficiencies in the studies of DCIS set up within the screening project in the United Kingdom. The Nottingham group have impressive results in their policy of managing DCIS outside the confines of the national DCIS trial.

Their policy includes a mandatory 1 cm clear margin around a DCIS excision, and using this policy they have had no local recurrences at all in a group of 90 patients followed for a minimum of 3 years (personal communication). Local recurrence after the management of DCIS will become an increasing problem and many of the characteristics are similar to those already observed with the occurrence of local disease after the treatment of invasive breast cancer. Unfortunately, many surgeons will regard DCIS as a more innocent disease than invasive cancer. However, the principles of local control by the attention to surgical technique and the judicious and selective use of radiotherapy are just as important as in invasive disease.

Case histories

Case 1 - Same quadrant IBTR after breast conservation and radiotherapy

A 64-year-old woman attended for her first NHS BSP invitation in September 1993. She was found to have an impalpable area of high risk microcalcification. Stereotactic fine needle aspiration biopsy (FNAB) showed grade 2 cancer cells. An ultrasound was normal. Wide local excision procedure (85 gm) and axillary dissection was performed as she wished to avoid mastectomy. The histology showed a 10 mm infiltrating duct cancer grade 2 associated with 32 mm of comedo DCIS extending for 15 mm beyond the invasive component. A cavity biopsy was negative, as were 9 lymph nodes. She was given post-operative radiotherapy to the breast and Tamoxifen 20 mgms daily. At a routine follow up appointment in April 1995 (disease free interval DFI = 19 months), impalpable local recurrence was detected by mammography (Figs 1 and 2). Stereotactic FNAB was positive for grade 2 cancer cells. 1500 gms of tissue were removed by mastectomy and revealed a 9 mm infiltrating duct cancer grade 2 without DCIS. Following surgery, Tamoxifen was switched to Megace 160 mgms daily.

This case represents same quadrant IBTR after standard breast-conserving therapy. It was probably related to residual multifocal breast cancer as predicted by the extensive intraduct component of the primary. The patient remains well 1 year after salvage mastectomy.

Case 2 - Multifocal local recurrence 10 years after breast conservation and radiotherapy

A 55-year-old woman attended for routine mammographic surveillance as part of the NHSBSP. A 1 cm spiculated mammographic lesion was found and this was new compared to previous follow up films (Fig 3). The lesion was impalpable and stereotactic FNAB was positive for grade 1 cancer cells. 11 years earlier in 1983 the patient had presented with a 4 cm lump in the same breast and this had been treated by wide local excision, axillary dissection, Tamoxifen, and radiotherapy. Due to Tamoxifen intolerance an oophorectomy was performed one year later. At the time of original presentation there had been 2 positive nodes and

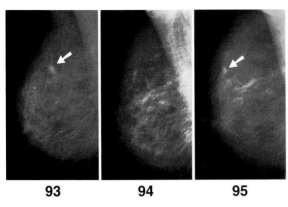

Fig. 1. Case 1. 45-degree oblique films from 1993, 1994 and 1995. Original cancer (arrowed) was a density associated with microcalcification (which doesn't project).
In 1995 the lesion (arrowed), absent in 1994, returned at the same site as the primary.

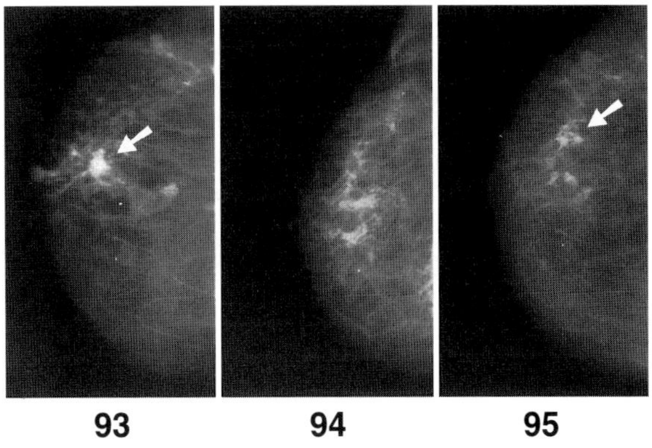

Fig. 2. Case 1. Cranio-caudal films from 1993, 1994 and 1995. Original cancer (arrowed) was a density associated with microcalcification (which doesn't project). In 1995 the lesion (arrowed), absent in 1994, returned at the same site as the primary.

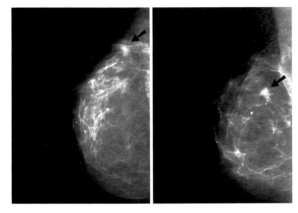

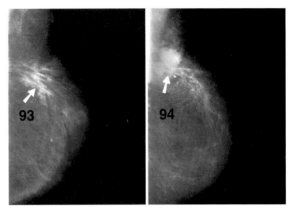

Fig. 3. Case 2. Two views of 1994 mammograms showing a spiculated density (arrowed) containing local recurrence 11 years after breast conservation and radiotherapy. The tumour lies close to surgical scarring. A separate tumour was found close to the nipple.

Fig. 4. Case 3. 45-degree oblique films from 1993 and 1994 showing tumour recurrence (arrowed) at site of previous scar (arrowed) from breast-conserving surgery and radiotherapy in 1986. In 1992 a contralateral tumour was treated.

the tumour was ER positive. After 10 years of routine follow up the patient had been discharged. At the time of her local recurrence in 1994, she was recommended to have a mastectomy. This revealed the presence of a 13 mm infiltrating lobular cancer, and LCIS close to the scar of her original operation and representing same quadrant local recurrence. In addition a separate 6 mm focus of infiltrating duct cancer was found underneath the nipple. Subsequent to mastectomy no further adjuvant strategy was used and the patient is well 2 years later.

This case represents a true second primary within the breast as well as same quadrant local recurrence. A disease free interval was 11 years which is characteristic of a new primary within the retained breast,

and in this patient there was also field change despite adjuvant radiotherapy.

Case 3 - Scar phenomenon local recurrence after breast conservation and radiotherapy

In November 1994 a 47-year-old woman was attending for routine follow up visits to the breast clinic having previously had bilateral breast cancer. On this occasion the surgeon had detected a lump in the left breast scar and needle aspiration cytology was positive for grade 2 cancer cells. Mammography showed an abnormality which had developed within the last year (Fig 4). In 1986 a left-sided cancer had presented and had been treated by wide local exci-

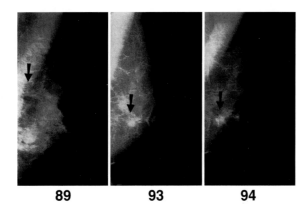

Fig. 5. Case 4. 45-degree oblique films from 1989, 1993 and 1994. In 1989 there was fine calcification with a small posterior density (which doesn't project). In 1993 and 1994 there was a developing spiculated density (arrowed) representing local recurrence.

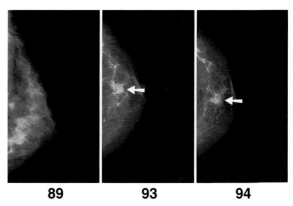

Fig. 6. Case 4. Cranio-caudal films from 1989, 1993 and 1994. In 1989 there was fine calcification with a small posterior density (arrowed). In 1993 and 1994 there was a developing density (arrowed) representing local recurrence.

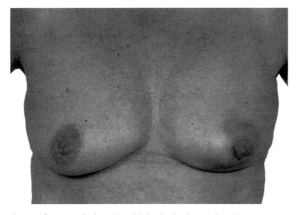

Fig. 7. Case 4. Deformity of left nipple due to local recurrence (discolouration is from FNAB).

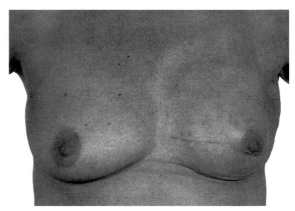

Fig. 8. Case 4. Cosmetic result after mastectomy and immediate reconstruction utilising a *latissimus dorsi* flap and implant. Notice radiotherapy field for electron therapy to zone of nipple.

sion, radiotherapy and tamoxifen. Nodes were not removed and the tumour was classified as a 25 mm grade 3 lesion. In 1992 contralateral right-sided breast cancer had developed and another breast preserving procedure was performed together with axillary dissection, radiotherapy and chemotherapy. The pathology of the right sided cancer was a 28 mm grade 3 cancer with 10 negative nodes. When the left sided cancer recurred in 1994 a mastectomy was performed and a 17 mm infiltrating duct cancer, grade 3, was found and 6 nodes were negative. There was no DCIS. Post-operatively she was given a further course of chemotherapy having had 1100 gms of breast tissue removed. The timing of the recurrent left-sided cancer suggests that it may be related to entrapment of circulating breast cancer cells from the 1992 right-sided breast cancer excision within the capillary network of the left breast scar.

Case 4 - Different quadrant local recurrence in breast treated by conservation therapy but no radiotherapy

In September 1989 a 41-year-old woman found a lump in her breast and investigations showed the presence of a solid lesion with mammographic features of high risk microcalcification. On clinical examination there was a lump and FNAB was positive for cancer with the presence of some necrosis suggestive of DCIS. A wide local excision was performed together with an axillary sampling procedure and the patient was given Tamoxifen. Histology showed a 25 mm zone of DCIS with multiple microinvasive changes. Six lymph nodes were negative. The patient remained well until local recurrence was diagnosed at annual follow up clinical review. A mammogram had revealed a 1.5 cm spiculated density close to the nipple and clinical appearance of the

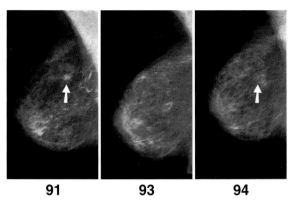

91   93   94

Fig. 9. Case 5. 45-degree oblique films from 1991, 1993 and 1994. Original tumour is arrowed as is the local recurrence.

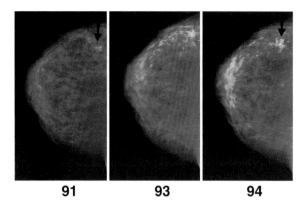

91   93   94

Fig. 10. Case 5. Cranio-caudal films from 1991, 1993 and 1994. Original tumour is arrowed as is the local recurrence.

nipple showed some distortion (Figs. 5-7). FNAB of the zone in question produced grade 1 cancer cells, and there was also one palpable lymph node. The patient chose to have a mastectomy combined with an immediate reconstruction utilising the latissimus dorsi flap (Fig. 8). The histology showed a 14 mm infiltrating duct cancer which was grade 2 and associated with one positive node out of 15. As the patient was now 46 and still pre-menopausal a post-operative course of CMF chemotherapy was given. Also associated with the tumour was a 13 mm high grade DCIS encroaching close to the nipple which was preserved but later irradiated.

The patient is well 18 months after salvage surgery and because she had an immediate reconstruction has not suffered any psychological side effects associated with recurrence of her disease.

Case 5 - Same quadrant IBTR after breast conservation without radiotherapy

In January 1992 a 52-year-old woman attended for a first mammographic screen and was asymptomatic. A stellate density was found in the upper outer quadrant of the right breast and the diagnosis of cancer was supported by an irregular ultrasound. FNAB was inadequate and the patient was recommended to have needle localisation biopsy and frozen section to establish the diagnosis. This was done and when positive a wide local excision was performed together with an axillary lymph node dissection. A 15 mm infiltrating duct cancer was found which was grade 1 and associated with 17 negative nodes. There was 20 mm margin of safety. Papillary DCIS was found extensively within the tumour and extending beyond it by only 1 mm. The patient had been given pre-operative tamoxifen 40 mgms daily for 33 days but this was discontinued after a clinicopathological conference. It was decided that no fur-

ther therapy was necessary. The patient was well until November 1994 (DFI = 34 months) when a second annual follow up mammogram and clinical examination revealed a recurrent cancer (Figs. 9 and 10). The recurrent spiculated density was in the bed of the original tumour resection and was associated with a 9 mm ultrasound mass. Clinical examination revealed an area of thickening in this zone without a definite lump. Needle aspiration cytology taken from this area produced grade 1 cancer cells. The patient was advised to have a mastectomy which revealed a 13 mm infiltrating duct cancer, grade 1 in organisation, with appearances very similar to the original. The rest of the breast was unremarkable. The patient has remained well 18 months later.

This patient had a consi derable loss of confidence when she had IBTR but is now much happier having had a mastectomy. A repeat breast-conserving procedure together with radiotherapy was offered to her at the time of local recurrence but she chose to have mastectomy and was not interested in a reconstruction.

Case 6 - Same quadrant IBTR after breast conservation without radiotherapy

A 72-year-old woman presented in May 1994 with a lump in her left breast. On clinical grounds this was a large cancer in a large breast. She was adamant she did not want to have a mastectomy. FNAB showed grade 1 cancer cells and a mammogram confirmed the diagnosis of a 3 cm spiculated density. 140 gms of breast tissue were resected and specimen X-ray showed a very wide and satisfactory margin. Histology revealed a 21 mm infiltrating duct cancer which was grade 2 in organisation. There was no vascular invasion or DCIS and the nearest margin was 7 mm. As she had extremely sensitive skin it was recommended that no radiotherapy be given and the patient was put on Tamoxifen 20 mgms daily. Exact-

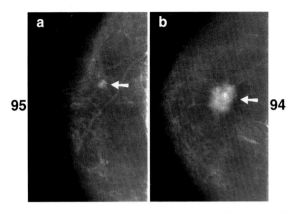

Fig. 11. Case 6. Cranio-caudal films from 1994 and 1995 showing recurrent tumour (a) recurring at site of previously excised primary (b).

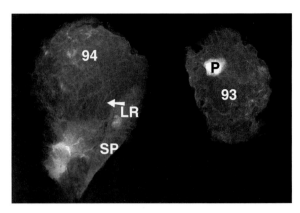

Fig. 12. Case 7. Right side 1993 primary excision (P), left side local recurrence arrowed (LR) lying in skin paddle (SP).

ly 1 year later, her first annual follow up mammogram showed a density in the scar which was diagnosed by ultrasound guided FNAB as local recurrence also grade 2 (Fig. 11). There was no palpable abnormality. The patient was switched from tamoxifen to megace and at her own request once again a mastectomy was avoided. This time a further 45 gm of tissue were resected and this revealed a 9 mm infiltrating duct cancer, grade 2 similar to the original lesion. Once again there was no DCIS or vascular invasion, and the nearest margin was 10 mm. Radiotherapy was given on this occasion. She remains well 1 year after the local recurrence but has recently switched from megace to arimidex 1 mgm daily due to excessive weight gain. Having had two breast conserving procedures the treated breast is now somewhat smaller than the other side, and she is contemplating a contra-lateral reduction for symmetry. It is possible that this local recurrence could have been prevented by giving radiotherapy after the first procedure, but overall nothing significant has been lost in the long term.

Case 7 - True scar recurrence after breast conservation without radiotherapy

In May 1993 a 73-year-old lady presented with a 3 week history of a lump in the right breast. On examination a 1 cm peripherally based lesion was found almost at the edge of the breast disc in the upper central portion. Needle aspiration cytology was positive for grade 1 cells. Mammography revealed a rounded density with a slightly irregular margin. A wide local excision and axillary dissection was performed and revealed a 14 mm infiltrating duct cancer, grade 1 with 8 negative nodes. There was no DCIS. Post-operatively there was quite a lot of seroma and slight wound infection which re-

mained thickened for some time. Exactly 1 year later the patient noticed some thickening in the scar which had developed 4 weeks after her last routine follow up clinical visit. A diagnosis of local recurrence was made by FNAB and 60 gm of breast was excised including the scar at the centre (Fig. 12). Her histology showed a 5 mm local recurrence similar to the original, but lying in the deep dermis extending into subcutaneous fat. There was no unstable tissue in the surrounding breast. The histological conclusion suggested that this could be regarded as dermal implantation from needle aspiration biopsy. Following wide local excision of the scar recurrence, the patient was given tamoxifen. She remains well 2 years later, without any active disease. Tumour implantation after needle aspiration is very rare after mastectomy, but may account for a considerable number of local recurrences after breast conservation if the needle track is not excised.

Detection of local recurrence

The optimum surveillance method for the detection of local recurrence following breast conservation remains uncertain. Diagnostic evaluation using the triple assessment of clinical, mammographic and cytological examinations is frequently difficult even with the addition of ultrasound, as post-treatment appearances due to surgical scarring and radiotherapy change can tend to obscure or mimic recurrent cancer.

The British Association of Surgical Oncology (BASO) guidelines have stipulated that local recurrence should occur with a rate of less than 10% within 5 years of breast conservation.[17] Furthermore, two thirds of all recurrences should occur within this time frame. It has been suggested that the patient be

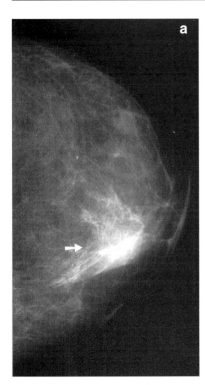
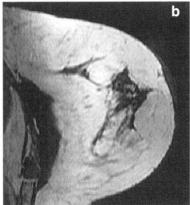
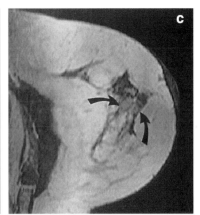

Fig. 13. Local recurrence detected by magnetic resonance imaging (MRI).
(a) shows cranio-caudal mammogram with
an area of increased density (arrowed)
suggestive of post-operative scarring only.
MR images pre-contrast (b) and
post-contrast (c) transverse T1-weighted
3D FLASCH (TR 18ms, TE 7ms, FA 40 degrees).
MR images show a 25 mm enhancing mass (curved arrows)
confirming local recurrence.

reviewed clinically every 6 months for 5 years, then annually thereafter, and that mammograms should be carried out on the ipsilateral breast on an annual basis. The Royal College of Radiology have noted that at 10 years there may be a 10 to 15% incidence of local recurrence after breast conservation. This may be especially so in younger patients or those with poorer prognosis.[18] They recognise that interpretation of follow-up mammography may be hampered by radiotherapy changes and surgical scarring. Only half of the local recurrences may be detected by planned clinical follow-up visits or mammography. They too have suggested mammography on the ipsilateral breast every year. The mammographic features that predict for breast tumour recurrence include micro calcifications, multifocality, and solid stellate densities close to the nipple.[19]

The treated breast is a rapidly changing organ and routine mammographic imaging should be deferred for at least 6 months after conservation therapy. By this time a lot of the oedema will have started to settle and many of the scar-related calcifications will not yet have formed. Nonetheless, there will still be quite a lot of fluid collection, skin thickening, scarring and fibrosis, which makes diagnosis difficult.[20]

Recent studies with gadolinium enhanced magnetic resonance imaging (MRI) of the breast have shown promising results in the differentiation of benign post-therapeutic changes from recurrent tumour with a sensitivity approaching 100%. Residual or recurrent tumour exhibits early strong homogenous enhancement after contrast injection, while sterile fibrosis shows no substantial enhancement. Confusion may occur up to 9 months after therapy as the scar has not matured and therefore might still enhance. A recent study looked at 28 difficult breasts after breast-conserving surgery and radiotherapy.[21] Local recurrence was present in 12 of these and were detected by MRI in 11. This form of imaging proved superior to mammography which only identified 6 cases. An example of MRI detected local recurrence is shown in Figure 13. The images show a 66-year-old woman with a suspected local recurrence 54 months after breast-conserving surgery and radiotherapy. The mammogram shows an increased area of density suggesting post-operative scarring whereas the MRI images show a 25 mm enhancing mass confirming the diagnosis of local recurrence.

Management of local recurrence

Having detected local recurrence in the conserved breast and given the patient appropriate counselling, further therapy is indicated. The overall strategy depends on the particular type of local recurrence encountered and the extent of primary therapy. Osborne and Simmons reviewed the role of salvage mastectomy for these patients and noted that it offered good disease control.[22]

Further loco regional recurrence occurred in 15% of women who were followed for a median period of five years after salvage mastectomy, and at ten years the disease-free survival was 50-60%. The success of salvage mastectomy is related to the size and extent of the recurrence, the disease-free interval, and the original lymph node status. It has generally been thought that immediate complications of salvage mastectomy must be higher than those of routine surgery because of working in previously irradiated skin, but this has not been found to be the case. When an immediate reconstruction is advocated after a previous breast conservation with radiotherapy, then it is necessary to use either a *latissimus dorsi* flap or a TRAM flap. Simple tissue expanders or prostheses by themselves are always associated with an inferior cosmetic result.

Kurtz *et al.* reported on 118 cases of local recurrence after breast conservation and radiotherapy.[23] Fifty per cent of these were treated by salvage mastectomy and the other half by a further breast conserving procedure.

As a group, there was a 72% five year survival and a 58% ten year survival. Survival was related to the disease free interval and the original stage of the cancer and was irrespective of the operation chosen to salvage the situation. These figures suggest a much better prognosis than local recurrence after initial mastectomy.

After seven years of median follow up, 20 of the 180 patients had a further local recurrence and this was more likely to occur in those treated by a further breast-conserving procedure rather than a salvage mastectomy. In order to perform a second breast-preserving procedure, strict follow up criteria are required. Kurtz advises a repeat wide local excision if the tumour is mobile, was originally lymph node negative and measures less than 2 cm. Approximately one third of patients fall into this group.

There is considerable interest at the moment in the role of chemotherapy prior to initial surgical treatment. This 'neo-adjuvant' approach may have the ability to reduce the bulk of the tumour to the extent that a breast-preserving procedure becomes a feasible physical exercise rather than a mastectomy. Success in this field has led to various groups showing interest in treating local recurrence with chemotherapy in order to be able to do a second breast-preserving procedure. Unfortunately, the previously treated breast will often have a marked zone of fibrosis due to surgery and radiotherapy, rendering the recurrent tumour relatively avascular and, therefore, a difficult area to penetrate.

There is very little information regarding the salvage of patients who have had breast-preserving surgery without radiotherapy. This group of patients are in an ideal position to have a second breast-preserving procedure plus delayed radiotherapy compared to their counterparts. Therefore, for small grade 1 node negative patients treated by wide local excision alone, all local options are still open for use. Providing patient confidence can be maintained, these patients should be able to avoid salvage mastectomy.

Future directions

The role of radiotherapy

As a result of the randomised controlled studies described above, it is now standard practice to advise women having breast-conserving surgery to go forward and have adjuvant radiotherapy to the retained breast. This will decrease the local recurrence rate. However, much of the local recurrence will depend on the extent of surgical removal, and therefore radiotherapy should never be given purely as a means to circumvent inadequate surgical technique. Holmberg has acknowledged that for most women after breast conservation there is no local recurrence at 5 to 10 years, and as radiotherapy does not improve overall survival, he questions whether it can be safely abandoned in subgroups of patients.[24] It remains uncertain whether radiotherapy reduces local recurrence rates by eliminating remnants of disease that remain *in situ*, or discourages local growth induced by growth factors and cytokines. There is also the possibility that radiotherapy could induce new tumour formation. Holmberg notes that the cost of preventing local recurrence at the 5 year mark is approximately the same cost as a life-year saved by giving chemotherapy to an older patient with breast cancer, and is greater than the cost of a life-year saved by screening. If radiotherapy were used selectively, then the cost of preventing local recurrence could be reduced from 4,100 to 2,600 dollars. In order to explore the selective use of radiotherapy after breast conservation, urgent research is needed to seek out low risk groups in whom radiotherapy can safely be avoided. In such a group of patients it would be acceptable to find 10% local recurrence at 10 years without use of radiotherapy which could then be employed as part of the salvage strategy.

Psychological implications

Relatively little is known about the psychological adjustment to breast-conserving therapy as compared to mastectomy. It was initially thought that breast conservation would be an added bonus for the patients as they were likely to suffer less psychiatric morbidity as a result of these interventions compared to those having mastectomy. However, as Fallow-field has shown, patients having breast-conserving therapy have just as much anxiety and depressive illnesses as those having mastectomy.[25] Whilst there is no overall difference in the chance of maladjustment to treatment which was present in approximately one third of patients, there was a difference in the greatest fear between those having mastectomy and breast conservation. For the mastectomy group it was problems associated with body image, whereas with breast-conserving therapy it was anxiety related to local recurrence that was predominant. Clearly further studies are required to assess the place of local recurrence in the mind of breast cancer sufferers. Some evidence suggests that patients offered a choice and given fuller explanations and counselling are better adjusted to the problems that could occur in their follow up.

BASO II trial

The BASO II trial is an important randomised controlled study to try and assess the use of selected radiotherapy after breast-conserving surgery. This was launched in 1991 and so far 314 patients have been randomised. Patients with either special type of breast cancer (e.g. tubular, cribriform, or mucoid) or grade 1 infiltrating duct lesions of less than 2 cm in size and with negative nodes can be entered into the study providing there is a clear margin and no vascular invasion. Randomisation is between control without any further treatment, or addition of tamoxifen 20 mgms daily for 5 years, radiotherapy to the breast itself, or tamoxifen and radiotherapy. Part of the trial recommends that there is a minimum of 5 mm of clear pathological margins around the excised lesion, and preferably 10 mm. It is hoped that 1200 cases will be accrued. Similar trials have been carried out in Europe as part of EORTC and also in Uppsala-Orebro.

Local recurrence within the screening programme

The screening project continues to find patients with small node negative grade I cancers, these occurring in up to 25% of the total screen detected group. These patients are ideally suited to be entered into the BASO II trial described above. Data from the South West Thames (West) screening area of England from 1989 to 1995 showed that 17% of 323 patients with DCIS had mastectomy and a similar percentage of 1408 patients had mastectomy for invasive disease.

This leaves a very large number of patients being treated by breast conservation, but not all of these are having radiotherapy. Patients and their surgeons are assuming that the reward for finding a small screen detected cancer is the avoidance of both mastectomy and radiotherapy. Thus 38% of 1165 patients with invasive cancer were treated by breast conservation without radiotherapy.

This includes 101 patients treated by breast conservation alone, and 339 who had surgery plus Tamoxifen. The follow up on all these patients will be monitored carefully, and the local recurrence rate eagerly awaited. This will add complementary data to the BASO II trial in determining which patients can avoid radiotherapy and be free of local recurrence. For patients with tumours less than 15 mm in diameter breast conservation is even more popular with 88% patients avoiding a mastectomy and 44% of these also are avoiding radiotherapy with a subgroup of 68 (9%) being treated by surgery without Tamoxifen.

Whilst it is possible there will be an explosion of local recurrence in these potentially undertreated patients over the next 5 years, it is hoped that the improved services for screen detected breast cancer and also symptomatic breast cancer made possible by the introduction of the National Breast Screening Programme and the formation of the National British Breast Surgical Society will help maintain standards at the highest level. This will include meticulous attention to surgical technique which should reduce the local recurrence rate to a minimum.

Conclusions

1. Local recurrence is expected to occur at a rate of 1% per annum in the conserved breast.
2. Inadequate surgical technique leads to an excess of local recurrence. This can be reduced by giving radiotherapy.
3. Adequate surgical resection combined with radiotherapy produces the lowest possible local recurrence rate.
4. Identification of patients in whom radiotherapy can safely be omitted is urgently required.
5. Local recurrence after inadequate surgery may identify patients in whom distant relapse is about to occur.
6. Mammography and clinical examination detect most local recurrences, but for difficult cases magnetic resonance imaging is recommended.
7. Local recurrence does not always need to be salvaged by mastectomy.
8. The psychological implications of local recurrence need further evaluation.

References

1. Early Breast Cancer Trialists Collaborative Group: The effect of radiotherapy and surgery in early breast cancer: an overview of the randomised trials. N. Engl. J. Med. 1995; 333: 1444-55

2. Fisher B. *et al.*: Reanalysis and Results after 12 Years of Follow Up in a randomised clinical trial comparing total mastectomy with lumpectomy with or without irradiation in the treatment of breast cancer. N. Engl. J. Med. 1995; 333: 1456-61

3. Fisher E.R. *et al.*: Ipselateral breast tumour recurrence and survival following lumpectomy and irradiation: pathological findings from NSABP Protocol B-06. Sem. Surg. Onc. 1992; 8: 161-166

4. Holland R. *et al.*: Histologic multifocality of Tis, T1-2 Breast Carcinomas. Implications for clinical trials of breast conserving surgery. Cancer 1985; 56: 979-990

5. Macmillan R.D. *et al.*: Breast conserving surgery and tumour bed positivity in patients with breast cancer. Br. J. Surg. 1994; 81: 56-8

6. Reid S.E. *et al.*: Role of cytokines and growth factors in promoting the local recurrence of breast cancer. Br. J. Surg. 1996; 83: 313-320

7. Rubin P. *et al.*: Tumour bed biopsy detects the presence of multifocal disease in patients undergoing breast conservation therapy for primary carcinoma. Europ. J. Surg. Oncol. 1996; 22: 17-22

8. Lockyer A.P. *et al.*: Factors influencing local recurrence after excision and radiotherapy for primary breast cancer. Br. J. Surg. 1989; 76; 890-894

9. Macmillan R.D. *et al.*: Local recurrence after breast conserving surgery for breast cancer. Br. J. Surg. 1996; 83: 149-155

10. Clarke D.H., Martinez A.A.: Identification of patients who are at high risk for loco-regional breast cancer recurrence after conservation surgery and radiotherapy: a review article for surgeons, pathologists, and radiation and medical oncologists. J. Clin. Oncol. 1992; 10: 474-483

11. Forest A.P. *et al.*: Scottish trial of conservation therapy. Breast 1995; 4: 232

12. Fisher B. *et al.*: 8 year results of a randomised clinical trial comparing total mastectomy and lumpectomy with or without irradiation in the treatment of breast cancer. N. Engl. J. Med. 1989; 320: 822-8

13. Veronesi U. *et al.*: Radiotherapy after breast preserving surgery in women with localised cancer of the breast. N. Engl. J. Med. 1993; 328: 1587-90

14. Veronesi U. *et al.*: Local recurrences and distant metastases after conserving breast cancer treatments: partly independent events. J. Natl. Cancer Inst. 1995; 87: 19-27

15. Sibbering D.M. *et al.*: Selection criteria for breast conservation in primary operable invasive cancer. The Breast 1995; 4: 232

16. Fisher E.R. *et al.*: Pathologic Findings From The National Surgical Adjuvant Breast Project (NSABP) Protocol B-17. Intraductal Carcinoma (Ductal Carcinoma *In Situ*). Cancer 1995: 75; 1310-9

17. Breast: guidelines for surgeons in the management of surgeons group symptomatic breast cancer in the United Kingdom Association of Europ. J. Surg. Oncol. 1995; 21: (Suppl A) 1-13. Surgical Oncology

18. Council of Royal College of Radiologists : use of imaging in the follow up of patients with breast cancer. Royal College of Radiologists, London 1995

19. Dalberg K. *et al.*: Mammographic features, predictors of early ipselateral breast tumour recurrences? Europ. J. Surg. Oncol. 1996; 22:483-490

20. Mendelson E.B.: Evaluation of the post operative breast. Radiol. Clin. N. America 1992: 30; 107-138

21. Mumtaz H. *et al.*: Breast MR for the assessment of recurrent breast cancer. Clin. Rad. (In press)

22. Osborne M.P., Simmons R.M.: Salvage surgery for recurrence after breast conservation. World J. Surg. 1994: 18; 93-97

23. Kurtz J.M. *et al.*: Results Of Salvage Surgery For Mammary Recurrence Following Breast Conserving Therapy. Ann. Surg. 1988: 207; 347-351

24. Holmberg L.: Breast conserving surgery without radiotherapy. Acta Oncol 1995: 34; 681-683

25. Fallowfield L.J.: Psychosocial adjustment after treatment for early breast cancer. Oncology 1990: 4; 89-100

Interval carcinomas

R. Warren

Interval carcinomas

A feature of all forms of screening for cancer is the occurrence of cases between the screening events. In the case of breast cancer this is a group of particular interest in more respects than one. These cases may be the ones missed by the screening examination and so they represent a valuable tool in the assessment of screening quality and can be compared between different programmes as an audit of screening effectiveness. These cancers may also include the faster growing cases that reach the size of clinical detection in the screening interval, and so the prognostic factors such as size, grade and nodal status may be different from the screen detected group.

Classification of cancers

If, as indicated above, the interval cancer rate is to be used to monitor screening performance and to be a surrogate predictor of screening effectiveness, it is essential to define the terms used and the categories of cancers that are to be considered. In the British National Screening Programme, considerable work was undertaken to make clear definitions and this material is available in a publication to guide the centres of the national programme.[1] As a result, it has been possible to analyse early the first signs of screening performance that have emerged and to suggest putting in place changes that will improve that performance.[2]

In this NHSBSP publication the following categories have been identified in relation to a screening programme:

1. Cancers in non-attenders

In women who have failed to attend, following an invitation for screening.

2. Cancers in lapsed attenders

In women who have attended for screening, and who either by their own choice, or as a result of exceeding the recommended age, do not attend on the next occasion.

3. Cancers in the uninvited

In women who have not yet been invited or have been suspended from screening or who are not called because of inaccuracy of the population register.

4. Interval cancers

In women who have been screened, and whose cancer arises clinically before the next invitation for screening. Clearly the rates will be affected by the woman's age and the screening interval.

5. Programme-provoked presentation

A few women present clinically after receiving an invitation for screening, or after screening and before assessment, and are difficult to categorise under the headings above.

It is likely that the screening intervention triggers the clinical presentation in a woman who has come to suspect that she has a breast lump.

Categories of interval cancer

In order for the audit of radiology to be useful, interval cancers have been categorised. For the British National Breast Screening Programme, the following categories have been defined:

1. *Cancers developed* in the screening interval (true interval cancers)

2. *False negatives.* For legal reasons these are not termed missed cancers
3. *Mammographically occult.* Cancers not visible on the mammogram at clinical presentation
4. *Cancers in follow up* non-attenders
5. *Unclassifiable.* Cases where there is no mammogram at the time of clinical presentation for comparison with the screening mammogram.

This categorisation is standard to the UK national programme, but has differed from some of the international publications in the literature quoted below. In particular, some of the papers recognise a group where the abnormality can be seen with hindsight, or on comparison with the clinical mammograms, but is considered so subtle as to be reasonably overlooked. "Missed with minor signs" is one description of this situation.[3,4,5] (From 1996 the UK NHS Breast Screening Programme added such a category).

Interval cancers as a means of monitoring screening performance

Several publications in the literature debate the use of interval cancer data in the assessment of screening performance.[2,6,7,8,9,11] There is no doubt that this material is useful.[10]

Radiological features of interval cancers

Interval cancers are a group composed of false negative screening cases, those arising *de novo* and those that are radiologically occult at the time of clinical diagnosis. It is not surprising that they may be radiologically different from those diagnosed by screening. Two publications address these differences.[12,3] In these papers the features are analysed, and tend to be the less specific ones such as asymmetrical density and parenchymal distortions. These cancers tend to be smaller and to lie in denser breast parenchyma than other cancers.

Histological features of interval cancers

In all analyses of interval cancers, some differences are found compared with the screen detected group, and with cancers presenting clinically without the intervention of screening. In all the series, carcinoma *in situ* is an unusual finding, and is typically a screen detected type. The few that arise as interval cancers may arise from serendipity. Lobular carcinomas are more frequent and this is probably because the radiological features reflect the typical histology which shows file-like infiltration of malignant cells that do not make a sharp edge, either histologically or radiologically. In some of the series the group was characterised by a subset of rapidly growing tumours with unfavourable prognostic characteristics.[3,5,13,14]

Do interval cancers grow faster than screen detected and clinically diagnosed cancers?

The literature is not consistent in the reply to this question. In some of the series there is a subset of cancer with bad prognostic features both by size, grade and nodal status and by DNA content which would suggest that a bad prognosis will ensue. In others the difference is less clear cut, and perhaps this illustrates how the interval cancers in both number and nature may indicate the effectiveness of the screening process. Logically the interval cancers should be matched against the trials with the most effective outcomes, and if their number and nature are similar, one might look to see equivalent mortality outcomes.[15,16]

Survival of interval cancer patients

As a result of the differences described in the last two paragraphs, it is believed that interval cancer patients have a poorer survival than women with screen detected cancers. This may equate with or exceed the mortality of those women who present clinically. That these findings are not constant between the different trials may support the view that the interval cancers are a predictor of screening performance.[17,18]

Can we draw conclusions from the literature?

Appended here is a full literature list relating to interval cancers which should be perused at source for a view of the final conclusions. Not all is known or understood of this interesting group of cancers. Without a doubt, to judge screening effectiveness, the effort of tracking this elusive group of cancers is rewarded, and some knowledge is gained of the outcome to be expected from screening. This knowledge remains incomplete because of the inconsistencies in the available data.[1-18,19,20]

From the patient's perspective, it is not surprising that when screening seems to have failed, women seek a different doctor, and it is for this reason that even obtaining knowledge of this group of cases is a detective game, which may be rewarded by incomplete information, as some cases will inevitably be handled by the non-experts who offer alternative care to the screeners and their surgical colleagues. From this group of cases may also come the information from which the best screening interval can be deduced.[21,1]

References

1. Patnick J., Muir Gray J.: Guidelines on the collection and use of breast cancer data. NHSBSP 1993; 26
2. Field S., Michell M., Wallis M., Wilson ARM.: What should be done about interval breast cancers? Brit. Med. J., 1995; 310:203
3. Ikeda D., Andersson I., Wattsgard C., Janzon L., Linell F.: Interval cancers in the Malmo mammographic screening trial: Radiographic appearance and prognostic considerations. AJR 1992; 159: 287-294
4. Van Dijck J., Verbeek A., Hendriks J., Holland R.: The current detectability of breast cancer in a mammographic screening program. A review of the previous mammograms of interval and screen detected lesions. Cancer 1993; 72: 1933-8
5. Peeters P., Verbeek A., Hendriks J., Holland R., Mravunac M., Vooijs G.: The occurrence of interval cancers in the Nijmegen screening programme. Br. J. Cancer 1989; 59: 929-932
6. Kopans D.: Mammography screening for breast cancer. Cancer 1993; 72: 1810-2
7. Paci E., Duffy S.: Modelling the analysis of breast cancer screening programmes: Sensitivity, lead time and predictive value in the Florence District Programme (1975-1986). Intern. J. Epidem. 1992; 20: 852-858
8. Kee F., Gorman D., Odling-Smee W.: Confidence intervals and interval cancers. Public Health 1992; 106: 29-35
9. Mosesen D., Meharg K.: Tumor registry audit of mammography in community practice. Amer. J. Surg. 1994; 167: 505-8
10. Baines C.: The Canadian national breast screening study: A perspective on criticisms. Ann Intern Med. 1994; 120: 326-334
11. Day N.E., Williams D., Khaw K.: Breast cancer screening programmes: the development of a monitoring and evaluation system. Brit. J. Cancer 1989; 59: 954-958
12. Reintgen D., Berman C., Baekey P., Nicosia S., Greenberg H., Bush C., Lyman G., Clark R.: The anatomy of missed breast cancers. Surg. Oncology 1993; 2: 65-75 258
13. Rosen A., Frisell J., Nilsson R., Wiege M., Auer G.: Histopathologic and cytochemical characteristics of interval breast carcinomas from the Stockholm mammography screening project. Acta Oncologica 1992; 31: 399-402
14. Yoshida K., Abe R., Itoh S., Taguchi T., Ohta J., Morimoto T. et al.: Comparisons of interval cancers of breast with other breast cancers detected through mass screening and in outpatient clinics in Japan. Jpn. J. Clin. Oncol 1990; 20: 374-379
15. Senie R., Lesser M., Kinne D., Rosen P.: Method of tumor detection influences disease-free survival of women with breast carcinoma. Cancer 1994; 73: 1666-1672
16. Frisell J., Rosen A., Nilsson B., Goldman S.: Interval cancer and survival in a randomised breast cancer screening trial in Stockholm. Breast Cancer Res. Treat. 1992; 24: 11-16
17. Moss S., Coleman D., Ellman R., Chamberlain J., Forrest, Kirkpatrick A., Thomas B., Price J.: Eur. J. Cancer 1992; 29A: 255
18. Brekelmans C., Collette H., Collette C., Fracheboud J., de Waard F.: Breast cancer after a negative screen: follow-up of women participating in the DOM screening programme. Eur. J. Cancer 1992; 28A: 893-895
19. Moskowitz M.: Interval cancers and screening for breast cancer in British Columbia. AJR 1994; 162: 1072-75
20. Burhenne H., Burhenne L., Goldberg F., Hislop T., Worth A., Rebbeck P., Kan L.: Interval breast cancers in the screening programme of British Columbia: analysis & classification. AJR 1994; 162: 1067-1071
21. Tabar L., Fagerberg G., Day N.E., Holmberg L.: What is the optimum interval between mammographic screening examinations? Brit. J. Cancer, 1987; 55: 547-551

Case 1. HGH Aged 58. Grade 2, invasive ductal carcinoma, 40 mm diameter, four out of six nodes involved. True interval cancer 22 months after screening.

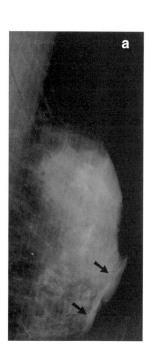
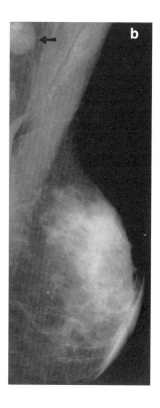
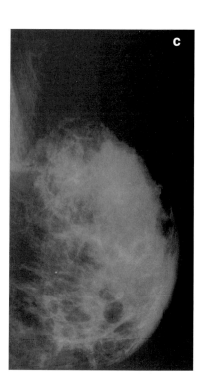

Fig. 1.**a**. MLO view, films of 1.5.91.Thickening of skin of areola seen with hindsight (arrows). **b**. MLO view, film of 5.8.92. Lymph node at axilla enlarged, seen with hindsight (bold arrow). **c**. MLO view, film of 30.6.94. At diagnosis, the films show gross lymphoedema of breast. **d**. CC view, film of 1.5.91. Areolar skin thickening. **e**. CC view, film of 30.6.94. Gross lymphoedema. **f-g**. Magnification view showing widespread fine calcification.

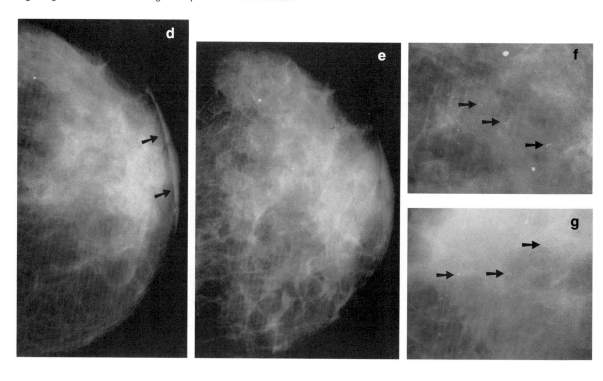

Case 2. TR Aged 55. False negative interval cancer, 8 months after screening 10mm, grade 2 invasive lobular carcinoma with lobular carcinoma *in situ*, one out of twelve nodes involved.

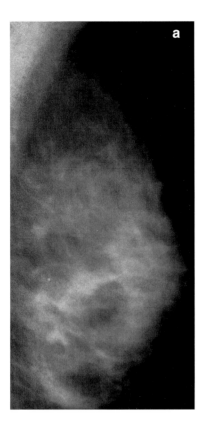

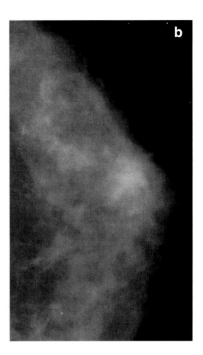

Fig. 2.**a**. MLO view, normal film of 12.12.89. **b** CC view, film of 12.12.89, probably abnormal with hindsight, but features very subtle. **c**. MLO view at diagnosis film of 23.8.90. Cancer marked with arrows. **d**. CC view at diagnosis film of 23.8.90. Cancer marked with arrows.

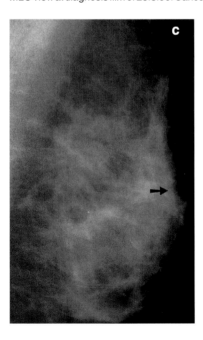

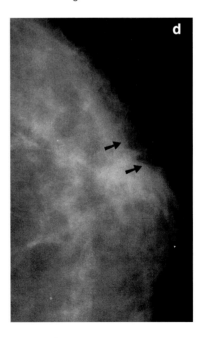

Case 3. RS Aged 62. True interval cancer, 14 months from screening. The technical quality of the first mammogram is poor, and it is possible that this tumour was present but in the part of the breast off the back of the mammogram. Grade 2, invasive ductal carcinoma, 24 mm diameter, one out of seven nodes involved, also non-invasive ductal carcinoma of comedo type.

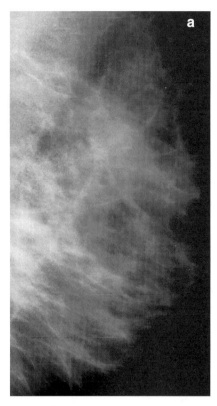
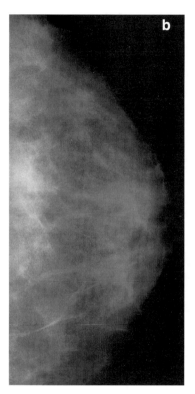

Fig. 3.**a**. MLO view of 12.12.89 normal examination. **b**. CC view of 12.12.89 normal result. **c**. MLO view at diagnosis 17.1.91. Large mass marked with arrow. **d**. CC view of 17.1.91. Widespread calcification marked with small arrowheads.

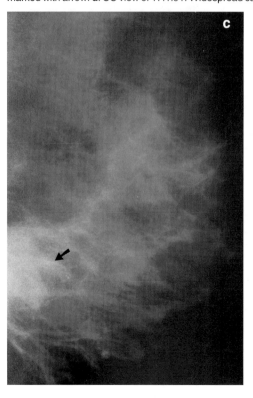
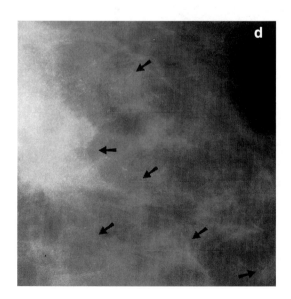

Case 4. IM Aged 62. True interval cancer 17 months from screening. Grade 2, invasive ductal carcinoma, 15 mm diameter, no nodal involvement.

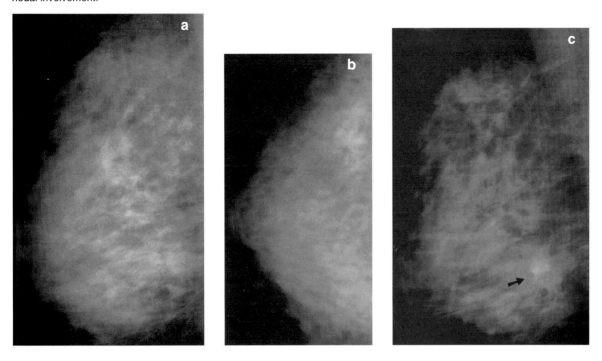

Fig. 4.**a**. MLO 28.6.88. Normal examination. **b**. CC 28.6.88. Normal examination. **c**. MLO 16.11.89. At diagnosis. **d**. CC 16.11.89. At diagnosis. **e**. MLO magnification view. 16.11.89. **f**. specimen mammogram.

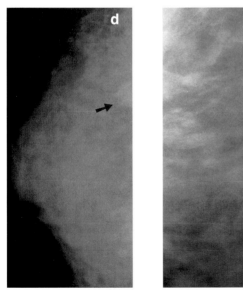
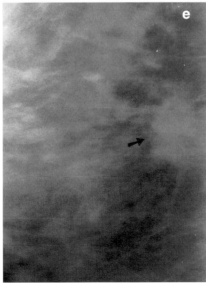
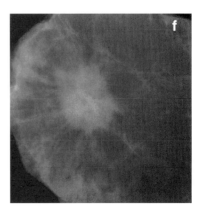

Case 5. CW Aged 63. True interval cancer 5 months after screening in yearly screening trial, second round. This case indicates the difficulty of screening even with a yearly interval in the dense breast. It is likely that this large tumour was present in the breast throughout the screening process, although not detectable on technically adequate mammograms. Grade 2, mixed invasive ductal and lobular carcinoma, 20 mm in diameter, four out of six nodes involved.

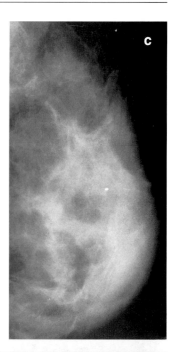

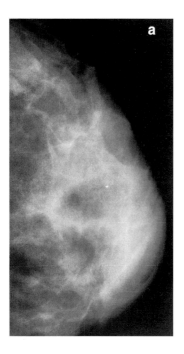

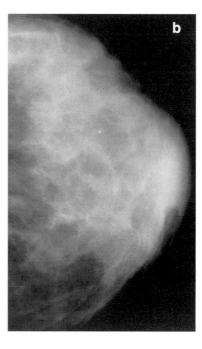

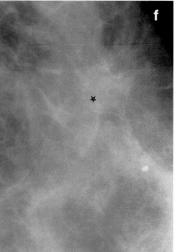

Fig. 5.**a**. MLO view of 6.2.90. Normal examination. **b**. CC view of 6.2.90. Normal examination. **c**. MLO view of 6.2.90. Normal examination. **d**. MLO view of 17.6.91. Parenchimal deformity (**arrow**). **e**. CC view of 17.6.91. Tumour mass marked with star at centre. **f**. MLO magnification view. Tumour mass marked with star at centre. **g**. CC magnification view. Tumour mass marked with star at centre.

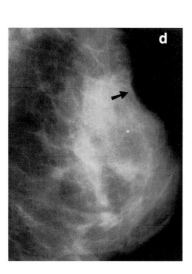

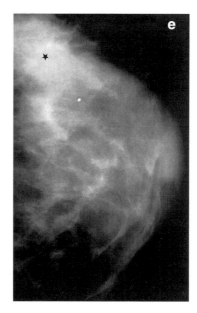

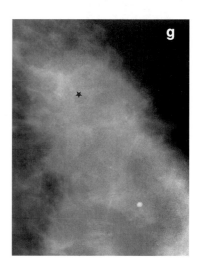

Case 6. BA Aged 62. False negative interval cancer 22 months after screening. 15 mm invasive ductal carcinoma with three out of eight lymph nodes involved.

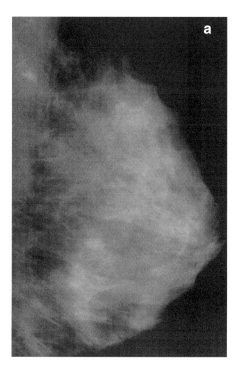
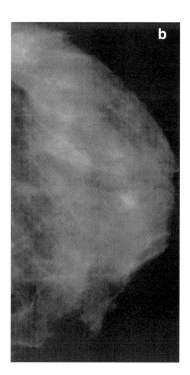

Fig. 6.**a**. MLO Screening films of 28.6.89. **b**. CC Screening films of 28.6.89. **c**. MLO Screening films of 26.5.92. The arrow shows the small tumour visible with hindsight. **d**. MLO Diagnostic film of 9.3.94. **e**. CC Diagnostic film of 9.3.94.

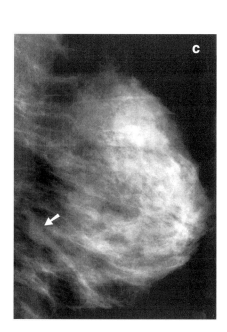
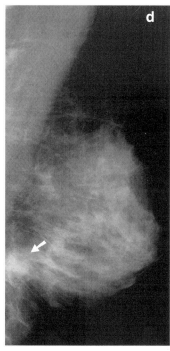
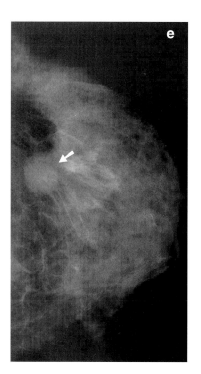

Case 7. VF Aged 56. False negative interval cancer 24 months from screening. This 8mm tumour was of invasive ductal type with one lymph node out of fourteen involved. The small tumour can be seen with hindsight and has been misinterpreted as a small normal lymph node on the original screening examination. Its position in this woman with tiny breasts rendered detection by the patient at a small size possible.

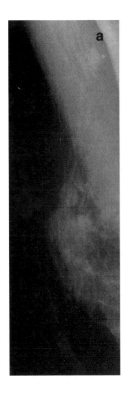
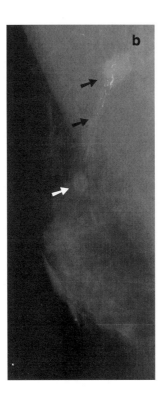

Fig. 7.**a**. MLO Screening film of 13.6.90.
b. MLO Diagnostic film of 18.6.92. Arrowheads mark the small tumour mass and the line of calcification. A full arrow indicates a lymph node, probably involved by tumour.

Case 8. AD Aged 52. True interval cancer 17 months from screening. The tumour was 20 mm in diameter, a grade 2 lobular carcinoma with two out of eleven lymph nodes involved.

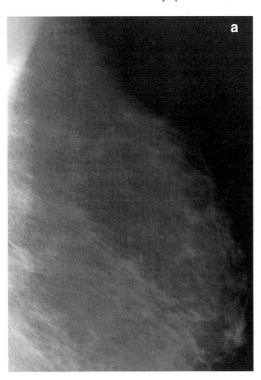
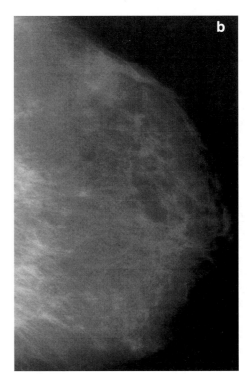

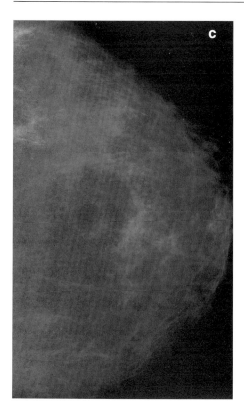

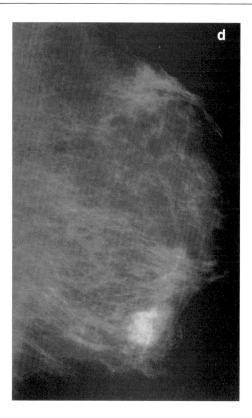

Fig. 8.**a**. Upper MLO of left breast Screening film of 3.4.90. **b**. Lower MLO of left breast. Screening film of 3.4.90. **c**. CC view of 3.4.90. **d**. MLO view, diagnostic film of 16.9.91. **e**. CC view of 16.9.91 **f**. Magnification view of tumour. MLO. **g**. Magnification view of tumour. CC projection.

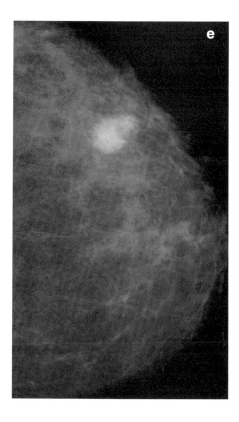

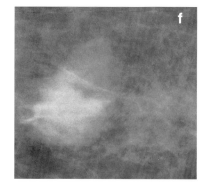

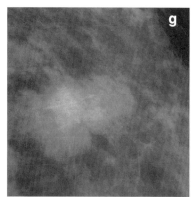

Final remarks

Medico-legal aspects

S. Levene

Preliminary

Breast screening and the subsequent management of patients have medico-legal implications which are worth considering against a background of the law of negligence generally.

First, some statistics that may give comfort: in 1978 it was estimated[1] that in America less than 1% of patients are injured by negligent care, and that only 10% of those patients seek the advice of a lawyer. No comparable study has been carried out in the UK, but there is no reason to think that patients in the UK are more litigious than those in America, and the proportion of injured patients seeking legal advice in the UK is likely to be well below 10%. In seeking to understand the legal process, it is also important to remember that:

1. The majority of potential claims against doctors are dropped before proceedings are commenced.
2. The overwhelming majority of cases that are commenced in which there has been negligence result in negotiated settlements rather than in contested trials.
3. The majority of contested trials end in a finding in favour of the defendant.
4. Less than 5% of medical defence budgets goes on payment to successful claimants: most of the money is spent on administrative costs and legal fees.

To illustrate this, one English firm's experience was that out of 24 medical negligence cases concluded in a nine-month period:

11 discontinued following investigation and either before or after the issue of protective proceedings;
10 concluded successfully after the issue of proceedings and before trial;
2 discontinued after the issue of proceedings;

1 taken to trial, where the Plaintiff lost.

Following the introduction of Crown Indemnity, it was predicted that cases would settle more readily and at an earlier stage in the litigation process. In fact, the course of litigation does not seem to have changed significantly. The fear of many doctors that Health Trusts and Health Authorities would take litigation decisions on purely commercial grounds, and that the Defence Unions were more protective than their employers, seems to have been groundless.

Negligence

The aim of this article is to give the legal background against which the practice of medicine is criticised by the law. The legal principles are the same whatever medical discipline is being criticised, though a court will take into account the fact that different disciplines might take a different approach to a problem. However, it is important to remember that the clinician under scrutiny is to be judged by his own speciality. So, a casualty officer who treats a neurological case on an emergency admission is to be judged by the standard of a casualty officer, not a consultant neurologist. This is recognised in the medical profession, and the courts took note of it in Sidaway v Board of Governors of the Bethlem Royal and Maudsley Hospital[2]:

"The language of the Bolam test clearly requires a different degree of skill from a specialist in his own special field than from a general practitioner. In the field of neurosurgery it would be necessary to substitute for the.. phrase "no doctor of ordinary skill", the phrase "no neurosurgeon of ordinary skill". All this is elementary, and... firmly established law."

To lawyers, "negligence" means a breach of the

duty of care that one person owes to another. This is not laid down by statute: the test is one that has been evolved by judges over the years. It must always be remembered that although the test *is* a legal one, it was evolved (and it is applied) in the light of expert evidence given to the courts by medical experts.

A medical practitioner is not obliged to achieve success: his duty is to exercise reasonable skill and care. The classic formulation of the test is found in Lanphier *v* Phipos[3]:

"Every person who enters into a learned profession undertakes to bring to the exercise of it a reasonable degree of care and skill. He does not undertake, if he is an attorney, that at all events you shall gain your case, nor does a surgeon undertake that he will perform a cure; nor does he undertake to use the highest possible degree of skill. There may be persons who have higher education and greater advantages than he has, but he undertakes to bring a fair, reasonable and competent degree of skill..."

The test is now known as the "Bolam" test, from McNair J's famous jury direction in Bolam *v* Friern Hospital Management Committee[4]:

"A doctor is not guilty of negligence if he has acted in accordance with a practice accepted as proper by a responsible body of medical men skilled in that particular art... Putting it the other way round, a doctor is not negligent, if he is acting in accordance with such practice, merely because there is a body of opinion which takes a contrary view."

The Bolam test works by looking for broad consensus in the medical profession, and allows practitioners to make advances in treatment and techniques without making every advance a bandwagon on to which they must all leap. It is also important to look at the doctor's specialisation or lack of it. In Hucks *v* Cole[5] the Court pointed out that the defendant "was to be judged as a general practitioner with a diploma in obstetrics" - though part of a doctor's ability lies in knowing when he is getting out of his depth, and when to refer a patient for more specialised advice. In the case of a junior hospital doctor, there are two possible tests, both taken from Wilsher *v* Essex Health Authority[6].

1. The higher test, which comes from Mustill LJ's judgment: *"The standard is not just that of the averagely competent and well-informed junior houseman (or whatever the position of the doctor) but of such a person who fills a post in a unit offering a highly specialised service"*, and

2. The lower test, which comes from Sir Nicholas Browne-Wilkinson's judgment: *"If the standard of care required of such a doctor is that he should have the skill required of the post he occupies, the young houseman or the doctor seeking to acquire specialist skill in a special unit would be held liable for shortcomings in the treatment without any personal fault on his part at all."*

The former test is the test generally used, and was recently confirmed by the Court of Appeal in Wilsher *v* Essex Area Health Authority[7]. In other words, the standard to be expected of a consultant who heads a team sets the standard for the work of the team as a whole. If it were otherwise, the experience of the treating doctor would become a relevant factor, and an inexperienced doctor, while more likely to make mistakes, would be less likely to be successfully sued. If a procedure is beyond the capacity of a junior doctor, it should not be entrusted to him, and if he finds himself out of his depth in the course of a procedure, he should seek the help of a more senior colleague. (This is one of the commonest criticisms in "birth trauma" cases.)

In Whitehouse *v* Jordan[8] Lord Denning sought to redefine medical negligence as something other than "an error of judgement." He proposed putting this question to the average competent and careful practitioner:

"Is this the sort of mistake that you yourself might have made?" If he answers 'Yes, even doing the best I could, it might have happened to me', then it is not negligent."*

When Whitehouse *v* Jordan went to the House of Lords, however, the judgment reaffirmed the Bolam test and deprecated the use of the term "error of judgment":

"It is high time that the unacceptability of such an answer be finally exposed. To say that a surgeon committed an error of clinical judgement is wholly ambiguous, for, while some such errors may be completely consistent with the due exercise of professional skill, other acts of omission in the course of exercising 'clinical judgment' may be so glaringly below proper standards as to make a finding of negligence inevitable... I would have it accepted that the true doctrine was enunciated in Bolam *v* Friern Hospital Management Committee."*

In the light of all this, it is clear that since a great deal of medical treatment, even if administered with all due skill and care, involves some degree of risk, mishaps will occur for which the patient has no remedy[9]. In Mahon v Osborne[10], Scott L.J. discussed the position of the surgeon, which has universal application to the law of negligence, as follows:

"It is not every slip or mistake which imports negligence and, in applying the duty of care to the case of the surgeon, it is peculiarly necessary to have regard to the different kinds of circumstances that may present themselves for urgent attention...."

Causation

The Court applies a different test to the issue of causation. This was considered in the case of Loveday v Renton[11], in which the Court had to decide whether pertussis vaccine could cause permanent brain damage in young children. The question was purely one of causation, and the Plaintiff argued that the court was only concerned to ascertain the general state of medical opinion on the question, not whether that opinion was well founded. Stuart-Smith L.J. disposed of the argument thus:

"It is fundamental to the Bolam test, which is concerned only with the issue of breach of duty, that if a doctor acts in accordance with the practice and opinion of a respectable and responsible body of medical opinion he is not guilty of negligence, even if another respectable and responsible body holds different views ... It is obvious that the court is not concerned to decide the merits of one practice as opposed to others, but only to determine if a respectable and responsible body of medical practitioners would have acted as the Defendant acted. But it is equally obvious that such a test cannot apply to the issue of causation, where the question is: Did the treatment, in this case vaccination, cause brain damage?

"Since by a parity of reasoning if there is a respectable and responsible body of medical opinion which holds the view that it is not proved that the vaccine causes brain damage, a Plaintiff must fail on causation ... the court has to determine the factual issue by weighing and evaluating all the evidence in the case and seeing whether at the end of the day the Plaintiff has discharged the onus of proof on all the evidence. That is the approach I propose to adopt."

The majority of claims arising out of the management of breast cancer founder on the issue of causation. The onus is on the Plaintiff to establish that a failure to diagnose, or a late diagnosis, made a significant difference to the patient's prognosis. Sup-

pose that a Unit has a policy of screening patients every three years, and negligently fails to call a woman for five years, or fails to detect a cancer on mammography. Either

a. the screening would not have picked up any abnormality (in which case there is no loss),
b. the screening would have picked up an abnormality, but the delay makes no difference to the prognosis (in which case there is again no loss), or
c. the woman's life, or breast, could have been saved if the diagnosis had been made earlier.

Only (c) would give rise to a claim for substantial damages, but even then the Plaintiff would have to prove that *no reasonable doctor would have delayed a screening for so long*. Thus, it would not be enough for a Plaintiff to show that a clinic was in breach of *its own* protocols (though this would help her): she must show that the delay was unreasonable by *any* standards.

There may be tension between the protocol of a screening clinic and the circumstances of an individual patient. Although it would be exceedingly difficult for a patient to establish that the protocol was one which no clinic could reasonably operate, it might well be easier to prove that the protocol was applied so rigidly that significant factors were ignored in a particular woman's case. Where a clinic decides it is inappropriate to screen a woman who is asking to be screened, the issue will be whether in *all* the patient's circumstances it was reasonable to refuse.

Innovative practice

Having ascertained the standard of care that a patient was entitled to expect, a Court then goes on to consider how the care provided to the Plaintiff measured up to that standard. Professional practice may change over time so that what was once accepted as the correct procedure is no longer considered to be respectable or responsible. In Bolam, McNair J. pointed out that a medical practitioner cannot

"obstinately and pigheadedly carry on with some old technique if it has been proved to be contrary to what is really substantially the whole of informed medical opinion".[12]

Thus, there is an obligation on doctors to keep up to date with developments -

"Otherwise you might get men today saying: 'I don't believe in anaesthetics. I don't believe in antiseptics. I am going to continue to do my surgery in the way it was done in the eighteenth century.' That would clearly be wrong".[13]

In his book "Professional Negligence", Professor Michael A. Jones says of the doctor's duty to keep up to date:

"There is an inevitable tension between the doctor's obligation to keep up to date, and the trite observation that doctors should not adopt any and every new idea until it has been proved to be both effective and safe. Doctors should not subject patients to untried methods of treatment unless the traditional approach has proved ineffective and the anticipated benefits are justified by the risks. On the other hand, despite the emphasis within many malpractice actions on complying with common practice, the Courts are careful to avoid the suggestion that findings of negligence may stifle innovation. A new technique may carry an unforseen danger, not withstanding the reasonable efforts of the profession to identify risks in advance, and this will not be held negligent."

It goes without saying that a doctor is only to be criticised by the medical standards at the time of his criticised act. See Roe v Minister of Health.[14] Contemporary literature is often of crucial importance, though it is possible to construct too flimsy a case for either the Plaintiff or the Defendant out of too extensive a literature search. Literature must be mainstream: doctors (even specialists) are too busy to read everything. It is always helpful to take standard textbooks as the starting point: if the criticised doctor departed from approved practice and cannot give a satisfactory reason why he did so, a wise Health Authority will not contest the claim:

"One must be careful when considering documents culled for the purpose of a trial, and studied by reference to a single isolated issue, not to forget that they once formed part of a flood of print on numerous aspects of industrial life, in which many items were bound to be overlooked. However conscientious the employer, he cannot read every textbook and periodical, attend every exhibition and conference, on every technical issue which might arise in the course of his business: nor can he necessarily be expected to grasp the importance of every single item which he might come across. Thus, if a works doctor regularly read the "Lancet" from cover to cover he would have seen the modest announcement of the V-51R ear plug in the edition of 28 April 1951 but it would be unrealistic to hold that all shipbuilders and repairers were thereafter on notice of the existence of plastic ear plugs whose manufacturers claimed an attenuation of 30 db."[15]

The fact that a procedure was standard is not necessarily the end of the matter, however. In Clarke v Adams,[16] the Plaintiff was severely burned during a course of heat treatment administered by a physiotherapist. Before the treatment he had been given the warning in the form approved by the Chartered Society of Physiotherapists, but the Court held that this warning was not enough to safeguard him.

What effect does the definition of negligence have on treatment? Does it stifle innovation, or penalise conservatism? In one sense it is bound to favour defensive medicine because a doctor is likely to feel that if a pioneering procedure, never before performed, goes wrong, he will be unable to call up a body of medical opinion in support. The Courts are aware of this problem, however, and are not only prepared to reject an established practice shown to be manifestly wrong, but to approve a practice that had never been tried before:

"I think that, in an appropriate case, a judge would be entitled to reject a unanimous medical view if he were satisfied that it was manifestly wrong and that the doctors would have been misdirecting themselves as to their duty in law."[17]

Nor is innovation precluded by the test. Because the burden is on the Plaintiff to prove that there has been negligence, he cannot simply point to his treatment and say that "innovation = not approved by a reputable body of medical opinion". See Hunter v Hanley.[18]

"It follows from what I have said that in regard to allegations of deviation from ordinary professional practice ... such deviation is not necessarily evidence of negligence. Indeed, it would be disastrous if this were so, for all inducement to progress in medical science would then be destroyed. Even a substantial deviation from normal practice may be warranted by the particular circumstances. To establish liability by a doctor where deviation from normal practice is alleged, three facts require to be established. First of all it must be proved that there is a usual and normal practice; secondly it must be proved that the defender has not adopted that practice; and thirdly (and this is of crucial importance) it must be established that the course the doctor adopted is one which no professional man of ordinary skill would have taken if he had been acting with ordinary care."

Landau v Werner[19] sounds a warning:

"A doctor might not be negligent if he tried a new technique, but if he did he must justify it before the

Court. If his novel or exceptional treatment had failed disastrously he could not complain if it was held that he went beyond the bounds of due care and skill as recognised generally."

In Roe v Minister of Health,[20] Lord Denning made specific mention of the need for the law not to stifle innovation:

"It is so easy to be wise after the event and to condemn as negligence that which was only a misadventure. We ought always to be on our guard against it, especially in cases against hospitals and doctors. Medical science has conferred great benefits on mankind but these benefits are attended by considerable risks. We cannot take the benefits without taking the risks. Every advance in technique is also attended by risks. Doctors, like the rest of us have to learn by experience; and experience often teaches in a hard way. Something goes wrong and shows up a weakness, and then it is put right ....

"We should be doing a disservice to the community at large if we were to impose liability on hospitals and doctors for everything that happens to go wrong. Doctors would be led to think more of their own safety than of the good of their patients. Initiative would be stifled and confidence shaken. A proper sense of proportion requires us to have regard to the conditions in which hospitals and doctors have to work. We must insist on due care for the patient at every point, but we must not condemn as negligence that which is only a misadventure."

Where a practitioner is embarking on a novel treatment, he is under a greater duty than usual to inform and warn the patient.

Disclosure of risks

The Bolam test governs all aspects of the practitioner - patient relationship, from initial information, through diagnosis and advice, to treatment and aftercare. In Sidaway[21] the House of Lords considered the duty of disclosure to a patient of the advantages and disadvantages or risks and benefits of a proposed course of treatment, and held that the issue of whether non-disclosure of a particular risk in a particular case should be condemned as a breach of the doctor's duty of care is an issue to be decided primarily on the basis of expert medical evidence, although a Judge might in certain circumstances come to the conclusion that disclosure of a particular risk was so obviously necessary to an informed choice on the part of the patient that no reasonably prudent medical man

would fail to make it. The House of Lords rejected the alternative view that different standards should apply to the disclosure of risks, as was the law in Canada. In upholding the Bolam test, Lord Bridge specifically referred to the following passage in the Canadian case of Reibl v Hughes:[22]

"To allow expert medical evidence to determine what risks are material and, hence, should be disclosed and, correlatively, what risks are not material is to hand over to the medical profession the entire question of the scope of the duty of disclosure, including the question whether there had been a breach of that duty. Expert medical evidence is, of course relevant to a finding of risks that reside in or are a result of recommended surgery or other treatment. It should also have a bearing on their materiality but this is not a question that is to be concluded on the basis of the expert medical evidence alone. The issue under consideration is a different issue from that involved where the question is whether the doctor carried out his professional activities by applicable professional standards. What is under consideration here is the patient's right to know what risks are involved in undergoing or foregoing certain surgery or other treatment."

It is not enough for a court to determine that a doctor did not give the patient appropriate warnings about a procedure or treatment. If the warning *was* inappropriate, what would the patient have done when given an appropriate warning?

The Court applies a subjective test in determining what the patient would have chosen if properly informed - see Ellis v Wallsend District Hospital.[23] This raises a difficulty, because a doctor's opinion that a course of treatment is desirable may lead him to soft-pedal the warnings, and the patient may well end up either saying "What would *you* advise, doctor?", or getting the subliminal message that the treatment is one of which the doctor approves.

Conclusion

Clinical considerations should guide clinical decisions. Even the most diehard Plaintiff's lawyer would not expect doctors to practice with one eye on the Bolam test - and in refining the test over the years the courts have tried to strike a balance between the need to protect patients and the need for the medical profession to have a free hand in taking clinical decisions. Properly considered, the law of negligence does not inhibit advances in medicine; nor does it foster conservative treatment for safety's sake.

References

1. Mills D.H.: Medical Insurance Feasibility study. *West J. Med.* 1978: 128:360-368
2. [1985] AC 871 at 897
3. [1835] 1 C & P 31
4. [1957] 1 WLR 582 at 587
5. [1993] MLR 393
6. [1987] QB 730
7. [1987] 2 WLR 425 esp. per Mustill LJ at 439-440
8. [1980] 1 All ER 650 at 658
9. See e.g. White v. Board of Governors of Westminster Hospital, (The Times, October 26, 1961), where the retina was accidentally cut. There are a series of cases following this line: Kapur v. Marshall (1978) 85 DLR (3d) 567, through to Ashcroft v. Mersey RHA [1983] 2 All ER 245, which was affirmed on appeal [1985] 2 All ER 96.
10. [1939] 2 KB 14
11. [1990] 1 MLR 117
12. [1957] 2 All ER 118, 122.
13. McNair J in Bolam
14. [1954] 2 QB 66
15. Mustill J. in Thompson v Smiths Ship Repairers (North Shields) Ltd [1984] QB 405 at 422
16. (1950) 94 SJ 599
17. Sidaway v Board of Governors of the Bethlem Royal and Maudsley Hospital [1985] AC 871
18. [1955] S.C. 200
19. (1961) 105 Sol Jo 1008
20. *Supra*
21. *Supra*
22. 114 DLR (3d) 1
23. [1990] 2 MLR 103)

The prevention of breast cancer: recent progress and future developments

T.J. Powles, J. Chang

Introduction

Breast cancer affects one in fourteen women in the United Kingdom and results in 150,000 deaths each year in Europe. Breast cancer remains the commonest cause of death in women aged 35 to 45 years (Cancer Statistics, 1988). Metastatic breast cancer is still incurable. Despite mammographic screening, modern surgical techniques and adjuvant chemo-endocrine therapy, approximately 50% of patients die of the disease. There has consequently been a search for a suitable agent for the prevention of breast cancer.

The design of chemoprevention trials

Before large-scale trials of chemoprevention involving healthy women are embarked upon, there must be a defined population at sufficiently high risk to counterbalance any potential short and long term toxicity of the chosen drug. Epidemiological factors which confer higher risk include increasing age, early menarche, late menopause, nulliparity

Table I. Risk factors for breast cancer.

Risk factor	Relative risk
Family history	
One first degree relative	2
Two first degree relatives	4
Relative with bilateral disease	5
Benign breast disease	
Biopsy proven	2
Atypical ductal/lobular hyperplasia	3-4
Lobular carcinoma in situ	10
Nulliparity/ 1st child >30 yrs	1.5

and first pregnancy at more than 30 years. The easiest high risk group to define includes women with a positive family history who have at least one affected relative (sister, mother, daughter). This risk is further increased with increasing numbers of affected relatives, relatives diagnosed under the age of 40 years or a relative with bilateral breast cancer (Table I).

Statistical considerations

A large sample size would be required to give adequate statistical power to produce a significant difference between the intervention and placebo arms. Hence, before multicentre studies could be designed, feasibility pilot trials were set up to assess the logistics of such a study and the level of compliance in a healthy population.

Suitable agents for chemoprevention

Tamoxifen

Tamoxifen is a non-steroidal triphenylethylene derivative with both oestrogenic and anti-oestrogenic properties.

This drug has been used since 1971 to treat in excess of 5 million women world-wide with all stages of breast cancer. It is highly effective in the treatment of metastatic breast cancer.[33] When used as adjuvant therapy, tamoxifen is effective in delaying relapse and prolonging survival in about 30% of women.[3]

The strongest argument for its use as a potential chemoprevention agent is the decrease in contralateral breast cancers in women on adjuvant tamoxifen. The overall analysis of 30,000 women showed a 39% reduction in contralateral tumours in women receiving tamoxifen as adjuvant therapy.[7]

Retinoids

Retinoids are natural and synthetic analogues of vitamin A. The clinical use of retinoids have been limited by mainly hepatic toxicity. Fenretinide or N-(4-hydroxy phenyl) retinamide is a new synthetic retinoid which has a more favourable toxicity profile. This drug has not led to an increase in hepatic abnormalities in phase I studies. There have been reports of impairment of dark adaptation with a 23% incidence of mild and 26% incidence of moderate impairment. Current studies allow a 3 day gap at the end of each month to minimise this side effect. Fenretinide is currently under investigation to evaluate the possible reduction in contralateral new primaries in women with resected early breast cancer.[5,13,32]

If found to be effective in preventing second primary cancers, fenretinide may be a potential agent in clinical trials involving healthy high risk women.

Synergism between tamoxifen and fenretinide has been found in Sprague-Dawley rats and this combination is currently under investigation as a phase I study in women with metastatic breast cancer.[6]

Gonadotrophin-releasing hormone agonists

Bilateral oophorectomy substantially reduces the incidence of breast cancer,[20] and therefore it may be possible that LHRH agonists in pre-menopausal wom-en may have a similar effect. The anticipated long term toxicity would be associated with chronic oes-trogen depletion, in particular accelerated bone loss and cardiovascular disease. It may be possible to give low doses of oestrogen replacement without losing any protective effect on the breast.[24] This type of regimen would be complicated to administer but may be necessary if tamoxifen was found to be ineffective in pre-menopausal women.

Diet

The role of high unsaturated fat intake remains controversial although an overview analysis of over 10,000 women has shown a correlation with breast cancer.[12] It would be difficult to set up a randomised study in ensuring compliance in the intervention arm and a standard high fat intake in the control arm.

Side effects and long term sequelae of tamoxifen

Acute toxicity

Compliance with tamoxifen is high with only 4% of adjuvant patients withdrawing from treatment because of acute toxicity. In a randomised pilot che-moprevention feasibility study of 2,000 healthy wom-en, acute toxicity was again found to be low with a corresponding high compliance of 77% in women on

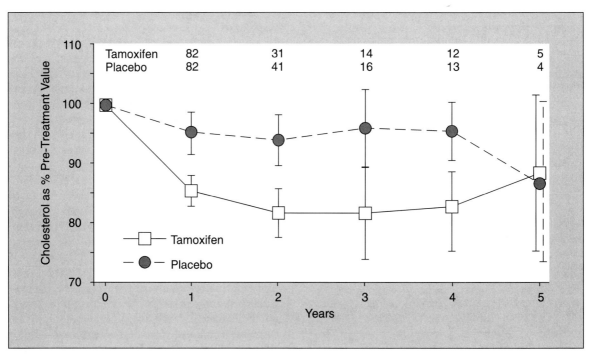

Fig. 1. Effect of tamoxifen on total serum cholesterol.

tamoxifen and 82% in women receiving placebo.[27] There was a significant increase in hot flushes (34% *versus* 20%) found predominantly in pre-menopausal women, vaginal discharge (16% *versus* 4%) and menstrual irregularities (14% *versus* 9%).

Serum cholesterol

As with adjuvant studies (Love *et al.*, 1990)[19] tamoxifen results in a reduction in total plasma cholesterol by 15% to 20% of pretreatment values when used in a prevention study and this change is sustained throughout treatment.[25-27]

These changes in plasma cholesterol are similar to the effects seen with oestrogen replacement therapy and suggest that tamoxifen has an oestrogenic effect on cholesterol metabolism in the liver.[2] This reduction in plasma cholesterol may account for the observed 60% reduction in fatal myocardial infarction in women on adjuvant tamoxifen.[22]

Coagulation factors

In a pilot prevention programme,[14] tamoxifen resulted in reduction of plasma fibrinogen, changes in antithrombin III and cross-linked fibrinogen degradation products. Any decrease in fibrinogen or degradation products might be expected to be associated with a decrease in arterial disease. Apart from one trial involving a small number of events,[7] there have been no reports from randomised trials of increased risk of thrombo-embolism in patients on tamoxifen.

Bone mineral density

Two randomised adjuvant trials in predominantly post-menopausal women have shown that tamoxifen given over 2 years is associated with an increase in bone mineral density.[17,19]

Recent published data using dual energy x-ray absorptiometry in a prevention study has shown significant protective effect in both the femoral neck and lumbar spine of post-menopausal women. In contrast, tamoxifen had an opposite effect in pre-menopausal women with significant reduction in bone mineral density in both femoral neck and lumbar spine during the first 2 years of tamoxifen medication.[28]

Gynaecological effects

Annual screening with transvaginal ultrasound has shown an increase in benign ovarian cysts in pre-menopausal women.[27] Adjuvant tamoxifen has not been associated with an increased risk of ovarian cancers (EBCTC, 1992).[9]

Tamoxifen in post-menopausal women results in endometrial hyperplasia with a consequent increased risk of endometrial cancer. At higher doses of 40 mg daily, the reported increased risk is about sixfold[9] compared to a 2 to 3 fold increased risk at a standard dose of 20 mg daily.[31] Screening for endometrial thickening with transvaginal ultrasound and colour doppler may identify women at risk of endometrial pathology.[16]

Other carcinogenic risks

Tamoxifen has been shown to form stable DNA adducts *in vitro*.[11,34] In some strains of rats but not in mice or hamsters, high levels of stable DNA adducts have been detected by ^{32}P-post labelling of rat livers. There has been no increase in adduct formation in liver tissue obtained from women on tamoxifen compared to placebo.[21] To date, in both adjuvant and preventative trials, the data at present indicates no evidence for increased risk in liver or other cancers (apart from the endometrial risk) in women on tamoxifen 20 mg daily. At 40 mg daily, the Scandinavian adjuvant trial suggests a possible increase in gastro-intestinal tumours.[29]

Other toxicities

High dose tamoxifen (180 mg/day) is associated with a characteristic retinopathy and keratopathy. At lower doses, one study has indicated evidence of retinopathy in 4 out of 63 patients[23] but this is not confirmed in other controlled studies.[18]

Acute hepatic toxicity[1] and agranulocytosis have been reported as anecdotal events.[4]

In summary, tamoxifen is well tolerated with high compliance and few acute side effects. There are favourable effects on total plasma cholesterol and bone mineral density in post-menopausal women. There is no concrete evidence for increase in thrombo-embolic events or clotting abnormalities. Pelvic screening with transvaginal ultrasound and colour doppler is recommended to detect any endometrial abnormalities.

Current ongoing clinical trials

The Royal Marsden pilot trial

This study was commenced in 1986 and aimed to evaluate the logistic, ethical and clinical problems related to a chemoprevention trial using tamoxifen in healthy women. Use of tamoxifen in a prevention setting required identification of high risk women volunteers and the development of stringent safety monitoring criteria and close clinical surveillance. This feasibility study is now complete having recruited 2500 women.

It has shown that healthy women can be accrued in tamoxifen trials and that the toxicity profile (acute side effects, bone, lipid and gynaecological assessment) is encouraging. The overall results indicate that the potential benefits, to date, outweigh any risks that may be associated with its use in a prevention trial.

NSABP breast cancer prevention trial

Favourable results from initial pilot studies have encouraged the establishment of multicentre trials in the USA, UK and Italy. The NSABP prevention study was commenced in 1992.[8-10] This double-blind, placebo-controlled trial is being conducted in 288 centres in the USA and Canada and a total accrual of 16000 women is planned. Preliminary results were releasey to the press recently.* Women taking tamoxifen daily for an average of four years had 45% fewer diagnosis of breast cancer. Tamoxifen use, however, also increased the risk of endometrial cancer, pulmonary embolism and deep vein thrombosis.

Other national studies

In the Italian trial, based at the Milan Cancer Institute, eligibility is limited to women who have previously undergone hysterectomy in order to eliminate any increased risk of endometrial cancer. In the UK, over 1400 healthy women have been included in a multicentre trial which also includes centres in Australia and Scandinavia. In view of the fears regarding the potential carcinogenic risk of tamoxifen, further recruitment into these national studies may become increasingly difficult.

Future developments

Tamoxifen analogues

Various synthetic analogues of tamoxifen such as toremifene, droloxifene and raloxifene have not been shown to be experimentally genotoxic[15] and are now in clinical development.

Of these agents, toremifene has been the most extensively used. Initial phase II studies indicate similar response rates and toxicity profile to tamoxifen.[30]

The absence of genotoxicity, together with its clinical and experimental profile make toremifene an attractive next candidate for feasibility testing in chemoprevention trials.

---

*: K. Smigel: News. J. Nat. Canc. Inst. 1998; 90: 647-648

Discussion

In breast cancer chemoprevention, there are a number of feasible candidates. Tamoxifen is the most extensively used with advantages in terms of efficacy in established disease, low acute toxicity and relatively low cost. There is controversy regarding the age at which to start intervention. Pre- and peri-menopausal women are most likely to benefit but this has to be balanced against potential risks and side effects in younger women.

The optimal duration of intervention is again uncertain and in most trials, tamoxifen is continued from 5 to 10 years. This long term exposure has necessitated stringent safety monitoring. The current evidence suggests that the benefits of tamoxifen are likely to outweigh the potential drawbacks, but pelvic screening with transvaginal ultrasound and colour doppler is recommended for post-menopausal women. The efficacy of tamoxifen as a chemopreventive agent for breast cancer will only be answered by long term follow up of women enrolled in these large multicentre clinical trials.

References

1. Blackburn A., Amiel S., Millis R., Rubens R.: Tamoxifen and liver damage. Br. Med. J. 1984; 289: 288
2. Bush T.L., Fried L.P., Barratt-Connor. Cholesterol lipoproteins and coronary heart disease in women. Clin. Chem. 1988; 34: B60-70
3. Cancer Research Campaign Breast Cancer Trials Group: The effect of adjuvant tamoxifen: the latest results from the Cancer Research Campaign Adjuvant Breast Trial. Eur. J. Cancer, 1992; 28A(4-5): 904-907
4. Ching C., Smith P.G., Long R.G.: Tamoxifen-associated hepatocellular damage and agranulocytosis. Lancet 1992; 339: 940
5. Costa A., Formelli F., Chiesa F., et al.: Prospects of chemoprevention of human cancers with the synthetic retinoid fenretinide. Cancer Res (suppl.) 1994; 54: 2032s-2037s
6. Costa A.: Breast cancer chemoprevention. Eur. J. Cancer, 1993; 29A (4): 589-592. EBCTCG: Systemic treatment of early breast cancer by hormonal, cytotoxic, or immune therapy. Lancet, 1992; 339: 1-15, 71-85
7. Fisher B., Contantino J., Redmond C., et al.: A randomised clinical trial evaluating tamoxifen in the treatment of patients with node-negative breast cancer who have oestrogen receptor positive tumours. N. Engl. J. Med. 1989; 320: 479-489
8. Fisher B., Constantino J., Redmond C.K., et al.: Endometrial cancer in tamoxifen-treated breast cancer patients: findings from the National Surgical Adjuvant Breast and Bowel Project (NSABP) B14. J. Natl. Cancer Inst. 1994; 86: 527-573
9. Fornander T., Hellstrom A.C., Moberger B.: Descriptive clinico-pathologic study of 17 patients with endometrial cancer during or after adjuvant tamoxifen in early breast cancer. J. Natl. Cancer Inst. 1993; 85: 1850-1855
10. Gail M.H., Brintom L.A., Byar D.P., et al.: Projecting individualised probabilities of developing breast cancer for white females who are examined annually. J. Natl. Cancer Inst. 1989; 81: 1879-1886
11. Han X., Liehr J.G.: Induction of covalent DNA adducts in rodents by tamoxifen. Cancer Research 1992; 52: 1360- 1363
12. Howe G.R., Hirollata T., Hislop G., et al.: Dietary factors and the

risk of breast cancer: combined analysis of 12 case-control studies. J. Natl. Cancer Inst. 1990; 82: 561-569

13. Jordan V.C.: Effect of tamoxifen (ICI 46,474) on initiation and growth of DMBA-induced rat mammary carcinomata. Eur. J. Cancer, 1976; 12: 41 9-424

14. Jones A.L., Powles T.J., Treleaven J., et al.: Haemostatic changes and thromboembolic risk during tamoxifen therapy in normal women. Br. J. Cancer 1992; 66: 744-7747

15. Kanga L., Nieman A.L., Blanco G., et al.: A new triphenylethylene compound, Fc- 1 1 57a.II Antitumour effect. Cancer Chemother. Pharmacol. 1986; 17: 109-113

16. Kedar R.P., Bourne T.H., Powles T.J. et al.: Effects of tamoxifen on the uterus oand ovaries of postmenopausal women in a randomised breast cancer prevention trial. Lancet 1994: 343: 1318-1321

17. Kristensen B., Ejiersten B., Dalgaard P., et al.: Tamoxifen and bone metabolism in postmenopausal low-risk breast cancer patients: a randomised study. J. Clin. Oncology, 1994; 12: 992-997

18. Longstaff S., Sigurdsson H., O. Keeffe M., et al.: A controlled study of the ocular effects of tamoxifen in conventional dosage in the treatment of breast carcinoma. Eur. J. Cancer Clin. Oncol. 1989; 25: 1805-1808

19. Love R.R., Newcomb P.A., Wiebe D.A., et al.: Effects of tamoxifen therapy on lipid and lipoprotein levels in postmenopausal patients with node negative breast cancer. J. Natl. Cancer Instit. 1990; 82: 1327-1332

20. MacMahon B., Feinlieb M.: Breast cancer in relation to nursing and menopausal history. J. Natl. Cancer Inst. 1960; 24: 733-753

21. Martin E.A., Rich J.R., White I.N.H,. et al.: ^{32}P-Post labelled DNA adducts in liver obtained from women treated with tamoxifen. Carcinogenesis, 1995; 16: 1651-1654

22. McDonald C.C., Stewart H.J.: Fatal myocardial infarction in the Scottish adjuvant trial. The Scottish Breast Cancer Committee. Br. J. Cancer, 1991; 303:435-437

23. Pavlidis N., Petris C., Briassoulis E., et al.: Clear evidence that low-dose tamoxifen treatment can induce ocular toxicity. Cancer, 1992; 69: 2961-2964

24. Pike M.C., Spicer D.V.: The chemoprevention of breast cancer by reducing sex steroid exposure: perspectives from epidemiology. J. Cell. Biochm. Suppl. 1993; 17G: 26-36

25. Powles T.J., Hardy J.R., Ashley S.E.: A pilot trial to evaluate the acute toxicity and feasibility of tamoxifen for prevention of breast cancer. Br. J. Cancer, 1989; 60: 126-131

26. Powles T.J., Tillyer C., Jones A.J., et al.: Prevention of breast cancer with tamoxifen - an update on the Royal Marsden pilot programme. Eur. J. Cancer, 1990; 26: 680-682

27. Powles T.J., Jones A.J., Ashley S.E., et al.: The Royal Marsden Hospital pilot tamoxifen chemoprevention trial. Breast Cancer Res and Treat l994; 3l: 73-82

28. Powles T.J., Hickish T., Kanis J.A., et al.: The effect of tamoxifen on bone mineral density measured by dual energy x-ray absorptiometry in healthy pre and postmenopausal women. J. Clin. Onco 1996; 14(1): 78-84

29. Rutqvist L.E., Johallson H., Signomklao U.l. et al.: Adjuvant tamoxifen for early stage breast cancer and second primary malignancies. J. Natl. Cancer Inst., l995; 87(9): 645-51

30. Valvaara R.: Phase II trials with toremifene in advanced breast cancer. Breast Cancer Res. Treat. 1990 (Suppl.); 16: s31-s35

31. van Leeuwen F.E., Benraadt J., Coebergh J.W. et al.: Risk of endometrial cancer after tamoxifen treatment of breast cancer. Lancet, 1994; 343: 448-452

32. Veronesi U., De Palo G., Costa A., et al.: Chemoprevention of breast cancer with retinoids. J. Natl. Cancer Inst. 1992; 12:93-97

33. Ward H.W.C.: Antioestrogen therapy for breast cancer. A trial of tamoxifen at low dose levels. Br. Med. J. 1973, 1: 13-15

34. White I.N., de Matteis F., Davies A. et al.: Genotoxic potential of tamoxifen and analogues in female Fischer F344/n rats, DBA/2 and C57BL/6 mice and in human MCL-5 cells. Carcinogenesis, 1992; 13: 2197-2203

Mammographic screening in women under age 50: a critical appraisal

I. Jatoi, M. Baum

Mammographic screening for women under the age of 50 continues to be a subject of intense controversy.[1] Although common practice in the United States, it is generally not recommended in Europe. The rift between the American and European views became apparent in February, 1993. The American Cancer Society (ACS) and the European Society of Mastology (EUSOMA) met in New York and Paris, respectively, to review the results of the various clinical trials on screening for younger women.

After reviewing the same data, the two organizations arrived at opposite conclusions: the ACS reaffirmed its longstanding recommendation of screening women starting at age 40 while EUSOMA recommended that screening be reserved for women above the age of 50. Perhaps this reflects a cultural bias: the European willingness to accept the results of clinical trials at face value, and the American reluctance to accept those trials which fail to support a common sense view. Nonetheless, although the ACS guidelines are generally followed in the United States, and the EUSOMA guidelines generally practiced in Europe, there are opponents and proponents of screening for younger women on both sides of the Atlantic. Recently, the National Cancer Institute of the United States (NCI) elected to make no recommendation on screening younger women, but instead issued the statement that "randomized controlled trials had not shown a statistically significant reduction in mortality in women under age 50".[2] Two other influential American organizations, the American College of Physicians and the United States Preventive Services Task Force do not recommend breast cancer screening for women younger than 50 years.[3]

Biases of clinical studies

More is known about screening for breast cancer than about screening for any other type of cancer.

Over the past 30 years, various methods have been used to study the efficacy of mammographic screening: case control studies, retrospective analyses, and prospective series. All these methods have potential shortcomings. In particular, there are three biases that must be considered in trials that examine the efficacy of screening mammography: lead time, length, and selection. An understanding of these is necessary before discussing the relevant clinical trials. Ultimately, the success of screening mammography should be measured by its ability to reduce mortality, not by its ability to extend survival from point of diagnosis.

Lead time bias is the interval between the diagnosis of cancer on mammography and the time when the cancer becomes apparent clinically. Lead time bias may make it appear that screening prolongs life when in fact it simply increases the period over which a disease is observed. Retrospective studies which compare survival between screened and unscreened populations fail to account for lead time bias and are therefore flawed. A good example is the comparison of the retrospective study of Stacey-Clear *et al.* with the Canadian prospective breast screening trials.[4,5] Both showed good five year survival for younger women who underwent mammographic screening. However, at seven years, the Canadian study showed a non-significant excess in mortality in the screened group, which could only be explained by assuming a lead time bias of up to four years.

Length bias relates to the fact that screening tends to detect those tumours with a better prognosis. Slower growing tumours (those with a better prognosis) exist for a longer period in the preclinical phase, and are therefore more likely to be diagnosed by mammographic screening. In contrast, the faster growing tumours exist for a shorter period of time in the preclinical phase, and are therefore less likely to be detected at screening. Thus, length bias invalidates comparisons of tumours detected by screening mammography with those detected by physical examination. The impact of length bias is best seen when cancers detected by screening are compared with interval cancers (cancers detected between screening sessions).[6] The interval cancers are not detected during screening, are often rapidly progressive, and carry a poor prognosis.

Those clinical trials which recruit volunteers contain a selection bias. Women who volunteer for screening are more likely to be health conscious, and have a lower all-cause mortality. The impact of selection bias was illustrated in a case-control evaluation of the effect of breast cancer screening in the United Kingdom, comparing attenders and non-attenders for screening.[7] By comparing populations from two separate districts (one a breast cancer screening district and the other a comparison district), breast cancer mortality was found to be relatively higher among non-attenders in the screening district. The investigators attributed this to selection bias.

Randomized prospective studies

All these biases can be excluded by comparing screened and unscreened populations in a randomized study with all-cause mortality as the end point, and cause-specific mortality as a questionable surrogate end point. There have been eight randomized prospective trials designed to evaluate the efficacy of mammographic screening, and of these, seven have evaluated its impact on mortality reduction in women less than 50 years of age: the Health Insurance Plan (HIP), Swedish two-county, Malmö, Stockholm, Goteborg, Edinburgh, and the first Canadian National Breast Screening Study (NBSS 1) (Table I). Only the Canadian National Breast Screening Study (NBSS 1) was specifically designed to evaluate mammographic screening in women under the age of 50, while the others studied the impact of screening on women of a broad age range.

The HIP was the first randomized control trial of mammographic screening for breast cancer (initiated in 1963), and it demonstrated a 25% relative reduction in mortality in screened women under the age of 50.[8] The study involved 62,000 women between the ages of 40 and 64 of the HIP medical insurance scheme of New York who were randomly assigned to either a study or control group of 31,000 women each. However, the HIP was not designed specifically to assess the potential benefits of screening younger women, and a benefit was not seen in women under the age of 50 until 10-18 years after entry in the study. This leads to an important question: would these women have obtained the same benefit if screening had started after the age of 50? It is also important to understand the design of the HIP study: screening was carried out with a physical examination as well as a mammogram. Ultimately, only 19% of breast cancers were detected exclusively by mammography, and the majority (57%) were detected by physical examination alone. Thus, the HIP cannot be used to justify mammographic screening of younger women. If anything, it suggests that physical examination may have an important role to play as a screening modality.

The Edinburgh Trial was a randomized clinical trial involving 45,130 women between the ages of 45 and 64 which was initiated in 1979.[9] Women in the

Table I. Randomized prospective studies of screening mammography, involving women less than 50 years of age.

Trial	Age at entry	Duration of follow up	Relative risk of death from breast cancer for women younger than 50 (95% confidence interval)
HIP	40-64	5	0.95 (0.51-1.78)
		10	0.77 (0.50-1.16)
		18	0.75 (0.52-1.09)
Swedish 2-counties	40-74	6	1.26 (0.56-2.84)
		8	0.92 (0.52-1.60)
		11	1.03 (0.65-1.63)
Malmö	45-69	12	0.51 (0.22-1.17)
Stockholm	40-64	8	1.04 (0.53-2.05)
Goteborg	40-59	7	0.73 (0.27-1.97)
Edinburgh	45-64	7	0.98 (0.45-2.11)
Canadian (NBSSI)	40-49	7	1.39 (0.84-2.21)

study group received screening mammography and clinical examinations while the control group received no screening. There were only 5,913 women less than 50 years of age enrolled in the study. After seven years, there was a non-significant mortality reduction of 17% (relative risk of 0.83, 95% CI: 0.58-1.18) among all women screened, but this benefit was almost completely confined to women over the age of 50. If the small number of younger women were considered alone, the relative risk of death in the screened group in comparison to the control group was 0.98 (95% CI: 0.45-2.11).

The overview of the combined Swedish trials, involving about 90,000 women under the age of 50, showed a 13% (95% CI: 37% to -20%) decrease in mortality for the study group of women between the ages of 40-49, after 12 years of follow up, but this was not statistically different from the control group.[10] Assuming that the risk of a 40-year-old developing breast cancer over 10 years is 1.0%, and her risk of dying of it is 0.5% (worst case scenario), then the Swedish overview would suggest that screening would result in an absolute risk reduction of 0.5% X 13%, or 0.065% in women between 40-49 years of age.

The Canadian National Breast Screening Study (NBSS I) is the only randomized prospective study specifically designed to address the efficacy of screening for women between the ages of 40-49, and has generated immense controversy in the medical literature and the lay press.[5] The total number of women enrolled in the NBSS I was 50,430. The NBSS I was designed with enough statistical power to detect at least a 40% reduction in mortality by screening. After seven years, there was a non-significant excess in mortality in the screened group, the relative risk in the screened group being 1.36 (95% CI: 0.84 to 2.21). In the NBSS I, the screened group received mammography and physical examination on an annual basis for 4 or 5 examinations while the control group received an initial physical examination upon entry and thereafter follow up by mail. In the NBSS II (women between the ages of 50-59), the study group women were offered physical examination and mammography while the control group was offered physical examination alone.

Whereas five other randomized prospective trials have demonstrated a significant reduction in mortality when women over the age of 50 are screened with mammography alone (compared to women who receive no mammography and no physical examination), the NBSS II demonstrated no such reduction in mortality, suggesting that mammography adds little to mortality reduction above and beyond the benefits of physical examination alone.

Thus, like the HIP, the NBSS suggests that physical examination deserves further consideration as a screening modality.

Critics of the NBSS have charged that in the first 2 years of the study over 50% of the mammograms were technically inadequate, and that neither the equipment nor the training of the radiologists were properly standardized.[11] However, these claims are probably unfounded. It should seem apparent that in a large study such as this, total standardization would be impractical, and that the NBSS represented the true technology and the skills of the radiologists of the communities at the time the study was undertaken. We also note with irony that no such criticisms were levelled against the HIP Study which used techniques and standards now considered obsolete, suggesting a double standard for those only willing to reinforce their prejudice!

The NBSS has also been criticized on the grounds that there was contamination of the control group: about 26% of the unscreened population had "diagnostic" mammograms to evaluate palpable breast masses.[12] The critics argue that mammography is not particularly useful as a "diagnostic" procedure, and that in a symptomatic woman, the benefit comes from screening the ipsilateral and contralateral breast for clinically occult cancer. Thus, some believe that the NBSS in fact compared screened women with other screened women, and that this might account for the lack of mortality reduction in the study group. However, it seems unlikely that such mammograms would serve to change significantly the outcome of such a large study. Given the standard practice of medicine in the world today, it would be impossible to run a trial in which women presenting with palpable breast masses were denied mammography, and proceeded directly with an excisional biopsy.

Perhaps the most definitive evidence on the impact of mammographic screening of younger women on mortality reduction will come from the large randomized controlled trial now underway in the United Kingdom.[13] In this study, women will be aged 40 to 41 at entry. A study group of 65,000 women will be offered mammography at the first visit and annually thereafter for 7 or 8 rounds, while a comparison group of 135,000 women will be offered the usual care with no screening. Upon reaching the age of 50, both groups will be offered regular screening. A follow up of 14 to 15 years is planned, and the study has been designed to give 80% power to detect a mortality reduction of 20%, assuming that 70% of the women accept the offer to undergo screening.

A recent meta-analysis on the efficacy of mammographic screening was undertaken by Kerlikowske et al., reviewing all the seven randomized prospective trials as well as one case control study (the Nijmegen project).[14] For women between the ages of

40 and 49, the Authors found that at 7 to 9 years of follow up, there was a non-significant increase of 2% (95% CI: -18% to 27%) in breast cancer mortality, whereas at 10 to 12 years follow up, there was a non-significant mortality reduction of 17% (95% CI: -35% to 6%). Could these differences be related to the menopause? Perhaps what we are seeing is an immediate benefit from screening post-menopausal women, and a delayed benefit to screening pre-menopausal women (no benefit until these women become post-menopausal). Thus, age may simply be an approximate reflection of menopausal status. Had the clinical trials categorized women based upon their menopausal status rather than age, a more significant difference between the younger and older women might have become apparent.

Why should mammographic screening be beneficial to older women but not younger women? This question is wide open to speculation. The epidemiology of breast cancer varies widely between the two groups, and this is primarily, although not exclusively, attributed to the menopause.[3] There are, for example, changes in the incidence of breast cancer that occur in most populations around the time of the menopause: a steep rise in incidence occurs until about the age of 45 to 55 and this is followed by a less rapid increase thereafter. Changes in tumour characteristics are also apparent: tumours of younger women have a lower proportion of oestrogen receptor positive tumours and a higher labeling index. There are also differences in risk factors for breast cancer that change with the menopause: in many studies, obesity is associated with a higher risk of postmenopausal breast cancer but a lower risk of pre-menopausal cancer. Thus, the difference seen in mammographic screening for younger and older women is consistent with previous observations on the epidemiology and biology of breast cancer.

However, speculation as to the specific reasons for the differences seen in mammographic screening continues to run rampant, and we can only mention a few. Van Netten has proposed an intriguing hypothesis based on observations from medico-legal necropsies showing that *in situ* breast carcinomas are not uncommon in younger women.[15] Although it has generally been presumed that infiltrating carcinoma of the breast may be derived from *in situ* carcinoma, the mechanism is unknown. Van Netten has suggested that tissue injury in areas of *in situ* carcinoma could be an important factor. Blows to the breast or severe compression could result in spillage or dislocation of *in situ* carcinoma cells into the surrounding stroma, where these cells could then interact with macrophages, resulting in invasion or distant spread. As much as 25 kg of compression is applied to the breast during mammography, and young women would be particularly vulnerable to this sort of trauma: as women grow older, the chances of accidental trauma to external organs such as the breast increase, and mammographic trauma becomes less of an issue. While such an explanation may seem far fetched, it is of interest that Egan found that breast cancer mortality was twice as high among women with mammographically dense breasts (DY and P2 groups of Wolfe's parenchymal patterns)[16] than in women with less dense breasts (N1 and P1 groups of Wolfe's parenchymal patterns), and Levallius has suggested that this could be due to the much greater compression force required during mammography of the more dense breasts.[17]

It has also been suggested that interval cancers (cancers arising between mammographic screens), may account for the difference in mortality reduction between younger and older women. Tabar has observed that in the Swedish Two-County study, the rate of interval cancers were much higher in the 40-49 age group than in the other age groups.[18] This finding is contrary to what one might expect: Adami has shown that breast cancers arising in women between the ages of 40-49 have the best overall prognosis, which would indicate a slower growth rate for cancers of this age group relative to those of older women.[19] This would lead one to expect a lower incidence of interval cancers in women between the ages of 40-49. Nonetheless, interval cancers appear to be a significant factor to consider in all screening programs. In the Nijmegen project, after seven rounds of screening, the interval cancer rate peaked at 24.9/10,000 whereas the rate of cancer detected by screening was between 29.5-38.9/10,000.[20] The high incidence of interval cancers recently documented in an NHS screening programme may well mean that the stated target of reducing breast cancer mortality in the U.K. by 25% by the year 2000 will not be met.[21]

Kopans has argued that there are insufficient numbers of women under the age of 50 in the world's screening trials, and that the trials therefore lack power to detect a statistically significant reduction in mortality.[12] He has estimated that a trial that could prove a 25% mortality reduction at 5 years for women between the ages of 40-49 would require about 500,000 women. Proponents of screening for younger women also argue that technology has improved over the years, and that mammographic equipment today is better able to detect earlier breast tumours.[22] Thus, they argue, the trials of the past are not indicative of what can be achieved using the more modern technology of today. Although these are valid criticisms, the bigger question is how to deal with the solutions. It would be very difficult to conduct a screening trial involving such a large number of women as has been proposed by Kopans. The biggest trial to date has been the Canadian study, involving over 50,000 women, and a trial involving 10 times this number of women will probably never be conducted. And, in regard to the technology issue: technology is constantly improving, but it would be impractical to conduct a new trial every time there is an improvement in mammographic technology. Furthermore, in the face of hazards to be described in the next section the onus of proof is on the proponents of screening who would have us accept the intervention on trust alone.

Hazards of screening

If there is no evidence that mammographic screening reduces mortality in younger women, then is it justifiable to continue to screen these women? It would seem not, because there are at least 5 harmful effects of mammographic screening: cost, lead time, radiation exposure, false positives, and over-diagnosis (Table II).[1]

Cost

In recent years, health care costs have increased dramatically, and governments around the world are attempting to reduce those costs. In light of this, attention has focused on the cost of mammographic screening of younger women, particularly as there is as yet no evidence to suggest that it is beneficial in reducing mortality from breast cancer. Eddy has estimated that, in the United States alone, the cost of screening women aged 40-50 will be over $402 million by the year 2000.[23] Recently, Kattlove analyzed the expense and benefits of mammographic screening of a hypothetical American health care organization of 500,000 individuals in which 360 new cases of breast cancer are diagnosed each year.[24] The most cost-effective guideline for such a health

care organization would be to restrict screening to women aged 50 to 69. This would save such a health care organization about $6.8 million when compared to screening other age groups.

Lead time

Mammographic screening detects breast cancer earlier, but if this is not accompanied by a reduction in breast cancer mortality, then the patient is given advanced notice of impending death, with no tangible gain. This has an adverse effect on the quality of life. This "lead time" is probably in the range of two to four years, meaning that many women will suffer needless worry and anxiety during this period.[1]

Radiation exposure

The risk of radiation exposure is of particular concern to the small group of patients who carry the gene for ataxia telangiectasia (about 1.4% of the population).[25]

These patients may be at increased risk of developing breast cancer as a result of low dose radiation, and the risk appears to be greater in younger women. Thus, the risk of screening these women may exceed any potential benefit. It has been suggested that women with a family history of ataxia-telangiectasia should seek alternatives to mammography, but most carriers will have no family history.

False positives

False positive results of mammographic screening are common, and result in unnecessary biopsies. In the United States, where litigation is of paramount concern, the incidence of false positives is much higher than in Europe, probably due to the unwillingness of radiologists to commit themselves to a benign diagnosis. In fact, analysis of data from the American breast cancer detection demonstration project (BCDDP) suggested that the positive predictive value of mammographic screening was only 10%, meaning that nine women had a false positive result on screening for every cancer found. On the other hand, European studies have indicated positive predictive values ranging from 30% to 60%.[26] These figures represent the positive predictive value of screening in all age groups. If women below the age of 50 were considered alone, the incidence of false positives would be much higher.

Over-diagnosis

Over-diagnosis of breast cancer is probably the most serious adverse consequence of mam-

Table II. Hazards of screening younger women.

Harmful Effect	Consequences
Cost	Increased expenditure on intervention of no proven value
Lead time	Advanced notice of impending death
Radiation exposure	Increased risk of breast cancer in women who carry the gene for ataxia-telangiectasia
False positives	Unnecessary breast biopsies
Over-diagnosis	Financial/emotional consequences of being falsely labelled as a cancer patient

mographic screening, and one that most profoundly affects the quality of life.[27] Peeters defines over-diagnosis as "a histologically established diagnosis of invasive or intraductal breast cancer that would never have developed into a clinically manifest tumor during the patient's normal life expectancy if no screening examination had been carried out".[28] Since the advent of screening mammography, there has been a rapid increase in the overall incidence of breast cancer with little or no corresponding change in breast cancer mortality. The most striking feature has been the sharp increase in incidence of ductal carcinoma *in situ* (DCIS), which in most instances is detected mammographically. In fact, prior to screening mammography, DCIS accounted for only 1-2% of all breast cancers but today 8% of such cancers and 22% of those detected by screening are identified as DCIS.[29]

There is now ample evidence to suggest that not every mammographically detected DCIS progresses to invasive cancer and that we are overdiagnosing breast cancer in many women. Nielsen has reported the results of 110 medicolegal autopsies of women between the ages of 20 and 54 dying of accidents: DCIS was detected in 15%, a prevalence four to five times greater than the number of overt cancers expected to develop over 20 years.[30]

Furthermore, in autopsies of women diagnosed with breast cancer, Alpers and Wellings have found DCIS in 48% of the contralateral breasts, even though only 12% of all breast cancer patients develop contralateral breast cancer after 20 years of follow up.[31] And in two separate studies, Rosen and Page reviewed benign breast biopsies and found several instances where DCIS had been overlooked by the pathologist.[32,33]

Thus, these patients received no additional treatment for the DCIS other than simple excision at the time of the original biopsy. Yet, only a small number of these women developed clinically manifest tumours after 15 to 18 years of follow up. These examples suggest that not all DCIS progresses to invasive cancer, and much of the increase in incidence of breast cancer attributed to mammographically detected DCIS may in fact represent over-diagnosis.

The consequences of over-diagnosis can be devastating. Women with DCIS are classified as cancer patients, and the diagnosis adversely affects their quality of life. In the United States, these women face severe financial challenges: outright refusal of health insurance coverage or coverage with inflated premiums, denial of life insurance, and difficulty in obtaining bank loans.[34,35] Many employers continue to discriminate against individuals with serious illnesses, even though the Americans with Disabilities Act of 1992 prohibits them from doing so (most employers are unaware of the Act).[36] A single patient with a mammographically detected DCIS can significantly raise a small company's health insurance premium, and many small companies are unwilling to accept such a financial burden. Just as important as the financial consequences of over-diagnosis is the feeling of uncertainty that goes with a diagnosis of cancer, and this affects the emotional well being of many women.

Conclusion

Harris has recently computed the potential risks/benefits of mammographic screening for a group of 1000 women between the ages of 40 and 49 in the United States.[37] Annual mammography for this group of women would require a total of 10,000 mammograms (he ignores the "6 month follow up" mammograms that are frequently ordered in the United States). This would result in about 300 women (30%) having false positive mammograms and unnecessary biopsies (the BCDDP data suggests that the incidence of false positives is much higher). During this period, 30 women would be reassured that they do not have breast cancer when in fact they do. Harris assumes a mortality reduction of 20% from screening and estimates that this will result in one women's life being prolonged from screening 1000 women, but only after the women approach the age of 60. He calculates that 125 breast cancers will be diagnosed during this period: if we accept this value, then we can assume that about 25 of these will be DCIS, and about half will be non-comedo DCIS, which in most instances probably would never develop into a clinically manifest tumour.

In the United States, as a result of the public advertisement campaigns launched by the American Cancer Society, there continues to be a large demand for screening women under the age of 50. In Britain, several companies provide private health insurance coverage for their employees, and this often covers the expense of mammographic screening for women under the age of 50 outside the NHS. Given the lack of data to support any benefit to screening younger women and the potential for harm outlined above, we believe that it is unethical to screen women under 50 without first obtaining proper informed consent. Thus, informed consent should be viewed as the middle ground in the continuing debate on whether or not to screen women under the age of 50.

References

1. Jatoi I., Baum M.: American and European recommendations for screening mammography in younger women: a cultural divide? B.M.J., 1993; 307: 1481-1483
2. Kaluzny A.D., Rimer B., Harris R.: The National Cancer Institute and guideline development: lessons from the breast cancer screening controversy. J. Natl. Cancer Inst., 1994; 86: 901-902
3. Elwood J.M., Cox B., Richardson A.K.: The effectiveness of breast cancer screening by mammography in younger women. Onlin J. Curr. Clin. Trials, 25 Feb., 1993 [Doc. No. 32]
4. Stacey-Clear A., McCarthy KA., Hall D.A., Pile-Spellman E., White G., Hulka C., et al.: Breast cancer survival among women under age 50: is mammography detrimental? Lancet, 1992; 340: 991-994
5. Miller A.B., Baines C.J., To J., Wall C.: Canadian national breast screening study. 1. Breast cancer detection and death rates among women aged 40 to 49 years. Can. Med. Assoc. J. 1992; 147: 1459-1476
6. Miller A.B.: Mammography in women under 50. Hem. Onc. Clin. of North America, 1994; 8: 165-177
7. Moss S.M., Summerley M.E., Thomas B.J., Ellman R., Chamberlain JOP. A case-control evaluation of the effect of breast cancer screening in the United Kingdom trial of early detection of breast cancer. J. Epidemiol. Community Health, 1992; 46: 362-364
8. Shapiro S., Venet W., Strax P., Venet L.: Periodic screening for breast cancer: the Health Insurance Plan project and its sequelae, 1963-86. Baltimore: Johns Hopkins University Press, 1988
9. Roberts M.M., Alexander F.E., Anderson T.J., Chetty U., Donnan P.T., Forrest P., et al.: Edinburgh trial of screening for breast cancer: mortality at seven years. Lancet, 1990; 335: 2416
10. Nystrom L., Rutquist L.E., Wall S., Lindgren A., Lindquist M., Ryden S., et al. Breast cancer screening with mammography: overview of Swedish Randomized trials. Lancet, 1993; 341: 973-978
11. Canadian study of breast screening under 50. Lancet, 1992; 339: 1473-1474
12. Kopans D.B.: Screening for breast cancer and mortality reduction among women 40-49 years of age. Cancer, 1994; 74: 311-322
13. Breast screening in women under 50. Lancet 1991; 337: 1575-1576
14. Kerlikowske K., Grady D., Rubin S.M., Sandrock C., Ernster V.L.: Efficacy of screening mammography. A meta-analysis. JAMA, 1995; 273: 149-154
15. VanNetten J.P., Morgentale T., Ashwood Smith M.J., Fletcher C., Coy P.: Physical trauma and breast cancer. Lancet 1994; 343: 978-979
16. Egan R.L.: Mammographic patterns and breast cancer risk. JAMA, 1980; 244: 287
17. Levallius B.: Screening mammography. Lancet, 1994; 343: 793
18. Tabar L., Faberberg G., Day N.E., Holmberg L.: What is the optimum interval between mammographic screening examinations? An analysis based on the latest results of the Swedish two-county breast cancer screening trial. Br. J. Cancer, 1987; 55: 547-551

19. Adami H.O., Malker B., Holmberg L., Persson I., Stone B.: The relationship between survival and age at diagnosis in breast cancer. N. Engl. J. Med., 1986; 315: 559-563
20. Field S., Michell M.J., Wallis M.G.W., Wilson A.R.M.: What should be done about interval breast cancers? B.M.J., 1995; 310: 203-204
21. Woodman C.B.J., Threlfall A.G., Boggis C.R.M., Prior P.: Is the three year breast screening interval too long? Occurrence of interval cancers in NHS breast screening programmes north western region. B.M.J., 1995; 310: 224-226
22. Sickles E.A., Kopans D.B.: Deficiencies in the analysis of breast cancer screening data. J. Natl. Cancer Inst., 1993; 85: 1621-1624
23. Eddy D.M., Hasselblad V., McGivney W., Hendee W.: The value of mammographic screening in women under age 50 years. JAMA, 1988; 259: 1512-1519
24. Kattlove H., Liberati A., Keeler E., Brook R.H.: Benefits and costs of screening and treatment for early breast cancer. Development of a basic benefit package. JAMA, 1995; 273: 142-148
25. Swift M., Morrell D., Massey R.B., Chase C.L.: Incidence of cancer in 161 families affected by ataxia-telangiectasia. N. Engl. J. Med., 1991; 325: 1831-1836
26. Reidy J., Hoskins O.: Controversy over mammography screening. B.M.J., 1988; 297: 932-933
27. Jatoi I., Baum M.: Mammographically detected DCIS: are we overdiagnosing breast cancer? Surgery, 1995; 118: 118-120
28. Peeters P.H.M., Verbeck A.L.M., Straatman H., et al.: Evaluation of overdiagnosis of breast cancer in screening with mammography: results of the Nijmegen programme. Int. J. Epidemiol., 1989; 18: 295-299
29. Moore M.M.: Treatment of ductal carcinoma in situ of the breast. Sem. Surg. Oncol., 1991; 7: 267-270
30. Nielsen M., Thomsen J.L., Primdahl S., Dyreborg U., Anderson J.A.: Breast cancer and atypia among young and middle aged women: a study of 110 medicolegal autopsies. Br. J. Cancer, 1987; 56: 814-819
31. Alpers C.E., Wellings S.R.: The prevalence of carcinoma in situ in normal and cancer associated breasts. Hum. Pathol., 1985; 16: 796-807
32. Rosen P.R., Braun D.W. Jr., Kinne D.E.: The clinical significance of pre-invasive breast carcinoma. Cancer, 1980; 46: 919-925
33. Page D.L., Dupont W.D., Rogers L.W., Landenberger M.: Intraductal carcinoma of the breast: followup after biopsy only. Cancer, 1982; 49: 751-758
34. Herold A.H., Roetzheim R.G.: Cancer survivors. Primary Care, 1992; 19(4): 779-791
35. McKenna R.J., Black B., Hughes R., et al.: American Cancer Society workshop on adolescents and young adults with cancer. Workgroup 2: insurance and employability. Cancer, 1993; 71: 2414-2418
36. Berkman B.J., Sampson S.E.: Psychosocial effects of cancer economics on patients and their families. Cancer, 1993; 72: 2846-2849
37. Harris R.: Efficacy of screening mammography for women in their forties. J. Natl. Cancer Inst., 1994; 86: 1722-1724

A critical appraisal of breast cancer screening for women aged 50 and over

J. Chamberlain

Introduction

The well-known association between stage at diagnosis of breast cancer and prognosis provided the impetus for a number of research studies aiming to find out if screening to diagnose breast cancer while it was still asymptomatic could reduce the number of women who died of the disease. The research findings are supportive of the conclusion that, for women aged 50 years or more when first screened, the chance of dying from breast cancer can be reduced to a limited extent. But controversy remains about whether the reduction in risk of death is sufficiently impressive to outweigh the physical and psychological disadvantages inherent in mass screening of well women, and the substantial resource costs of public health screening programmes. This chapter reviews these issues and discusses the policies which different authorities have adopted.

Size of benefit shown in research trials

The reduction in risk of death from cancer achievable by screening cannot be inferred from short-term indicators like the yield of cancer found nor its stage distribution, nor even the survival of screen detected cases compared with symptomatic cases. All of these indicators are subject to doubts and biases which spuriously favour a positive effect from screening. The only valid way of assessing the reduction in risk of death is to compare the subsequent cancer death rate in a population for whom screening has been provided with that in a control population without a screening programme.[1]

Ideally this comparison should be the end-point of a randomised controlled trial in which eligible disease-free subjects are randomly allocated to an offer of screening (routinely repeated as necessary), or to a control group, both groups being followed up for several years thereafter to record all deaths. We are fortunate that in the case of breast cancer several such randomised controlled trials of screening have been conducted during the past 30 years.

The Health Insurance Plan (HIP) Trial

This study, devised by Shapiro and his colleagues[2] and started in 1963, was a model for population-based randomised controlled trials of preventive medical interventions, and the same methodology, differing only in organisational details, has been followed in all subsequent trials of breast cancer screening. Sixty-two thousand women aged 40 to 64 who were insured for comprehensive health care with the Health Insurance Plan of Greater New York, were randomly allocated to an intervention group, or a control group. Women in the intervention group were invited to attend a screening clinic where they underwent two-view mammography and physical (clinical) examination of the breasts. Routine repeat invitations were sent annually in three successive years, after which screening ceased. Two-thirds of invited women accepted the first screen falling to 45% for the final screen.

Women in the control group just received their normal medical care. Details of all breast cancers, all breast cancer deaths, and all other deaths were recorded in both intervention group and control group over an 18-year period.

Within 5 years of the women's entry to the trial (the date of first invitation for screening, or equivalent date in the control group) it started to become apparent that there were fewer breast cancer deaths in the intervention group than the controls. Up to 10 years of follow up the reduction in deaths was concentrated entirely among women aged 50 or over at entry, although subsequently a suggestion of benefit also appeared in the younger age group. By 18 years the risk of breast cancer death in an intervention group woman relative to a control group woman was 0.79 (95% Cl 0.62 to 0.99); in women aged 50 and over at entry to the trial it was 0.80 (95% Cl 0.59 to 1.08).

The Swedish two-counties Trial

This study which started in the late 1970s, exploited recent improvements in mammography to test the effect on breast cancer mortality of screening using only a single medio lateral oblique view mammogram at each visit, with no physical examination.[3] One hundred and thirty-five thousand women, aged 40 and over and resident in Kopparberg and Ostergotland Counties were randomly allocated according to the parish in which they lived to an intervention group (78,000) or a control group (57,000). Women aged 50 and over in the intervention group were invited for routine mammography at average intervals of 33 months. In women aged 40 to 74 the average acceptance of screening was 89%, and mortality analyses are restricted to this age group.

After follow up of 11 years, for women aged 50 to 74 at entry, the odds ratio of an intervention group woman dying from breast cancer relative to a control group woman was 0.75 (95% Cl 0.65 to 0.87),[3] the reduction being evident, although not statistically significant, even in women aged 70 to 74 at entry.[4]

The Malmö Trial

At about the same time a further trial was started in Malmö, Sweden, in which 42,000 women aged 45 to 69 were randomised by birth cohort to an intervention group, offered screening by two-view mammography at 18 to 24 month intervals or a control group; 74% of intervention group women accepted screening.[5] Unlike other trials which chose age 50 as a cut-off point to distinguish older women from younger in mortality analyses, the Malmö investigators divided their population into those aged 55 and over, or under 55. In those aged 55 and over there was a non-significant mortality reduction (O.R. 0.79 95% Cl 0.51 to 1.24) after nine years. Approximately 25% of control group women were known to have had mammography during the course of the trial.

The Stockholm Trial

In 1981 a further trial was started in Stockholm in which 60,000 women aged 40 to 64 were randomised by birth cohort into an intervention group (40,000) who were invited for single-view mammography at 2-yearly intervals, or to a control group (20,000). Compliance with the screening invitation was 80%. After an average of 7.4 years, among women aged 50

to 64 at entry the risk of breast cancer death in the intervention group relative to the controls was 0.57 (95% Cl 0.3 to 1.1).

The Goteborg Trial

Another Swedish trial in the city of Goteborg, starting in 1982, randomised 50,000 women aged 40 to 59 into an intervention group of 21,000 offered screening by 2-view mammography at 18-month intervals or into a control group of 29.000. This trial has not yet independently reported its mortality findings, but they are included in an overview, discussed below, of all Swedish trials.[7] Among women aged 50 to 59 at entry, the risk of an intervention group woman dying of breast cancer relative to a control group woman was 0.91 (95% Cl 0.53 to 1.55).

The Edinburgh Trial

Starting in 1979, 45,000 women aged 45 to 64 were randomised, according to the general practitioner with whom they were registered, into an intervention group of 23,000 and a control group of 22,000. Women in the intervention group were invited for screening every year for 7 years. In the first, third, fifth and seventh screening rounds they were offered mammography and physical examination, while in intervening rounds they were offered physical examination alone. Sixty-one per cent of women accepted their first invitation, and non-responders were not re-invited in subsequent years. After 10 years of follow-up, the overall reduction in risk of breast cancer death was 18% (R.R. 0.82, 95% Cl 0.61 to 1.11); in women aged 50 to 64 at entry it was 15% (R.R. 0.85 95% Cl 0.63-1.13).[8]

Meta-analyses

The findings of those individual trials for women aged 50 or over at entry are summarised in Table 1. Although there is reasonable consistency showing a beneficial effect in women over 50 or 55 it is only in the Swedish two-counties trial that the results are statistically significant. There are a number of differences between the trials affecting their interpretation. Morrison[9] cites the relevant factors as differences in screening methods, available technology, frequency of screening, quality of screening, compliance, "contamination" by screening in the control group, duration of observation and sample size. Given the relatively low mortality from breast cancer in an initially disease-free population of middle-aged women, a short duration of follow up and a small sample size constrain some of the individual studies, which inevitably have wide confidence intervals on

Table I. Risk of breast cancer death in intervention group women aged 50 or more at entry, relative to control group women in six randomised controlled trials.

Trial	Relative Risk	95%Confidence Intervals
HIP[2]	0.80	0.59 to 1.08
Two-Counties[3]	0.75	0.65 to 0.87
Malmo[5*]	0.79	0.51 to 1.24
Stockholm[6]	0.57	0.30 to 1.1
Goteborg[7]	0.91	0.53 to 1.55
Edinburgh[8]	0.85	0.63 to 1.13

Women aged 55+

Table II. Risk of breast cancer death in intervention group women aged 50 or more at entry, relative to control group women in three meta-analyses.

Meta-Analysis	Relative Risk	95% Confidence Intervals
Nystrom et al.[7]	0.71	0.57 to 0.9
Elwood et al.[10]	0.66	0.55 to 0.79
Wald et al.[11]	0.76	0.69 to 0.88

their estimates of effect. These can be lessened by meta-analyses or statistical overviews in which findings from several trials are pooled and analysed together.

A number of meta-analyses have been published in recent years. An overview of all the Swedish trials[7] assessed breast cancer mortality by linking identification details of all women enrolled in the trials with Swedish National Mortality Statistics. An independent committee reviewed the pre-death case notes of all women with breast cancer who had died, without knowledge of whether each women was in intervention group or control group. Their conclusion was that women aged 50 to 69 in the intervention group experienced 19% fewer breast cancer deaths than women in the control group (RR 0.71 95% Cl 0.57 to 0.9). There was little evidence of benefit in women aged 70 to 74 at entry (RR 0.94 95% Cl 0.60 to 1.46).

The period of follow up in the Swedish overview varied from 5 years to 13 years. Elwood et al.[10] standardised duration of follow up to 7 years (thus excluding the Goteborg trial) and included the HIP and Edinburgh trials in the analyses. For women aged 50 to 64 or 69, the combined estimate of reduction of breast cancer mortality was 34% (RR 0.66 95% Cl 0.55 to 0.79). Wald et al.[11] also included the HIP and Edinburgh trials but took data for the longest duration of follow up then reported (ranging from 5 years for Goteborg to 18 years for HIP). Their conclusion for women aged 54 to 64 or 74 at entry was a breast cancer mortality reduction of 24% (RR 0.76, 95% 0.69 to 0.88). Thus all the meta-analyses, summarised in Table II, find a statistically significant mortality reduction in women aged 50 and over. De Koning et al.[12] took data from each of the individual Swedish screening trials and used it in a simulation computer model (MISCAN) to predict reductions in

breast cancer mortality. This model takes account of various performance indicators of screening (participation, frequency, etc), which the meta-analyses do not. When this was done the predicted mortality reduction in the combined trials for women aged 50 to 69 at entry was 11% greater than had been previously estimated.

From all the available evidence it thus seems clear that breast cancer mortality can be reduced by a quarter to a third among women aged 50 to 69 who are invited to regular routine breast screening. It should be noted that overall reduction in breast cancer mortality includes breast cancer deaths in the women who did not accept their screening invitations. Because such women have their counterparts in the control group, it is necessary to include them for a fair unbiased comparison. But it is clear that the proportionate reduction amongst women who accepted screening must be greater. Thus the statistical estimate of risk reduction in these trials gives a measure of the public health benefit which screening would confer on a whole population's mortality risk; the benefit to an individual screened woman would be greater than this when expressed as a proportion, although not necessarily in absolute terms since acceptors of screening tend to be at lower underlying risk of breast cancer death.[13] Day[14] has estimated that the risk reduction in a woman aged over 50 who accepts screening is 39%.

Screening by physical examination

All of the randomised controlled trials discussed above have used mammography as a screening test, although in the HIP trial and in Edinburgh it was supplemented by physical examination. It is clear from the Swedish trials that mammography on its own is effective in reducing mortality, but could physical examination on its own have a similar effect?[15] This is a most important question for developing countries, in many of which breast cancer mortality is increasing rapidly but which do not have the resources or skills for mammography. In the HIP trial, 45% of screen detected cancers were found by physical examination alone and it is reasonable to conclude that some of the observed benefit was achieved by their detection. But advances in mammography since the 1960s have improved its sensitivity such that in the Edinburgh trial only 6% of screen detected cancers were found by physical examination alone.[16]

The only trial so far published which addresses the question of the efficacy of physical examination is the Canadian National Breast Screening Study.[17] Among women aged 50 to 59 the aim of the trial was not to assess whether screening had any benefit (which was taken to be already proved), but to measure the size of any incremental mortality reduction conferred by the addition of mammography to physical examination in the screening procedure. Consequently 39,500 women, who had volunteered for the trial, were randomly allocated to a group offered annual screening by mammography plus physical examination or to a group offered annual screening by physical examination alone. Despite the fact that the incidence of interval cancers was lower in the mammographic arm of the trial, after 8 years of follow up there was no difference in breast cancer mortality between the two groups (RR 0.97 95% CI 0.62 to 1.52).

This particular trial has been criticised on the grounds of poor quality mammography (although none of the other trials published similar data on quality measurements), and small sample size. The latter problem may have been exacerbated by the fact that the volunteer subjects in this trial had a very much lower underlying cancer mortality than the average Canadian population, and longer follow up accumulating more breast cancer deaths is necessary to give the trial statistical power.

Even then it will not be possible to infer the size of mortality reduction which could be achieved by physical examination alone.

What is really needed is a randomised controlled trial, with provision of screening by physical examination alone in one arm, and no screening at all in the control arm. Such a trial is now planned in the Philippines (Parkin M., and Thomas D.B.; personal communication).

Research-based evidence on the disadvantages of screening

Like many preventive medical interventions breast screening has a number of unwanted side effects which mainly affect those people who are not beneficiaries - *i.e.* women who, in the absence of screen-

ing, would not develop or would not die from breast cancer. It is therefore obligatory on authorities promulgating screening to be informed about the frequency and the severity of these side effects, in order to reach a balanced judgement on whether the screening programme is likely to do more good than harm.

The disadvantages may be subdivided into those inherent in the screening procedure itself, those resulting from false positive test results, those resulting from over diagnosis of borderline lesions of little biological significance, those resulting from false negative test results, and finally, the opportunity costs of screening.

Disadvantages of the screening procedure

Psychological effects

It has been postulated that inviting women to be screened heightens anxiety both by making women aware of their vulnerability and, in those who do not accept the invitation, by inducing feelings of guilt. However there is no evidence to support these hypotheses.

One study, using a well-validated psychological questionnaire, found no difference in psychiatric morbidity between women attending for screening and an age-matched sample of the general population.[18] Similarly no difference in psychiatric morbidity has been found between attenders and non-attenders for screening.[19]

Discomfort

The breast compression needed to obtain a clear mammographic picture of the whole breast causes discomfort in some women. Studies of screened women in the US[20] and in the UK[21] suggest that around a third of women experience some transient discomfort but in only 5% or less does this amount to pain. Moreover, the UK study found that women regarded mammography as less unpleasant than other preventive procedures such as dental check-ups and cervical smears.

Radiogenic induction of cancer

A potential hazard from mammography has caused considerable concern because of evidence from nuclear bomb survivors and from women who in the past received large doses of medical X-irradiation to their chests, who subsequently had an excess incidence of breast cancers. Extrapolating from the very high doses received by these women to the very small doses of current mammography it has been estimated that for every million women screened at age 50, 21 breast cancers would be induced.[22] This compares with an underlying lifetime incidence of some 80,000 breast cancers. If, say, 50,000 of these cases were destined to die from their cancer, and if screening reduced these deaths by 25%, the ratio of deaths avoided to cancers induced would be nearly 600 to 1. This favourable balance for women over 50 is reassuring, but one sub-group of women, those carrying the ataxia-telangiectesia gene are at greater risk both of breast cancer and of radiogenic neoplasia, and mammographic screening may therefore be inadvisable for them, even after age 50.

Disadvantages of false positive test results

Women who are recalled for diagnostic work-up because of a positive screening test result inevitably experience anxiety about breast cancer, and have to undergo various further medical investigations, some of which entail physical morbidity. For the 9 out of 10 women who are eventually found not to have cancer this psychological and physical morbidity has been unnecessary. But measurement of the excess number of women investigated as a result of screening requires knowledge of how many women who consult with breast problems in the absence of a screening programme will require such investigation. Evidence is lacking except for biopsy rates in some of the earlier controlled trials. In the UK Trial of Early Detection of Breast Cancer for example[23] it was shown that the absolute rate of benign biopsies in a population offered screening was 7 times greater than in a control population during the prevalence screening period, falling to 1.5 times greater during later screening rounds.

The current approach to diagnostic work-up of a positive mammogram, discussed elsewhere in this volume, has reduced benign biopsy rates to less than 1 per 1000, which is lower than the annual rate in the control populations a decade earlier.

Despite many anecdotes about extreme anxiety caused to women recalled for further tests, when psychological morbidity has been studied using validated methods it has been found that anxiety is less in women referred from screening than among symptomatic "worried well women"[24] and is short-lived.[25]

Over-diagnosis of "biologically benign" breast cancers

Included among women with screen detected cancer is an unknown proportion in whom the cancer would not otherwise have been diagnosed in the woman's lifetime. Up to 20% of screen detected cancers are ductal carcinoma in situ (DCIS) whose natural history is still unclear. Autopsy studies of the breasts of women who have died of other causes have shown that DCIS and even some cases of invasive cancer may be undiagnosed during life. One study[26] found a prevalence of DCIS of 14% among women aged under 55, greater than the expected cumulative lifetime incidence of breast cancer. On the other hand, follow up of untreated (misdiagnosed) DCIS has shown that over a period of 10 years one quarter go on to develop invasive, sometimes metastatic, breast cancer.[27] Thus there is a dilemma, similar to that in screening for cervical and prostate cancers, of knowing how to manage patients with a condition which has the potential either to progress or to remain latent.

Giving these women the label of "a breast cancer patient" brings with it the physical morbidity of treatment and the psychological morbidity of anxiety in themselves and their family, as well as other possible disbenefits such as inability to obtain insurance. These side effects apply to some extent to all women with screen detected cancer because they are made aware of their disease earlier than would be the case without screening, and hence may suffer these side effects for longer. However, one study of psychological morbidity in breast cancer patients who were disease-free one year or more after diagnosis found that there was less anxiety and depression among the breast cancer patients than among age matched control women from the same population, and that there was no difference in morbidity between women whose cancer had been diagnosed by screening and those who had presented with symptoms.[28]

False negative screening results

It is obvious that false negative screening results in women who subsequently present with interval cancers are a serious disadvantage to any screening programme. The incidence of interval cancers, and the possible reasons for them, are described in detail elsewhere in this volume. The diagnosis of an interval breast cancer is presumed to have been delayed and it is sometimes postulated that because the woman concerned has had the reassurance of an earlier negative mammogram she may ignore symptoms and present with a cancer that is even more advanced at diagnosis than it would have been if she had not been screened. However, in controlled trials of screening there is little evidence that the prognosis of interval cancers is any different from that of control group breast cancers. There has been no psychosocial research into women's reactions to diagnosis of interval cancers, but anecdotal evidence, including many examples of litigation, suggests that they sometimes feel distressed, angry and resentful that their cancer was not diagnosed at screening.

Resource costs of screening programmes

In private health care the provision of screening is determined by (often uninformed) consumer demand, and the cost, in the final analysis, is controlled by what the individual will pay. But for public health programmes, the health authority which provides the service has to use limited public funds which would otherwise have been spent on different projects. These so-called "opportunity costs" of Breast Screening Programmes are more transparent in the public than the private sector and have occasioned much comment. Because the ultimate aim of public screening programmes is to reduce population breast cancer mortality rates, the authority has to spend resources on maximising uptake and ensuring that screening is accessible to the whole eligible population. It has a responsibility not only to provide high quality screening for all but also to provide diagnostic services for women with positive screening results, and to ensure availability of treatment.

Several countries have made estimates of the costs of their public screening programmes, but, even if all expressed in a standard currency, these cannot be compared because of differences in national health care organisation, funding and salaries.

A UK estimate, derived from earlier economic research in Edinburgh and updated to 1993, suggests that the average cost per woman screened (including the costs of an invitation and recall system, the costs of screening, and the costs of providing diagnostic assessment for those screening positive) is £22.60.[29]

The importance of Quality Assurance

The balance between benefit and harm can be tipped by a number of factors relating to the quality of the screening programme. Factors which will increase the benefit (i.e. reduce the number of breast cancer deaths) include: ensuring a high participation rate from the eligible population; ensuring a high sensitivity so that detectable cancers are not missed; organising the frequency of routine rescreening to minimise the incidence of interval cancers; and ensuring prompt effective treatment for the cancers found. Factors which will decrease the harm include: measures to maintain specificity (i.e. reducing false positives); provision of prompt diagnosis for women with positive results, including counselling to reduce anxiety; regular monitoring of radiological equip-

ment and radiation dose; and provision of dedicated, efficient and sympathetic staff in screening clinics. The latter applies particularly to radiographers who are the only professional group in contact with every screened woman, and on whom most responsibility lies for consumer satisfaction with the programme.

Resource costs, and their availability, are clearly major determinants of how much effort should be spent on these quality issues and which of them should have priority. Cost-effectiveness analyses, measuring the marginal extra cost per unit of benefit (e.g. life-year gained) by changes to improve the programme are recommended,[30] although so far have seldom been used in policy decisions.

Often it is found that a change to enhance benefit may have an unwanted side effect in increasing harm and/or cost. One notable exception to this is the finding from a randomised controlled trial that the use of 2-view mammography instead of 1-view mammography not only improves sensitivity, increasing the percentage of screen detected cancers by 24% but also improves specificity, reducing the positive rate by 15%.[31] Although the cost of 2-view screening was higher than 1-view, this was almost counterbalanced by the reduction in diagnostic investigation costs of false positives, and the marginal cost per extra cancer detected (albeit an imperfect proxy for life-years gained) was similar to the average cost of 1-view mammography.

Translating research into practice

Most large-scale public breast cancer screening services which have been set up in recent years have acknowledged the need to achieve the same quality standards as obtained in the research trials which proved benefit. Targets of interim indicators of screening performance have been set, which will maximise benefit and minimise harm, and information systems have been established to ensure that each screening programme can compare its performance with others.

In the Netherlands, for example, findings from the first 600,000 women aged 50 to 69 invited to participate in a national screening programme showed that targets for attendance, detection rates and stage distribution of breast cancers were being met, and when used in a computer simulation indicated that the expected mortality reduction would be achieved.[32]

Within the UK, the National Health Service Breast Screening Programme (NHSBSP) was set up following the recommendations of an expert advisory group which examined the evidence on breast cancer screening becoming available in the mid-1980s.[33] This advisory group, drawing largely on the findings of the Swedish Two-County trial, together with the Edinburgh and UK trials, recommended that all women aged between 50 and 64 should be routinely invited for screening by single oblique view mammography every 3 years. A number of screening programmes should be set up each providing for a defined population of women, and each programme should aim for a participation rate of at least 70%, a referral rate at first screening of no more than 7%, a biopsy rate no more than 3% and a breast cancer detection rate of at least 5 per 1000. Subsequently further targets were added, one specifying that the detection rate of invasive cancers of 10 mm diameter or less should be at least 1.5 per 1000 women screened, and another specifying upper limits for the incidence of interval cancers in each of the three years between screens.

Analysis of data for the three-year period from April 1990 to March 1993,[34] by which time 94 screening programmes had been set up, and over 4 million women had been invited, shows that the initial performance targets were being met. The acceptance of screening was 70.6%, 6.4% of women were referred following their first screen, 0.9% were biopsied and the cancer detection rate was 6 per 1000. There was variation between programmes but approximately three-quarters of programmes were meeting or exceeding these targets, giving optimism that the national screening programme will achieve its stated aim of a 25% breast cancer mortality reduction in women invited for screening, without causing an excessive burden of false positives.

However the optimism must be tempered with caution because overall detection of the small (10 mm diameter or less) invasive cancers which are the prime target of screening was only 1.3 per 1000, and only 30% of programmes met the target of a 1.5 per 1000 detection rate. Moreover data now becoming available on interval cancers indicates that these are occurring at double the rate expected from the Swedish Two-Counties trial.[35] Changes to improve this situation include routine use of 2-view instead of 1-view mammography which, as already seen, increases sensitivity and specificity without increasing cost,[31] and possibly reducing the interval between routine screens, on which data from a randomised controlled trial will soon be reported.

Routine monitoring of performance indicators of the screening programme is essential for its quality to be maintained, and its resource use to be foreseen.

Evidence-based policy decisions

Explicit recognition of the need for rationing of health services has followed the ever-increasing burden which technological advances place on limited health budgets. This recognition in turn has fuelled a demand for "evidence-based medicine" to inform purchasers of health services about the outcomes of their expenditure, and to enable them to decide on priorities. In contrast to the great majority of medical care which is unevaluated, breast cancer screening is one area where evidence on both its pros and cons exists in plenty. But it is apparent that this has not led to universal agreement about whether or not it should be provided.

Many expert groups advising national policymakers in developed countries have concluded that regular mammographic screening for women aged 50 to 69 is a priority area, and national programmes now exist in the UK, the Netherlands, Finland and Iceland. Regional or provincial programmes are provided in Sweden and Canada, and many more are under development, or being tested in pilot schemes, in Australia, New Zealand, France, Germany and several other European countries.

The report of the UK advisory committee[33] acknowledged that the cost-effectiveness of breast screening was less than that of several other medical procedures. Nevertheless the Government took a decision to fund it, injecting a sum of money from its Central Reserves to launch the programme. Presumably the decision to provide screening, in the UK and other countries, was based on the perceived priority of breast cancer as a high-profile disease and a relatively common cause of death, as well as on evidence from well-designed randomised controlled trials that the future number of breast cancer deaths in women of the eligible age-range could be reduced by around one-quarter.

In countries with lower breast cancer mortality rates, screening would logically have lower priority. For example using the MISCAN simulation model it has been estimated that the cost per life-year gained by screening women in Spain would be more than twice that gained by screening women in the Netherlands or the UK.[36]

Disagreement with provision of breast cancer screening has been intermittently voiced by a number of eminent and well-informed specialists.[37,40] Some place great emphasis on the psychological and physical harm incurred by women with false positive results, although, as seen earlier, research has not found these to be serious problems. Another argument against screening is the dilemma about overdiagnosis, and management of ductal carcinoma *in situ* which can only be resolved by randomised controlled trials of treatment. But the main case against screening is concerned with its expensive use of resources, coupled with a belief that the size of mortality reduction in practice will be less than that found in the research trials. Roberts[33] and Baum[40] argue that the resources used in screening should be redeployed into provision of open-access super specialist clinics for women with symptoms. But this would be a switch of resources from a use where there is evidence of benefit, to a use which past research has not shown to be effective. As part of the UK Trial of Early Detection of Breast Cancer, two specialist breast centres set up open-access clinics coupled with an education programme to encourage breast self-examination. After ten years there was no evidence that women provided with these facilities had lower breast cancer mortality than women in control populations.[13]

Assessment of how the balance tips between benefit on the one hand and harm and cost on the other will always be subject to the value judgement of the observer, and a diversity of views on value is to be welcomed. But now that widespread screening is in place, it is only by continuing it and monitoring it carefully for 10 to 20 years that its true effect in practice can be measured. Caution will have to be exercised to allow for changes in breast cancer mortality due to other factors such as changes in incidence and improved outcomes from therapy.[40] Knowledge of its effectiveness in practise can then contribute to more enlightened debate about continuation, modification or abandonment of the screening programmes.

References

1. Chamberlain J.: Evaluation of Screening for Cancer. In: Veronesi U, Peckham M. (Eds.) *Oxford Textbook of Oncology.* Oxford University Press, 1995; Vol. 1, pp. 185-198

2. Shapiro S., Venet W., Strax P., Venet L.: The Health Insurance Plan Project and its sequelae, 1963-1986. Baltimore, Johns Hopkins University Press, 1988

3. Tabar L., Fagerberg G., Duffy S.W., Day N.E., Gad A., Grontoft O.: Update of the Swedish Two-Gounty Program of Mammographic Screening for Breast Cancer. *Radiol. Clin. North. Am.,* 1992; 30: 187-210

4. Chen H-H., Tabar L., Fagerberg G., Duffy S.: The effect of breast screening after age 65. J. *Med Screening,* 1995: 2; 10-14

5. Andersson I., Aspegren K., Janzon L. *et al.*: Mammographic screening and mortality from breast cancer: the Malmo mammographic screening trial. *B.M.J.,* 1988; 297: 943-994

6. Frisell J., Eklund G., Hellstrom L., Lidbrink E., Rutqvist L-E., Somell A.: Randomised study of mammography - preliminary report on mortality in the Stockholm trial. *Breast Cancer Research & Treatment,* 1991; 18: 49-56

7. Nystrom L., Rutqvist L.E., Wall S. *et al.*: Breast cancer screening with mammography: overview of Swedish randomised trials. *Lancet,* 1993; 341: 973-978

8. Alexander F.E., Anderson T.J., Brown H.K. *et al.*: The Edinburgh randomised trial of breast cancer screening: results after 10 years of follow-up. *Br.J. Cancer,* 1994; 70: 542-548

9. Morrison A.S.: Screening for Cancer of the Breast. *Epidemiologic Reviews,* 1993; 15: 244-255

10. Elwood J.M., Cox B., Richardson A.: The effectiveness of breast cancer screening by mammography in younger women. *Online J. Curr. Clin. Trials,* 1993; DOC. No. 32

11. Wald N.J., Chamberlain J., Hackshaw A.: European Society of Mastology Consensus Conference on Breast Cancer Screening, Paris, 4-5 February 1993: Report of the Evaluation Committee. *Clin. Oncol.,* 1994; 4: 261-268

12. de Koning H., Boer R., Warmerdam P.G., Beemsterboer P.M.M., van der Maas P.J.: Quantitative Interpretation of Age-Specific Mortality Reductions from the Swedish Breast Cancer Screening Trials. *J. Nat. Cancer Inst.,* 1995; 87: 1217-1223

13. UK Trial of Early Detection of Breast Cancer Group. Breast cancer mortality after 10 years in the UK trial of early detection of breast cancer. T*he Breast,* 1993; 2: 13-20

14. Day N.E.: Screening for Breast Cancer. *Br. Med. Bull.,* 1991; 47: 400-415

15. Mittra 1. Breast screening: the case for physical examination without mammography. *Lancet,* 1994: 343; 342-344

16. Moss S.M., Coleman D.A., Ellman R., Chamberlain J., Forrest A.P.M., Kirkpatick A.E, Thomas B.A, Price J.L.: Interval cancers and sensitivity in the screening centres of the United Kingdom trial of early detection of breast cancer. Eur. J. Cancer, 1992: 29A (2), 255-258

17. Miller A.B., Baines C.J., To T., Wall C.: Canadian National Breast Screening Study 2. Breast Cancer Detection and Death Rates among Women aged 50 to 59 years. *Can. Med. Ass. J.,* 1992; 147: 1477-1488

18. Dean C., Roberts M.M., French K. Robinson S.: Psychiatric morbidity after screening for breast cancer. *J. Epidemiol. Community Health,* 1986; 40: 71-75

19. Hunt S.M., Alexander F., Roberts M.: Attenders and non-attenders at a breast screening clinic: a comparative study. *Public Health,* 1988; 102: 3-10

20. Stompar P.C., Kopans D.B., Sadowsky N.L. *et al.*: Is mammography painful? A multicentre patient survey. *Arch. Int. Med.,* 1988; 148: 521-524

21. Rutter D.R., Calnan M., Vaile M.S.B., Field S., Wade K.A.: Discomfort and pain during mammography: description, prediction and prevention. *B.M.J.,* 1992; 305; 443-445

22. Gohagen J.K., Darby W.P., Spitznagal E.L., Monsees B.S., Tome A.E.: Radiogenic breast cancer effects of mammographic screening. J. *Natl. Cancer Inst.,* 1986; 77: 71-76

23. UK Trial of Early Detection of Breast Cancer Group. Specificity of screening in United Kingdom trial of early detection of breast cancer. *B.M.J.,* 1992; 304: 346-349

24. Ellman R., Angeli N., Christians A., Moss S., Chamberlain J., Maguire P.: Psychiatric morbidity associated with screening for breast cancer. *Br. J. Cancer,* 1989; 60: 781-784

25. Bull A.R., Campbell M.J.: Assessment of the psychological impact of a Breast Screening Programme. *Br. J. Radiol.* 1991; 64: 510-515

26. Nielsen M., Thompson J.L., Primdahl S., Dyreborg U., Anderson J.A.: Breast cancer and atypia among young and middle-aged women: a study of 110 autopsies. *Cancer,* 1987; 751-758

27. Dupont W.D., Page D.L.: Breast cancer risk associated with proliferative disease, age at first birth, and a family history of breast cancer. *Am. J. Epidemiol.* 1987; 125: 769-779

28. Ellman R., Thomas B.A.: Is psychological wellbeing impaired in long term survivors of breast cancer? J. *Med. Screening,* 1995; 2: 5-9

29. Fraser M.N., Clarke P.R.: Cost-effectiveness of breast cancer screening. *The Breast* 1992; 1: 169-172

30. Brown J. Economics Aspects of Cancer Screening. In: Chamberlain J., Moss St. (Eds.) E*valuation of Cancer Screening.* London Springer Verlag, 1995; 175-186

32. de Koning H. Fracheboud J., Boer R. *et al.*: Nationwide breast cancer screening in the Netherlands: support for breast cancer mortality reduction. *Int. J. Cancer* 1995; 60: 777-780

33. Forrest A.P.M. *et al.*: Breast cancer screening. Report to the Health Ministers of England, Wales, Scotland and Northern Ireland. HMSO, London, 1986

34. Moss S.M., Michell M., Patnick J., Johns L., Blanks R., Chamberlain J.: Results from the National Health Service Breast

Screening Programme, 1990-1993 *J. Med. Screening,* 1995; 2 (4): 186-190

35. Field S., Michell M.J., Wallis M.G.W., Wilson A.R.M.: What should be done about interval cancers? *B.M.J.* 1995; 310; 203-204

36. van Ineveld B.M., van Oortmarssen G.J., de Koning H.J., Boer R., van der Maas: How cost effective is breast cancer screening in different EC countries? *Eur. J. Cancer* 1993; 29A (12): 1663-1668

37. Skrabanek P.: False premises and false promises of breast cancer screening. *Lancet* 1985; ii: 316-319

38. Roberts M.M.: Breast Screening: time for a rethink. *B.M.J.* 1989; 1153-1155

39. Wright C.J., Mueller C.B.: Screening mammography and public health policy: the need for perspective. *Lancet* 1995; 346: 29-32

40. Baum M.: Screening for breast cancer, time to think - and stop. (Letter). *Lancet* 1995; 346-347

Subject Index

Aberration of Normal Development
    and Involution (ANDI) 143-145
Acceptability of a screening test 18
Adenoid cystic carcinoma 194
Adenomyoepithelial lesions 122
Adenosis 88, 144
Adjuvant chemotherapy *vs* ovarian
    ablation 229
- *vs* tamoxifen *vs* chemotherapy 229
- polychemotherapy 228
- tamoxifen therapy 35
- therapies 39, 233
- - of breast cancer 226
Advanced Breast Biopsy Instrumentation
    (ABBI) 133-136
Alzheimer's Disease 56
American Cancer Society (ACS) 205
- College of Surgeons, the National
    Cancer 205
Angiogenesis in breast carcinoma 158
Antibiotics in diagnostic biopsies 127
Apex Biopsy 215
Apocrine cells 122
- metaplasia 143, 145, 162
Artefacts simulating calcification 88
Asymptomatic women 132
Atypical Ductal Hyperplasia
    (ADH) 93, 152, 164-167
- lobular hyperplasia (ALH) 167, 172
- proliferative diseases 152
Axilla, management of 214-218
Axillary dissection 56, 210, 214, 226
- nodes 179
- surgery, extent of 214

Basic Screening 43
- - mammographic unit 45
Benign breast disease 65
- - lesions 139, 191
- calcifications 199
- fibroadenoma 53
- microcalcifications 71
- phyllodes tumour 68, 70
- tumours 147
Biological models of breast cancer 34
Biology of breast cancer 34
Biopsies, pathological assessment 161
Blue domed cyst 145
Blunt duct adenosis 144
Bone mineral density 267
Borderline lesions 161, 165
Boston group 172
Breast cancer 29
- - Adjuvant Chemo Hormone Therapy
    Co-operative Group 229
- - - therapy 226-230
- - biological models 34
- - biology 34
- - deaths 23
- - Detection Demonstration Project 205
- - epidemiology of screening 17-28

- - gene 29-33
- - history of 49
- - , increase in 151
- - male 30
- - minimal, surgical treatment 205-213
- - mortality reduction 27
- - prevention 265-269
- - screening disavantages 280
- - - for women aged 50 and over 277-283
- - -, organisation 42-48
- - Trialists Collaborative Overview 229
- carcinoma, behaviour of 152
- - invasive 176-188
- carcinomas 109
- - small 109-114
- Care Nursing Service 56
- - support group 58
- conservation, local recurrence
    after 231-244
- cytopathology 189-195
-, development of the 139
- disease 152
- lesions, circumscribed 84
- local radiotherapy in breast conservating
    surgery 226
-, normal structure of 64, 139-150
- sarcoma 194
- Screening Centres 176
- - and Genetics 29
- -, cost of 274
- - Programme 34, 39, 42, 47, 58, 75
    117, 125, 176, 186, 245
- - service 130
- - Units 176
- self-examination (BSE) 19, 21
- surgery 100
- conserving surgery for DCIS 235

Calcification in ducts 90
- in the lobule 88
Calcifications classification 87
Canadian National Breast Screening Study
    (NBSS 1) 20, 271
Cancer and Steroid Hormone Study
    Group (CASH) from 31
- Committee of the College of American
    Pathologists 162
- detection rate 23
- Research Campaign trial (CRC) 216
- like lesions 72
Cancers, classification 245
- in lapsed attenders 245
- in non-attenders 245
- in the uninvited 245
Carcinogenic risks 267
Carcinoma, circumscribed 83
- *in situ* (CIS) 39, 133, 161, 165,
    167, 246
- of low malignant potential 133
Categories of interval cancer 245
Chemoprevention 265

- trials 265
Chemotherapy, results 228
Chronic mastitis 72
Circumscribed breast lesions 84
- breast masses 79-85
Coagulation factors 267
Colloid carcinoma 54
Colo-rectal cancers 152
Colorado mass screening programme 37
Comedo Mastitis 142
Complex sclerosing lesions (CSL) 146
Conservative surgery 219
Core Breast Biopsy (CBB) 125
Correlation with Histological Types 191
Cost of screening 274
Cystosarcoma phyllodes 149
Cysts 66, 145
Cytological correlation in breast 189

Day surgery 127
DCIS
    see Ductal carcinoma *in situ*
Detection of local recurrence 240
Diagnostic biopsies 125
- criteria in invasive carcinoma 172
- difficulties 121
Differential diagnoses 64, 79
- diagnosis of benign breast lesions 64-74
Digital system 134
Disadvantages of screening 280
Distant metastases 24
DNA index (ploidy) 38
Duct ectasia 142
Ductal carcinoma *in situ* (DCIS) 31, 39,
    90, 91, 101, 103, 133, 158, 161,
    164, 168, 180, 181
- and expression of biological markers 173
- and micro-invasion 172
- disease 143
- high grade (comedo) 168
- low grade (non comedo) 168-169

Early breast cancer diagnosis 110
- - - Trialists 227, 229
- - - Collaborative Group 35, 229, 231
Edinburgh Trial (EBSB) 37, 271, 278
Epidemiology of screening for breast
    cancer 17
Epithelial hyperplasia 144, 164
Equipment Requirements 46
- - computer system 46
- - film processing equipement 46
- - mammographic equipement 46
- - ultra-sound equipement 46
European Society of Mastology
    (EUSOMA) 271
Excision of impalpable lesion 127
- - palpable lesion 127
Excisional Biopsy 125

Extensive intraduct component (EIC)   232
Extent of axillary surgery   214

False negative screening results   281
- positive diagnosis   121
- - test results   281
Family Health Services Authority   50
- history of breast cancer   49
Fat necrosis   87, 143
Fibroadenolipomas   83, 94
Fibroadenoma (FA)   67, 96, 110, 121, 126,
    145, 147-148, 191
- , medullary carcinoma   66
Fibroadenomatoid hyperplasia   145
Fibrocystic change   152, 162
Fine needle aspiration (FNA)   54, 110,
    133
- - - cytology   117-124, 125, 176
Fisher's group   35
Focal hyperplasia   133
Foreign bodies   87
Forrest Report   18
- Working Group   43, 45
Frequency of Screening   43

Galactocoele   94
Gene BRCA1   29, 152
- BRCA2   29, 32, 152
Genes predisposing to
    breast cancer   30
General practitioner,
    the role of   49-50
Genetic tests   32
Genetics and breast screening   29
Golgi apparatus   167
Gonadotrophin-releasing hormone
    agonists   266
Goteborg study   271
- trial   278
Granular cell tumours   122
Guy's trial   35
Gynaecological Adjuvant Breast
    Group   229
- effects   267

Haemangiomas   94
Halsted radical mastectomy   234
Halstedian concept   214
- paradigm   34
Hazards of screening   274
Health Insurance Plan (HIP)   19, 271
- - - - Trial   277
Histological correlation in breast
    cytopathology   189
- grade   187
- - of tumours   187
Hormone replacement therapy
    (HRT)   102, 151
Hyperplasia with atypical features   133

ICRF Breast Unit of Guy's Hospital   229
Impalpable breast abnormalities   129-132
- - lesions, localization   131

- lesion, excision of   127
Importance of resection margins in
    conservative surgery   219-225
Incidence of breast cancer by age   24
Incisional biopsy   125
Indian ink marking   178
Indicator of patient survival   153
Infiltrating lobular carcinoma   183
Inflammatory carcinoma   102
Intermediate grade DCIS   170
International Collaborative Trial on
    tamoxifen   32
Interval carcinomas   186, 245-255
Intracystic papillary carcinoma   170
- papilloma   68
Invasive breast cancer   163
- carcinoma   161, 176-188, 209
- - - -, classification   180
- cribriform carcinoma   184
- ductal carcinoma   180
- lobular carcinoma (ILC)   100, 106, 196
- tumours   25
Invitation to be screened   43

Lactating breast   140
Lesion increasing in size   126
- with a premalignant potential   162
Li-Fraumeni syndrome   152
Lipoma   69
Lobular Carcinoma   123, 179
- in situ (LCIS)   89, 152, 161-175, 265
- variants   183
- neoplasia (lobular carcinoma in situ)   205
Local radiotherapy in breast conserving
    surgery   226
- recurrence after breast conservation   231
- - - - conserving surgery for DCIS   235
Lymph node metastasis   93, 187
- - stage   156
Lymphatic infiltration   232
- invasion (LVI)   211
Lymphoma   194

Macroscopic examination   177
Male breast cancer   30
Malignancy, radiological prediction of   77
Malignant calcifications   86
- lesions   192
Malmö mammographic screening trial   20,
    271, 278
Mammary gland   139
Mammograms, method of reading   61
Mammographic lesion   129
– screening   270-276
– screening in women under age 50   270
Mammography   151, 198
Management of local recurrence   241
Management of the axilla   214-218
Marsden grading   118
Mass screening programme in Colorado   37
Mastectomy   57, 127, 171, 180
Mastitis   70
- acute   72
- , chronic   72
Medico-legal aspects   259-264
Medullary carcinoma   54, 70,
    123, 185, 197

- carcinoma   54, 123
Metastatic carcinoma   123
- tumours   123
Method of reading mammograms   61
Micro-invasive carcinoma of breast   186
Microcalcification   76, 86-90, 100,
    126, 136
- composition   98
Microcystic disease   89
Microcysts   140
Microgranular adenosis   144
Milan Cancer Institute   268
- randomised control trials   233
- Trials of Conservation   234
Mild ductal hyperplasia   164
Minimal breast cancer   153
- invasive breast cancers   210
- - - carcinoma   153
Mixed carcinoma of breast   185
Models to breast screening   36
Moderate and florid hyperplasia without
    atypia   164
Molecular markers of prognosis   158
Morphological markers of prognosis   158
Mortality reduction in randomised
    trials   22
- - in the study group   20, 272
Mucinous (colloid) carcinoma   184
Multifocal invasive tumour   184
Multiple papillomas   163
- Round Masses   81

National Breast Screening Programme   75
- - - Radiology Quality Assurance   27
- Coordinating Group for Breast Screening
    Programme   176
- Health Service Breast Screening
    Programme   25, 51, 176
- - - - Project in the United Kingdom   231
- Surgical Adjuvant Breast and
    Bowel Project   230
- - - - Program (NSABP)   216
Natural history of breast cancer   17
NBSS see Canadian National Breast
    Screening Study   31
NHSBSP National Health Service Breast
    Screening Programme   125
- guidelines   27
- in UK   27
NIH Consensus Conference   227
Nijmegen project   273
Nipple discharge   69
No special type" (NST)/ductal
    tumours   154
Node positive   229
Non-comedo intraductal
    carcinoma   197
Non-invasive (in-situ) cancers   24
- investigative techniques   18
Non-neoplastic conditions   142
Normal breast   64, 139-150
Nottingham protocol   231
- Prognostic Index (NPI)   157
- scheme   190
- studies   235
- Tenovus Primary Breast Carcinoma
    Series   154, 155
- breast cancer prevention trial   268
Nurse's Health Study   151

Obliterating Chronic Mastitis   142
Oestrogen receptor (ER)   157
Oral contraceptives   151
Ovarian ablation   228
- cancer   29

p53 gene   30, 31
- proteins   173
- tumour suppressor gene   152
Paget's disease   142, 167, 186
Palpable lesion, excision of   127
Papillary carcinoma   185
- tumours   122
Papilloma   69, 148
Patchefsky's study   171
Pathogenesis of local recurrence (LR)   231
Pathology Reporting in Breast Cancer
      Screening   176
Patient desire   126
- survival   153
Perimenopausal women   162
Phyllodes tumour (cystosarcoma
      phyllodes)   149
- tumours   123
Plasma Cell Mastitis   142
Post-menopausal women   67, 229
- operative mammography   97
- radiation therapy   97
Pre-menopausal women   229
Preventative mastectomy   32
Prevention of breast cancer   265-269
Prognostic factors of a breast tumour   23
- indicators   151, 152
- -, use of   156
Programme design   42
- provoked presentation   245
Proliferative disease without atypia
      (PDWA)   164

Quadrant local recurrence   232
Quadrantectomy (QUART)   210
– ,axillary dissection and radiotherapy   35

Radial scar   75-79, 93, 126
Radiation exposure   151
- therapy   151
Radiographer, the role of the   51-52
Radiological false positive reports   197
- prediction of malignancy   77
Radio-pathological correlation   196
Radiotherapy   122
- technique   226
Randomised controlled trials, evidence
      for mortality   19
- - - of breast cancer screening   21
Randomized prospective studies   271
Recall decisions   63
Recalling the women   63

Reduction in mortality   25, 37, 39
- from population screening   39
Reductions of mortality from
      breast cancer screening   39
Reifenstein disease   30
Retinoids   266
Risk factors for breast
      cancer   21, 151-160
- - for local recurrence   232
- - of positive margins   224
- - from ionising radiation   18
- - prognostic indicators and
      staging   151-160
Risks/benefits of mammographic
      screening   275
Role of radiotherapy   242
Round Masses, multiple   81
- -, solitary   81
Royal Marsden pilot trial   267

Sarcoma   193
Scar phenomenon   232
- , the radial   75-78
Sclerosing adenosis   145, 162, 198
Sclerotic carcinomas   123
Scottish Cancer Trials Breast Group   229
Screening for breast cancer   17, 270
- modality to reduce mortality   40
- process   43
- procedure, disadvantages   280
- programme, clinical aspects   49
- test, acceptability   18
Sebaceous gland calcification   87
Serum cholesterol   267
Simple breast cyst   110
Size of benefit shown in research
      trials   277
Small expanding lesions   126
- primary tumour   39
Solitary Round Masses   81
Spiculated masses   126
Spicules of cancer lesions   200
St. Gallen Conference   228
Staging   151
- of breast cancer   155
- - lymph node disease   154
Stellate lesions   75-78
Stockholm study   271, 278
Sweden, randomised controlled
      trial   20, 37
Stromal calcifications   87
- component   148
- involution, aberration of   145
- lesions   123
Support Services   44
- -, education   44
- -, quality assurance   44
- -, training   44
Surgical treatment of minimal breast
      cancer   205
Survival curves for breast cancer   40
- of interval cancer patients   246

- probability   26
Swedish trials   20, 37, 271, 272
- two-counties trial, 19, 271, 273, 278
Symptomatic breast cancer   158
- mammography and screening   61
- tumours   153, 158

Tamoxifen   157, 227, 229, 265, 266
- analogues   268
- vs Tamoxifen + chemotherapy   230
Target Population   42
Technique of ultrasound   112
Terminal Ducto-Lobular
      Units (TDLU)   140, 161, 162
TNM staging method   155
- -system   217
Total mastectomy   32
- with lumpectomy   35
Toxicities   267
Traumatic fat necrosis   143
Tubular carcinoma   184, 198
Tumour bed biopsy   179
- characteristics   23
- histological grade   153
-, histological type   154
- necrosis   158
- recurrence   106
- size   153
- , staging   155
- type and grade   233
Tumorectomy (TART)   210

UK National Health Service Breast
      Screening Programme
      (NHS)   25, 27, 125, 153
- CCCR Breast Screening Frequency
      Trial   18
- - familial ovarian cancer study   30
Ultrasound and breast screening   110
- in breast diagnosis   109-114

Vascular calcification   87
- invasion (VI)   156, 232
- /lymphatic invasion   187

Well differentiated carcinomas   123
WHO Classification   176
Widespread mixed calcification   126
Women at Higher Risk   43
World Health Organisation
      (WHO)   34

Yorkshire Breast Cancer Group   153